EXOTIC PET BEHAVIOR

Birds, Reptiles, and Small Mammals

ABOUT THE AUTHORS

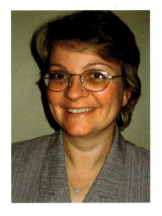

Teresa Bradley Bays, DVM, graduated from Kansas State University School of Veterinary Medicine in 1990. She completed preceptorships at Sea World of Florida and St. Louis Zoological Park before graduation, followed by a 1-year internship at Riverbanks Zoological Park in Columbia, South Carolina. She joined Belton Animal Clinic and Exotic Care Center in 1993, became part owner in 1997, and full owner in 2002. It is a five-doctor practice that has a 30% exotics caseload and that recently moved to a new 7300-square-foot facility that also supports Animal Urgent Care of Cass County. She is the author of numerous articles concerning exotic animal medicine and surgery, several chapters for *Veterinary Clinics of North America/Exotic Animal Practice*, and is a national speaker. She is a past president and 7-year board member of the Association of Reptilian and Amphibian Veterinarians and is currently president of the Missouri Academy of Veterinary Practitioners. As a wife, mother, business owner, and active member of her community, life is always busy!

Dr. Lightfoot received her DVM from the University of Missouri. She completed an externship at the St. Louis Zoological Park, and has been practicing in Florida since 1980. Dr. Lightfoot is a Charter Member of the ABVP–Avian specialty and is currently Regent for this specialty. She has served as the staff veterinarian for the Suncoast Seabird Sanctuary since 1987. Dr. Lightfoot served on the Florida Board of Veterinary Medicine from 1995 to 1999 and served as chair from 1997 to 1999. She has authored numerous articles on avian and exotic species and is an editor of the avian veterinary text *Clinical Avian Medicine* (in press). She has been an editor for *Seminars in Avian and Exotic Pet Medicine* since its inception. Teresa frequently lectures on avian and exotic medicine and surgery, both nationally and internationally. Dr. Lightfoot is the recipient of numerous awards, including the Association of Avian

Veterinarians Gold Star Award in 1998, the Florida Veterinarian of the Year award for 2000, the 2001 Exotic Veterinarian of the Year awarded by the International Conference on Exotics, and the Dr. Ted Lafeber 2002 Avian Practitioner Award.

Dr. Lightfoot has special interests in diagnosis and treatment of avian systemic mycoses and avian neoplasia. Her current research includes studying methods of captive raising and their effects on psittacine developmental behavior.

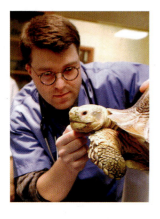

After Dr. Jörg Mayer graduated from the Veterinary University in Budapest, Hungary, in 1997, he completed an internship in zoological medicine at the Roger Williams Park Zoo in Providence, Rhode Island. At the end of the internship Dr. Mayer joined a research team to go into the cloud forest of Papua New Guinea to study wild and captive tree kangaroos for 2 months. Dr. Mayer received a M.Sc. degree in Wild Animal Health from the Royal Veterinary College and the Zoological Society of London, England, in 2000 before he started in his current position as the Director of the Exotic Service at Cummings School of Veterinary Medicine at Tufts University. He also holds a secondary appointment as Clinical Assistant Professor in the Department of Environmental and Population Health at the Tufts University School of Veterinary Medicine.

Exotic Pet Behavior

Birds, Reptiles, and Small Mammals

Teresa Bradley Bays, DVM
Belton Animal Clinic and Exotic Care Center, Inc.
Belton, Missouri

Teresa Lightfoot, DVM, DABVP—Avian
Florida Veterinary Specialists
Tampa, Florida

Jörg Mayer, Dr. med.vet., M.Sc.
Cummings School of Veterinary Medicine at Tufts University
Department of Exotic Animals
North Grafton, Massachusetts

With 4 Contributing Authors

SAUNDERS
ELSEVIER

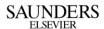

11830 Westline Industrial Drive
St. Louis, Missouri 63146

EXOTIC PET BEHAVIOR: BIRDS, REPTILES, ISBN-13: 978-1-4160-0009-9
AND SMALL MAMMALS   ISBN-10: 1-4160-0009-7
Copyright © 2006 by Saunders, an imprint of Elsevier Inc.

All rights reserved. No part of this publication may be reproduced or transmitted in any form or by any means, electronic or mechanical, including photocopying, recording, or any information storage and retrieval system, without permission in writing from the publisher. Permissions may be sought directly from Elsevier's Health Sciences Rights Department in Philadelphia, PA, USA: phone: (+1) 215 239 3804, fax: (+1) 215 239 3805, e-mail: healthpermissions@elsevier.com. You may also complete your request on-line via the Elsevier homepage (http://www.elsevier.com), by selecting "Customer Support" and then "Obtaining Permissions".

> **Notice**
>
> Knowledge and best practice in this field are constantly changing. As new research and experience broaden our knowledge, changes in practice, treatment and drug therapy may become necessary or appropriate. Readers are advised to check the most current information provided (i) on procedures featured or (ii) by the manufacturer of each product to be administered, to verify the recommended dose or formula, the method and duration of administration, and contraindications. It is the responsibility of the practitioner, relying on their own experience and knowledge of the patient, to make diagnoses, to determine dosages and the best treatment for each individual patient, and to take all appropriate safety precautions. To the fullest extent of the law, neither the Publisher nor the Authors assume any liability for any injury and/or damage to persons or property arising out or related to any use of the material contained in this book.
>
> The Publisher

ISBN-13: 978-1-4160-0009-9
ISBN-10: 1-4160-0009-7

Publishing Director: *Linda Duncan*
Publisher: *Penny Rudolph*
Developmental Editor: *Shelly Stringer*
Publishing Services Manager: *Patricia Tannian*
Senior Project Manager: *Sarah Wunderly*
Book Designer: *Jyotika Shroff*

Printed in China

Last digit is the print number: 9 8 7 6 5 4 3 2 1

♦ ♦ ♦

To my husband Martin, and to my daughter Nicole and stepsons Zachary and Isaiah, for their patience and support (and for making me laugh) during this more than 2-year project.

I am thankful for the many blessings that have been bestowed on me and for the lessons that I continue to learn in this journey called life.

Teresa Bradley Bays, DVM

♦ ♦ ♦

To my husband, Chris Lane, my mother, Bea Lightfoot, my brother, Tom Lightfoot, and my sons, Cory, Derek, Richard, and Matt. Without our convoluted family dynamics, I would not have developed such an interest in normal and abnormal behavior.
I love you all dearly.

Teresa Lightfoot

♦ ♦ ♦

To my parents, Christel and Walter. Their love, belief, and support made it possible for me to be a veterinarian caring for the smallest and most fragile patients today.

Ich möchte dieses Buch meinen Eltern, Christel und Walter, widmen. Ihre Liebe, Ihr Glaube und Ihre Unterstützung hat es für mich möglich gemacht, ein Tierarzt zu sein, der sich um die Kleinsten und die Zerbrechlichsten Patienten kümmert.

Jörg Mayer

♦ ♦ ♦

Contributors

Teresa Bradley Bays, DVM
Belton Animal Clinic and Exotic Care Center, Inc.
Belton, Missouri

Elizabeth I. Evans, DVM
Assistant Professor
Biology Department
Rockhurst University
Kansas City, Missouri

Peter G. Fisher, DVM
President
PetCare Veterinary Hospital
Virginia Beach, Virginia

Dan H. Johnson, DVM
Practice Owner
Avian and Exotic Animal Care, P.A.
Raleigh, North Carolina
Adjunct Assistant Professor
Department of Clinical Sciences
North Carolina State University, College of Veterinary Medicine
Raleigh, North Carolina

Teresa Lightfoot, DVM, Dipl. ABVP
Florida Veterinary Specialists
Tampa, Florida

Jörg Mayer, Dr. med.vet., M.Sc.
Cummings School of Veterinary Medicine at Tufts University
Department of Exotic Animals
North Grafton, Massachusetts

Carina L. Nacewicz, DVM
Seattle, Washington

FOREWORD

There is a growing trend toward ownership of exotic or unusual pets, and the experience of guardianship can be fascinating and educating for the owner, providing a glimpse into the world of a novel species. Caring for such creatures requires knowledge of the behavior of the species in order to provide proper husbandry in a captive environment.

Behavior and affiliations of exotic animals, as well as of more common domestic pet animals, are shaped by nature and nurture. Nature directs from its hard-wired bastions, while nurture (learning) fine tunes and shapes the final behavioral output and reactions. In species such as dogs and cats, their nature and the influence of learning is well known. Maternal and peer influence is important to normal behavioral development, and behavior can be shaped to advantage during certain well-defined critical (more accurately termed "sensitive") periods of learning. The behavior of the exotic species detailed in this book should be viewed in light of the normal behavior (nature), the influence of early interactions (maternal, peer, or otherwise), and the situation the animal is likely to encounter within the confines of captivity for each species.

Some owners research a species prior to purchase and are reasonably well-equipped to look after it, but others do not. Both types of owners may at some point seek out a veterinarian for advice. It is essential that they receive correct information concerning the proper health and welfare of their small charge. They must know which species are social and are best kept housed with conspecifics, and which should be housed individually. Some species have special requirements with respect to light, heat, and humidity, and others have specific nutritional needs. Also, the behavior of an animal can be an indication of its well-being or lack of same, and these behaviors are, for the most part, unique to each species.

Understanding an animal's behavior increases owner enjoyment and appreciation of their exotic pet and helps the owner recognize potential problems. Recognizing normal and abnormal behaviors can be interpreted as a crude form of communication, albeit mostly one-way. If owners do not understand normal behavior, they will not recognize abnormal behavior that may indicate a medical problem.

Veterinarians must recognize unusual behavior of various species and be prepared to convey pertinent information, appropriate recommendations, or treatments. The authors of this highly informative compilation have gone to great lengths to detail the behaviors of selected exotic pets. With this knowledge veterinarians will be able to guide their clients in the proper care for these animals.

Whether an owner is asking about an anorectic reptile, a rabbit that may be in pain, or the courtship behavior of a psittacine, veterinarians should be able to supply the answer. The authors of this important text cover these questions and numerous other behavioral issues related to many exotic species. Veterinarians will find this text beneficial as a behavioral reference as well as enormously interesting reading.

Nicholas H. Dodman, BVMS, DACVB, DACVA
Professor
Cummings School of Veterinary Medicine at Tufts University
North Grafton, Massachusetts

The study of animal behavior, or ethology, to ensure good health and improve welfare is a long tradition in veterinary medicine, starting originally with food-producing animals. Discerning readers will realize that the impact of a behavior on the human observer is not necessarily a function of its impact on the animal. Failing to do this, we get an anthropomorphic idea of animal consciousness in which the so-called "objective" measure becomes the test giving the wanted answer; if it fails, we seek other "objective" markers until we achieve a set of measurements that supports our subjective impression. Applied as such, the study of animal behavior is no longer based on objective data, but on manipulated opinions.

Unlike what is considered to be anthropomorphic, the scientific idea of animal consciousness has allowed us to appreciate the ability of each animal to express species-specific behavior in the environment in which it is placed. Any discomfort produced by husbandry or disease may be detected through anomalies in the expression of this behavior, or by examining preferences expressed by the animal when offered a free choice. Applied animal behavior is an objective approach to achieving good health and well-being in animals, avoiding either a mechanistic or an emotional evaluation of an animal's quality of life. Without knowing what is normal we cannot recognize what is abnormal or appreciate how animals express pain and suffering.

Information on behavior of exotic animals is widely scattered in many journals, so the publication of a single volume summarizing what is known is significant. This book represents a major advance in the field of exotic animal medicine as it will help veterinarians meet the needs of clients demanding the highest standards of care for their animals.

Thomas M Donnelly, DVM
The Warren Institute
Ossining, New York
Formerly Adjunct Professor and Associate Professor
New York State College of Veterinary Medicine
Cornell University
Ithaca, New York

PREFACE

In 1994 a dwarf rabbit patient changed my life forever (TBB). It was a 4-year-old intact female that had been seen by two other veterinarians because she was not eating or defecating and her abdomen was distended. After three enemas at the other practices, her "constipation" still hadn't improved. When she presented at our hospital she had not had the benefit of radiographs or other diagnostics, just the "red bag" technique. She died from the severe hydrometra (see Figure 1-4 in text) that caused her abdominal distention, severe dyspnea, weight loss, anorexia, and gastrointestinal stasis. It was then I realized that she died because, at that time, veterinarians often did not know what normal behavior was for rabbits and therefore did not recognize the abnormal behaviors that help to guide diagnostics and treatment. It was then that I decided to become more active in researching and disseminating information on behavior in exotics.

This book is a result of that effort and includes information on chelonians, snakes, lizards, psittacines, rabbits, guinea pigs, rats, mice, gerbils, hamsters, chinchillas, fennec foxes, hedgehogs, ferrets, sugar gliders, and short-tailed opossums. Each chapter includes social and antisocial behaviors, sensory behaviors, communication behaviors, elimination behaviors, eating behaviors, locomotor behaviors and activity, grooming behaviors, and reproductive behaviors. Medical implications of abnormal behaviors and pain-associated behaviors are also discussed. Several chapters highlight how behavior is affected by captivity and hospitalization. Tables and sections provide practical and invaluable information for rabbits (litter training, behavioral enrichment, curbing negative behaviors, common postures and vocalizations, and tips for bonding), guinea pigs (common postures and vocalizations), ferrets (litter box tips, controlling biting behaviors, and environmental enrichment) and psittacines (species-specific behaviors). Client education handouts are included for the miscellaneous small mammals.

Behavior is an intricate subject with many facets. It is associated with all aspects of anatomy, physiology, and pathology, making it an onerous task to stay on topic. Behavior is also not a static subject and the ability to capture normal and abnormal behaviors in still photographs is difficult. Add to that the tremendous number of exotic species that are presented to today's veterinarian and this subject becomes formidable. The editors and authors have taken this seemingly impossible task and created this text that is designed to provide an overview of behaviors seen in reptiles, psittacines, and small mammals. It is presented in order to aid the veterinary practitioner in addressing the needs of the entire patient and to provide a knowledge base that will allow the practitioner to answer clients' questions with confidence. The authors join together to wish you the best in your quest to further your knowledge regarding exotic patients and their treatment.

Teresa Bradley Bays, DVM
Teresa Lightfoot, DVM
Jörg Mayer, Dr. med.vet., M.Sc.

Acknowledgments

The understanding, support, and never-ending encouragement of my entire staff has been incredible (even when they thought I was more crazed than usual!). I am particularly thankful for those who have supported and encouraged me through good times and bad in my most recent growing-up years, including Ellen Esterkin, Ruth Liebau, RVT, Marcia Kristman, RVT, Michelle Ambler, Pam Olsen, Kelli Johnsen, CVT, VTS (ECC), Elizabeth Evans, DVM, Kaylee Beal, Jack Olsen and Dani Anderson. Thank you to Robin Rysavy and Kathy Smith for helping me to see beyond the disease to the entire patient and who taught me a lot about rabbits and the life they lead.

Many thanks to Drs. Teresa Lightfoot and Jörg Mayer for all of their help, knowledge, and patience throughout this process and to all of the authors for the precious time spent away from their families to make this book a reality. Thank you to Ray Kersey for asking me to work on this project and to Shelly Stringer, Sarah Wunderly, and Stacy Beane of Elsevier for their help and encouragement to make this a book we are all proud of.

Teresa Bradley Bays

My thanks to and admiration for Teresa Bradley for the incredible amount of effort, time, and knowledge she has poured into this text. Kudos to Jörg Mayer for his valuable insights, experience and prompt responses when time was critical.

Teresa Lightfoot

I would like to thank my partner Janet for understanding how important this project was for me and for accepting my sitting at the computer for hours and hours during the preparation, writing, and editing of this book. I would also like to thank my co-editors for such great and easy cooperation and communication throughout the 2-year process of "giving birth" to this book.

Jörg Mayer

Contents

1. Rabbit Behavior — 1
Teresa Bradley Bays

- Introduction — 1
- Natural History, Behavior, and Domestication — 1
- Sensory Behaviors — 2
  - Vision and Behavior — 2
  - Touch and Behavior — 3
  - Hearing and Behavior — 3
  - Olfactory Behaviors — 3
- Communicative Behaviors — 4
- Social and Antisocial Behaviors — 7
- Reproductive Behaviors — 12
  - Male Reproductive Behaviors — 12
  - Female Reproductive and Maternal Behaviors — 13
- Neonatal and Juvenile Behaviors — 15
- Eating Behaviors — 17
- Elimination Behaviors — 20
  - Urinary Behaviors — 23
- Locomotor Behaviors and Activities — 24
- Grooming Behaviors — 29
- Rabbits in Outdoor Enclosures — 31
- Behavioral Enrichment — 31
- Medical Implications of Abnormal Behaviors — 34
- Rabbits and the Hospital Environment — 38
- Pain Management Considerations — 41
  - Behaviors Associated with Pain — 41
- Hypnosis — 42
- Euthanasia and Adoption — 42

2. Psittacine Behavior — 51

Teresa Lightfoot
Carina L. Nacewicz

Introduction	**51**
Wild Bird Behavior	**51**
Species Differences	52
Time Allocation and Behaviors	52
Communication	53
Vocalization	53
Body Language	54
Foraging Behaviors	54
Intraspecies Contact and Species Variations	54
Parenting	56
Captive Psittacine Development	**57**
Socialization	58
Stimulation	59
Behavior Modification	60
Identifying and Creating the Proper Human-Psittacine Relationship	63
Husbandry Considerations	**65**
Caging	65
Bathing	65
Nutrition	66
Photoperiod	66
Grooming: Nail, Beak, and Wing Trimming	67
Disease Considerations	**68**
Neurologic Disease	68
Miscellaneous Neuropathies	70
Pain-Associated Behaviors	71
Captive Behavior and Training	**71**
Behavior Analysis	71
Modification Techniques	72
Problem Behaviors or Syndromes	**74**
Dominance	74
Biting	77

Phobias or Neuroses	78
Cockatoo Prolapse Syndrome	79
Feather Destruction	81
Environmental and Nutritional Factors	82
Psittacine Behavior in the Animal Hospital	**89**
Home-Court Advantage	89
Aggressive Amazons and Other Psittacines in the Animal Hospital	89
Intelligence, Cognition, and Communication in Parrots	**96**
Social and Cognitive Similarities to Great Apes	96
Perireferential Communication and Categoric Class Formation	97
Sentinel Behavior	97

3. Reptile Behavior   103

Jörg Mayer—Turtles and Snakes
Teresa Bradley Bays—Lizards

Introduction	**103**
Developmental Aspects of Behavior	**104**
Environmental Aspects of Behavior	**105**
Social and Antisocial Behaviors	**108**
Agonistic Behaviors	112
Taming and Training	**122**
Sensory Modalities and Behavior	**123**
Vomeronasal Organ, Olfaction, and Behavior	123
Vision and Behavior	125
Hearing, Vocalization, and Behavior	125
Gustation and Behavior	127
Reproductive Behaviors	**127**
Male Reproductive Behaviors	129
Female Reproductive Behaviors	130
Behavior of Hatchlings and Juveniles	**131**
Eating Behaviors	**132**
Elimination Behaviors	**138**
Locomotor Behaviors and Activities	**139**
Grooming Behaviors	**141**

Sneezing	142
Coloration and Behavior	142
Thermoregulatory Behaviors	143
Hibernation and Estivation	146
Burrowing Behaviors	147
Behaviors Associated with Pain	148
Behavioral Enrichment	148
Medical Implications of Abnormal Behaviors	151
Euthanasia	155

4. Ferret Behavior   163

    Peter G. Fisher

Natural Behavior and Domestication	163
Sensory Behaviors	166
Vision and Behavior	166
Hearing and Behavior	166
Olfactory Behaviors	167
Communication Behaviors	168
Olfactory Communication	168
Vocalizations	170
Visual	171
Locomotor Behaviors and Activity	172
Elimination Behaviors	173
Urine Licking Behaviors	174
Reproductive Behaviors	174
Male Reproductive Behaviors	175
Female Reproductive Behaviors	176
Social and Antisocial Behaviors	177
Grooming Behaviors	179
Feeding Behaviors	180
Prey-Catching Behaviors	181
Exploratory Behaviors	182
Play Behaviors	184
Environmental Enrichment	188
Aggressive Behaviors	189

Conspecific Aggression	189
Aggression and Biting Behaviors	193
Sleep Behavior	**197**
Medical Implications of Abnormal Behavior	**199**
Adrenal Disease	200
Insulinoma	202
Behaviors Associated with Pain	**203**

5. Guinea Pig Behavior — 207

Teresa Bradley Bays

Natural History, Behavior, and Domestication	**207**
Social and Antisocial Behaviors	**208**
Taming and the Bonding Process	**210**
Sensory Behaviors	**212**
Visual Behaviors	212
Vocalization Behaviors	212
Auditory Behaviors	213
Locomotor Behaviors and Activities	**213**
Grooming Behaviors	**216**
Eating Behaviors	**219**
Elimination Behaviors	**223**
Reproductive Behaviors	**224**
Male Reproductive Behaviors	224
Female Reproductive Behaviors and Parental Care	225
Neonatal Behavior	**226**
Behavioral Enrichment	**226**
Medical Implications of Abnormal Behavior	**228**
Hospitalization, Stress, and the Sick Guinea Pig	**231**
Behaviors Associated with Pain	**234**
Guinea Pigs and Euthanasia	**236**

6. Small Rodent Behavior: Mice, Rats, Gerbils, and Hamsters — 239

Elizabeth I. Evans

Introduction	**239**
Sensory Behaviors	**240**

Communicative Behaviors	241
Social and Antisocial Behaviors	243
Reproductive Behaviors	246
Male Reproductive Behaviors	246
Female Reproductive Behaviors	247
Eating Behaviors	250
Elimination Behaviors	251
Locomotor Behaviors and Activities	251
Grooming Behaviors	253
Temperature Sensitivity	256
Medical Implications of Abnormal Behaviors	256
Behaviors Associated with Pain	258

7. Miscellaneous Small Mammal Behavior   263

Dan H. Johnson

Chinchillas	**263**
Natural History and Behavior	263
Sensory Behaviors	263
Communicative Behaviors	265
Social and Antisocial Behaviors	265
Reproductive Behaviors	267
Eating Behaviors	271
Elimination Behaviors	271
Locomotor Behaviors and Activities	272
Grooming Behaviors	272
Medical Implications of Abnormal Behaviors	274
Behaviors Associated with Pain/Euthanasia	278
How Behavior Relates to Captivity	278
Fennec Foxes	**281**
Natural History and Behavior	281
Sensory Behaviors	281
Communicative Behaviors	282
Social and Antisocial Behaviors	283
Reproductive Behaviors	285
Eating Behaviors	286

Elimination Behaviors	287
Locomotor Behaviors	287
Grooming Behaviors	288
Medical Implications of Abnormal Behaviors	289
Behaviors Associated with Pain	289
How Behavior Relates to Captivity	289
Hedgehogs	**293**
Natural History and Behavior	293
Sensory Behaviors	294
Communicative Behaviors	295
Social and Antisocial Behaviors	295
Reproductive Behaviors	296
Eating Behaviors	298
Elimination Behaviors	299
Locomotor Behaviors and Activities	299
Grooming Behaviors	300
Medical Implications of Abnormal Behaviors	301
Behaviors Associated with Pain	302
How Behavior Relates to Captivity	303
Prairie Dogs	**305**
Natural History and Behavior	305
Communicative Behaviors	306
Social and Antisocial Behaviors	306
Reproductive Behaviors	308
Eating Behaviors	309
Elimination Behaviors	310
Locomotor Behaviors and Activities	310
Grooming Behaviors	310
Medical Implications of Abnormal Behaviors	312
Behaviors Associated with Pain	317
Behavioral Enrichment	317
How Behavior Relates to Captivity	318
Short-Tailed Opossums	**320**
Natural History and Behavior	320
Sensory Behaviors	320

Communicative Behaviors	320
Social and Antisocial Behaviors	321
Reproductive Behaviors	322
Eating Behaviors	324
Elimination Behaviors	324
Locomotor Behaviors and Activities	325
Grooming Behaviors	325
Medical Implications of Abnormal Behaviors	326
Behaviors Associated with Pain	326
How Behavior Relates to Captivity	326
Sugar Gliders	**328**
Natural History and Behavior	328
Sensory Behaviors	328
Communicative Behaviors	328
Social and Antisocial Behaviors	330
Reproductive Behaviors	331
Eating Behaviors	332
Elimination Behaviors	333
Thermoregulatory Behaviors	333
Locomotor Behaviors and Activities	333
Grooming Behaviors	334
Medical Implications of Abnormal Behaviors	335
Behaviors Associated with Pain	338
Behavioral Enrichment	339
How Behavior Relates to Captivity	339

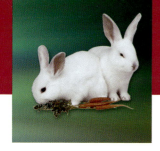

CHAPTER 1

TERESA BRADLEY BAYS

Rabbit Behavior

Introduction

Knowing the specifics of rabbit anatomy and physiology and how these differ from those of other mammals is imperative for veterinarians who treat exotics. Rabbits, like other exotic species, cannot be treated successfully by extrapolating from cat or small dog medical principles. Equally important is the need to become familiar with normal and abnormal behavior in order to provide the best health care possible for rabbit patients.

Understanding abnormal behavior in rabbits will enable practitioners to better interpret common presenting signs and owner complaints. With this information, veterinarians can better communicate and educate rabbit owners so that they may be able to detect problems in their pet rabbits earlier. This is especially important in light of the major shift that has occurred in the status of the rabbit from backyard child's pet to member of the family, often living freely in the house.

Natural History, Behavior, and Domestication

Domestic rabbits are the descendants of the European rabbit, *Oryctolagus cuniculus*, from Western Europe and Northwestern Africa, and have been kept as domesticated pets since the early sixteenth century.[12,16] Many of the behaviors that we see in wild rabbits are mimicked in our pet rabbits.

Rabbits live in large groups in warrens or burrows that are dug in sandy, hilly terrain, and they rarely venture far from the safety of the warren. They are primarily nocturnal, moving away from their burrows at dusk to forage. They have a highly developed social hierarchy and as a prey species have evolved for flight rather than fight.

The males are very territorial, and females will aggressively protect their nests. Pregnant females will dig burrows away from the warren, as the males can be aggressive toward and even kill the offspring. When the kits are small, the doe will carefully cover the nest burrow each time she leaves it.

Although rabbits have been domesticated for more than 2000 years,[85] the behavior of rabbits was relatively ignored until the pioneer observations of Southern[88,89] in the British Isles. Then, in the 1950s, the Australian government initiated an extensive rabbit research program in which the reproductive and general social behavior of the Australian wild rabbit was intensively studied.[43,73-76] However, in contrast with the aim of improving the well-being of laboratory rabbits, the goal of the Australian program was to find suitable methods for eliminating the wild rabbit population, which was vastly overabundant and creating an agricultural nuisance.[68,70]

Until the 1990s, studies of rabbit behavior focused almost exclusively on wild rabbits, in natural colonies,[22,59,79,82,89] and in experimental colonies.[71,90] There were relatively few investigations conducted on the behavior of single rabbits in cages or small pens.[54,55,61,65,90] The studies showed, however, that the behavior of wild and domestic rabbits is very similar.

The major behavioral difference between wild and domestic rabbits is their response to confinement. Wild rabbits do not adapt well to cages, often fail to breed, and exhibit abnormal behavior not seen under natural conditions. Other wild lagomorphs such as hares are resistant to domestication and cannot be successfully raised in cages. Taming of wild rabbits should therefore not be attempted, as it is very stressful to them and seldom successful. In contrast, domestication of rabbits has resulted in an animal with a more placid disposition with humans and that is not stressed by confinement, retaining most of the other behavioral repertoires of its wild ancestors.[6] Selective breeding has created over 100 recognized breeds, although many domestic rabbits are the result of hybrid breeding.

Sensory Behaviors

Vision and Behavior

A rabbit's eyes are placed laterally, and the cornea is very large, allowing for an extensive circular field of vision[16] like that possessed by most grazing herbivores. This positioning of the eyes, however, does not provide visualization of the area beneath the mouth. Rabbits that have vision problems may move their heads from side to side or up and down as if to focus in order to scan the area around them.[9] This scanning behavior is most evident as a visually impaired rabbit is carried around in a room.

Touch and Behavior

The lips and the vibrissae in the area beneath the mouth are sensitive enough to distinguish various food items as the rabbit grazes. Because of this sensitivity and because rabbits are obligate nasal breathers, rabbits do not like to have their noses touched. This should be taken into consideration during examinations and when medicating or teaching clients to medicate their rabbits. Rabbits generally do not like to have hands placed beneath their noses (as one might do when greeting a strange dog). Doing so may cause the rabbit to startle. Rabbits also have long sensory hairs above their eyes and around their noses.[36]

Hearing and Behavior

The ears of rabbits are very large and highly vascular, allowing for amplification and location of sound, providing an acute sense of hearing,[48] and thermoregulation. The ears constitute approximately 12% of the body surface area.[23] The ears are often held at odd angles, and the rabbit may shake its head and scratch at its ears with the rear feet if infection or mite infestation is present.

Olfactory Behaviors

Scent-marking is a common behavior of rabbits, whereby their scent glands are used to mark both animals and inanimate objects. Rabbits are strongly territorial, and both sexes release scent signals in the urine and from specialized skin glands found over the body. The anatomic location and morphology of these glands, and the behaviors used to disperse the secretions, have been investigated for the chin, anal, inguinal, and Harderian glands.

Chin glands, which are specialized submandibular glands opening onto the underside of the chin, are used by rabbits to mark almost any physical feature in their environment (see additional information on chinning in Communicative Behaviors). The pair of pocketlike perineal glands known as the inguinal glands and the harderian glands, located around the eye, are both believed to release pheromones that may serve as sexual attractants in both sexes.[5] The size of the glands and degree of marking are androgen dependent and related to the level of sexual activity. Males mark more frequently than do females, dominants of both sexes mark more frequently than do subordinates, and dominants mark most in the presence of subordinate rivals. Under natural conditions, both bucks and does in their own territory, surrounded by their own odor and that of their clan, win two thirds of all aggressive encounters.[74] Lehmann has suggested that scent-marking of individual animals in a group may represent a form of group identification.[55]

Large, fibrous fecal pellets can act as a vehicle for these anal gland secretions. Besides the apparently random distribution of pellets throughout their home range, rabbits also deposit pellets at special "dung-heap" or "latrine" sites.[5] Bell believes that latrine maintenance may serve several functions: the recognition of own or familiar odors at these sites may have a "confidence-enhancing" effect; the "strangeness" of any odors may inform an intruder that the area is occupied; latrines serve as loci for the indirect exchange of olfactory information among members of the same social grouping and contribute to the regulation of population density by inhibiting reproduction in socially subordinate animals.

Female rabbits will mark their kits with chin and inguinal gland secretions and are openly hostile to young that are not their own.[27] They will normally harass young from their own colony, but will actually pursue and kill young from other colonies. Even kits of a doe, smeared with the odor from other rabbits, are attacked and killed.[69] Minimally, does will reject strange kits that do not smell the same as the rest of the litter. Successful cross-fostering therefore not only requires having healthy kits with the energy to suckle but also camouflaging their scent by rubbing in the nest bedding and placing them at the bottom of the litter pile.[26,48]

Enhancement of olfactory cues during mating and nursing has been successfully exploited by rabbit breeders to increase reproductive performance and yields. However, the reproductive component of social olfaction is only one part of a rabbit's scent-marking repertoire, and a significant part of normal behavior involves maintaining what Bell[6] has described as an "optimum odor field."

Communicative Behaviors

A highly intelligent species, the rabbit is very aware of its surroundings and will initiate play and chase games with other rabbits as well as with people. It has been shown that rabbits can recognize other rabbits as well as individual people.[24] Deaf rabbits have been known to respond to hand signals from their owners.[57] A list of common behaviors that rabbits use to communicate can be found in Box 1-1.

Rabbits are in general very quiet pets, but they do on occasion vocalize. A high-pitched, repetitive scream denotes severe terror or pain. This sound is very much like a human baby crying. Fear may also be denoted without vocalization, by a motionless, crouched position with feet beneath the body, the head extended, ears flattened against the head, and eyes bulging.[10] Grunts, growls, and snorts are sometimes used to express anger or annoyance, especially in those guarding their territory or those influenced by

BOX 1-1   Common Rabbit Postures, Behaviors, and Vocalizations

Purring or tooth purring—A sound made by lightly and quickly grinding and vibrating the teeth as the whiskers quiver; a sign of contentment.

Oinking or honking—A sound made to gain food or attention or during courtship.

Clicking—A happy sound often made after a welcomed treat is given.

Wheezing or sniffing—Nasal sounds made by "talkative" rabbits; can be distinguished from abnormal respiratory sounds because they are intermittent and stimulated by interaction with the rabbit.

Whimpering or low squealing—A fretting noise that is made when one picks up a rabbit that is reluctant to be handled; made more often by pregnant and pseudopregnant does.

Chinning—Rubbing the secretions from the scent glands under the chin on inanimate objects and people to mark possession. Glands are more developed in males than females.

Nudging or nuzzling—The nose is used to nudge a person's hand or foot, or the rabbit may pull on a pant leg to signal a desire for attention. When enough petting has been done the rabbit may push the hand away.

Head shaking, ear shaking, body shudder—A shake of the head or body in response to an annoying smell or unwanted handling; often occurs as a rabbit settles down and becomes relaxed enough to begin eating and grooming.

Courting or circling—Can be a sexual or social behavior whereby a rabbit circles another rabbit or the feet of a human while softly honking.

Scratching at the floor—A rabbit may scratch at the floor with its forepaws in order to get a person's attention or to be picked up.

Nipping—Not always done in anger, this can mean "move over" or "put me down."

Presentation—The head is extended forward with the feet tucked under the body and the chin placed on the floor in order to present oneself as subordinate for petting from humans or to be groomed by another rabbit.

Flattening—A fear response wherein the rabbit flattens its abdomen onto the floor with ears laid back against the head; the eyes may be bulging.

Thumping—A sharp drumming of the hind feet as a warning or an alert to other rabbits of danger; often accompanied by dilation of the pupils and seeking of refuge.

Teeth grinding—A slower, louder teeth crunching, sometimes seen with bulging of the eyes and usually indicating discomfort, pain, or illness.

Snorting or growling—A warning sound, either hissing or a short barking growl, that occurs with aggression or fear and is often seen with the ears flattened against the head and the tail up and in the grunt-lunge-bite sequence.

(Continued)

> **BOX 1-1** **Common Rabbit Postures, Behaviors, and Vocalizations—cont'd**
>
> **Isolation**—A rabbit that normally seeks attention from its mates and human companions that isolates itself and is less active should be checked for illness.
>
> **Kicking**—If a rabbit feels insecure when being picked up it will kick violently in an effort to escape. The hindquarters *must* be supported to prevent trauma to the spine or legs. A rabbit should be placed hind end first into a cage in order to help prevent injuries caused by kicking.
>
> **Aggression**—Strained, upright stance with tail stretched out and ears laid back in defensive posture; the rabbit may also kick high and backwards.
>
> **Loud, piercing scream**—Similar to a human baby crying; signaling pain and fear, as when the rabbit is caught by a predator.
>
> **Scanning**—A rabbit with impaired vision may move its head from side to side to scan the area around it.

Adapted from Bradley TA: Rabbits: understanding normal behavior, *Exotic DVM Magazine*, 2(1):19-24, 2000, and Bradley TA: Rabbits: medical implications of selected abnormal behaviors, *Exotic DVM Magazine* 2(4):27-31, 2000.

hormones. Occasionally a honking or oinking sound will be made to gain food or attention or during courtship. A loud squealing sound may be made when rabbits are picked up and begin to fret.

An alert rabbit will have its ears forward, or the ears may be positioned laterally. A menacing expression is denoted by the ears being pulled back. An erect tail can indicate excitement or anticipation or may occur if a rabbit is threatened. Tail twitching may be noted during courting and often is accompanied by urine spraying (see Male Reproductive Behaviors). When presenting itself to be petted, a rabbit will assume a subordinate position with the feet tucked under the body, the head extended forward, and the chin on the floor.[10]

Rabbits may lick their human companions as a form of grooming them and as a sign of affection. Nipping is not always done in anger and may be done to indicate the need for attention or a desire for the handler to put the rabbit down or for another rabbit or human companion to move over. If a rabbit nips too hard, the handler should respond immediately with a high-pitched yelp (as a littermate might do during too-rough play fighting) to deter the behavior.[81]

Rabbits will "thump" by stomping their rear feet when angry and as an alarm to other rabbits; the thumping can be accompanied by dilated pupils, and the rabbit will often also seek refuge. When other rabbits hear the sound, they become quite still. Rabbits may also assume a strained upright stance with the tail stretched out and ears pulled back that indicates readiness to attack. Such rabbits may kick high and backward if a fight occurs. A short barking growl, hissing, or snorting sound may be made to denote aggression and is often noted in the grunt-lunge-bite sequence. Staff members should handle these agitated rabbits carefully, as an angry rabbit can be quite contentious and can inflict injury on the handler (by lunging, kicking, biting, and scratching) or on itself when resisting.

A low-pitched hum as well as a chatter of the teeth can indicate pleasure and contentment. This is referred to as "tooth purring" by the layperson and can be quite loud. During tooth purring the teeth vibrate lightly and quickly while the whiskers are quivering. Actual teeth grinding or bruxism is a slower, louder tooth crunching, often accompanied by bulging eyes and usually indicating discomfort, pain, and illness. Bruxism is especially noted when gastrointestinal pain is present.

Like people and other pets, some rabbits are more vocal than others. New rabbit owners with more vocal rabbits will often present their rabbits to clinicians because of wheezing or congestion. This wheezing or sniffing sound can be distinguished from upper airway disease in that it is intermittent and occurs only when the rabbit is being handled.

To communicate their presence, intact male rabbits will mark their territory by depositing strong-smelling feces at the periphery of their space. Rabbits may also mark with urine and by "chinning" their environment. They rub the scent gland located beneath the chin to deposit a strong-smelling secretion on inanimate objects including furniture, carpets, and household items (see chinning under Olfactory Behaviors). The chemical composition of chin gland secretions includes 34 volatile components, primarily aromatic and aliphatic hydrocarbons, and differs in animals from different geographic locations.[40]

The chinning behavior occurs earlier in females than in males, and the frequency increases throughout development because of an increase in sex steroid secretions.[35] Does that are pregnant or pseudopregnant exhibit lower rates of chinning than females in any other part of the reproductive cycle.[34] The chin gland secretions help to maintain dominance hierarchies in the wild, and dominant rabbits have the additional compound 2-phenoxyethanol, which is a fixative that allows the scent to persist longer in the environment.[41]

Social and Antisocial Behaviors

Rabbits are the only leporids that live in large stable groups or warrens, sometimes numbering several hundred animals.[79] This social nature was not lost during domestication, and rabbits tend to fare better in groups of two or three rather than as solitary pets (Figure 1-1). Unfortunately, until

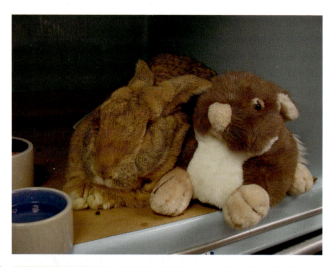

Figure 1-1
Bonded mates come in all shapes and sizes. A rabbit that is kept as a single pet often benefits from the "companionship" of a stuffed toy—as long as that toy is not consumed! (Courtesy Jörg Mayer.)

the 1990s this aspect of their sociobiology was neglected by researchers and lay owners alike. Part of the reason was the development of intensive husbandry techniques for breeding domesticated rabbits. This required good infectious disease control, and because these diseases are spread by contact, rabbits were kept isolated from one another in singly housed cages. With the development of specific-pathogen–free rabbits for laboratory research and the virtual absence of infectious rabbit diseases in most animal facilities, isolation of rabbits from one another is no longer the critical practice it once was.

Another reason for housing rabbits singly involved the false belief among rabbit producers that the euphemistically "conventionally housed" rabbit had the greatest growth performance.[17] Critical analysis of the growth performance for singly housed rabbits has shown that these animals have a higher amount of intraabdominal fat, abnormal musculoskeletal development associated with their restricted locomotion, and increased carcass damage because of "nervous" confinement-associated behaviors.[28]

Abnormal repetitive behavior is commonly seen in caged rabbits and includes pawing at the corners of cages, wire-biting, overgrooming, overeating, and playing with the water supply. Studies showed that rabbits group-housed in small social groups exhibited behaviors that included

Rabbit Behavior

increased exercise and social contact and that individuals exhibited preferences for microenvironments within the enclosures (Figure 1-2).[94] Rabbits also engage in "amicable" activities such as lying together, grooming, and nuzzling. Rabbits that isolate themselves from the group should be checked for medical problems. It has been shown that subordinate rabbits exhibit elevated heart rates that adjust to a lower level if the same rabbit achieves a more dominant position.[30] Rabbits often mount one another as a show of dominance, often facing the head of the subordinate.[10] This can happen regardless of the gender of the dominant or subordinate rabbit and in both intact and altered rabbits.

It has been found that rabbits that are handled in the first week postpartum are less apt to show signs of fear of humans than ones that are not handled.[8,80]

Aggression among young males at puberty makes it impossible to keep males in groups in pens. The space for one male to run away is not available, and serious injuries follow if the rabbits are not separated. However, aggression is minimal among groups of female rabbits grouped at a young age. This does not hold true for older females singly housed since a young age and then group-housed later in life. Their situation is analogous to that of males.

Introducing a new rabbit should always be done slowly and carefully and with direct adult supervision. The supervisors should be prepared to

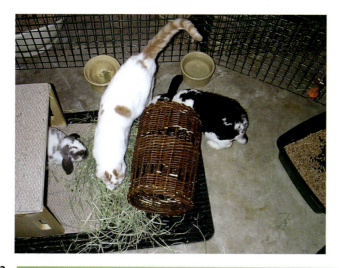

Figure 1-2
Rabbits can get along well with other pets as long as direct adult supervision is provided and a carefully supervised bonding time is allowed. (Courtesy Darice Heishman.) (See Box 1-2)

separate the rabbits if they begin to fight. Many owners wear heavy gloves or put tennis shoes on their hands so they are better protected from being bitten if they have to separate two fighting rabbits.

As with other species, introductions are best performed in neutral territory where neither of the rabbits feel at home (Box 1-2). A dry, clean bathtub may be used, as it is unfamiliar and a little slick and therefore somewhat challenging to the rabbits. Greens and hay can be offered to distract them as well. Placing them in a box or clothes basket and taking them for a long car ride (or circling in an empty parking lot) may also help with bonding, as they tend to comfort each other in the strange surroundings rather than to fight. The bonding process takes time and patience; however, these efforts can be well rewarded, because rabbits are naturally a highly social species. Bonding will be evidenced by mutual grooming and nose-to-nose, nose-to-body, and full-body contact.[7]

BOX 1-2   Suggestions for Bonding Rabbits

- Remember that not all rabbits can get along. Bonding takes time and patience, and direct adult supervision is necessary to prevent injuries.
- Because of rabbits' instinctive social behavior, a social hierarchy or pecking order needs to be established when rabbits that are new to each other are brought together. Some fighting and grouching should be expected. Preparations should be made to be able to separate fighting rabbits, because they can truly hurt each other. Supervisors can wear heavy leather gloves or put tennis shoes on their hands to allow them to separate the rabbits without getting hurt themselves.
- When rabbits begin to reach sexual maturity they will become hormonally driven and more territorial. Arrange to have them spayed or neutered before this becomes a problem.
- Start by placing cages near each other so that the presence of a new rabbit is established. Do not place cages too close to each other, because injuries can occur through the wire sides.
- Allow one rabbit out at a time into a rabbit-safe area. After some time replace that rabbit in its cage and then let the other rabbit into the same area. This allows them to get used to each other's scent.
- Introductions should be made in neutral territory such as a room that neither rabbit has been in. This will decrease the need to defend an established territory. It may also make the rabbits more interested in the new environment as well as less secure and therefore more likely to need each other's reassurance.

BOX 1-2   Suggestions for Bonding Rabbits—cont'd

- Putting both rabbits in harnesses on leashes will also allow them to see each other without getting too close at first. After several times and when they seem less hostile to each other, they can be allowed to get closer to each other, but be prepared to separate them if they fight.
- If bite wounds occur they should be treated by a veterinarian, because they can become infected or abscessed.
- Continue these visits in neutral territory. Eventually they can be let together in the neutral territory. Although some fighting may occur, they may eventually learn to tolerate each other and often will become bonded housemates.
- Owners can also try to place the rabbits in a clean, dry bathtub with some hay and greens as a distraction. This is slick and neutral territory, and the "new" experience may lead them to comfort each other. Alternatively, they can be placed in a laundry basket on the floor of a car and driven around in tight circles in an empty parking lot. By facing a stressful situation together they may again find comfort in each other and be less likely to fight. In both situations they need to be directly supervised by an adult wearing protective gear.
- Some rabbits never get along with each other. Owners should be prepared for this eventuality by understanding that a new rabbit to the household may need to have its own cage and space in the house if it never becomes bonded to the existing rabbit(s).
- Other suggestions for bonding techniques and ideas may be obtained on the National House Rabbit Society web site at www.rabbit.org.

It should be remembered that not all personalities get along well, just as with people. If rabbits are not able to be bonded, it is important to make sure that their enclosures are not kept too close to each other, as severe injuries can be inflicted on rabbits through cage wires. Clients should be counseled that multiple enclosures or separate rooms or areas might be needed if bonding is not successful.

Young rabbits that do well in a home may become aggressive and destructive as they reach sexual maturity. At as early as 3 to 4 months of age, does often become more aggressive to people and to other rabbits and pets, they can have intense mood swings, they mount companions, they spray urine, and they may begin digging and nesting. Bucks also become more aggressive at about 4 to 5 months of age and spray urine and may also mount objects, people, and other pets. Both males and females that were previously litter-box trained begin to urinate and defecate randomly to mark their territory. Clients should be counseled to have their rabbits altered, preferably before the onset of sexual maturity, in order to decrease these behaviors (see Male Reproductive Behaviors and Female Reproductive and Maternal Behaviors).

With time and patience rabbits may also get along with other pets including cats, birds, guinea pigs, and dogs. For example, rabbits were found to show no fear of cats if they were exposed to them before being weaned.[80] Their interactions should never be unsupervised, however, as instinct is a prominent driving force in all species. Any signs of aggression should indicate that predator (cats and dogs) and prey (rabbits and guinea pigs) species may not get along, and close interaction should be prevented. Although they can often cohabitate well with guinea pigs, rabbits can harbor *Bordetella bronchiseptica* subclinically, and this organism is pathogenic in cavies. Alternatively, guinea pigs may harbor *Pasteurella* and represent a source of infection to rabbits.

Reproductive Behaviors

The time that rabbits reach sexual maturity is more a function of size than of age. For instance, small breeds mature at approximately 4 to 5 months of age, medium breeds at approximately 4 to 6 months, and large breeds at approximately 5 to 8 months of age. In general, does mature earlier than bucks.

Male Reproductive Behaviors

Sexual behaviors of male rabbits include urine spraying and "chinning" objects to mark them with the scent glands that are located under the chin. The buck will sniff at, lick, nuzzle, groom and follow the doe and exhibit tail flagging. Enuration, or spraying of a jet of urine on the female, is another courtship behavior. Bucks will also mount and hump inanimate objects, other pets, and humans and will circle the doe or other "object of affection," often while making a soft honking sound (Figure 1-3).

Males in the presence of unfamiliar females exhibit sexual behaviors regardless of whether or not the females are receptive.[92] If the female is receptive, mating occurs quickly. The male grasps the female by biting the nape of her neck, and ejaculation occurs shortly after intromission. When mating is complete, the buck falls over on his back or on his side after mounting the doe, and he may emit a sharp cry. Males may take part in the caring of the young.

Neutered male rabbits tend to make better pets, as they are less territorial and they will mark less with both urine and feces. Neutered rabbits also tend to fight less with other rabbits. Behavioral changes stemming from decreased hormonal influence often are not apparent for 30 days or

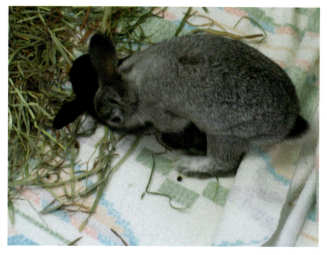

Figure 1-3
Juvenile male rabbits that are just becoming sexually mature. Mounting can be a show of dominance between intact and altered rabbits of either gender. The dominant rabbit often mounts the head of the subordinate rabbit. (Courtesy Teresa Bradley Bays.)

more after neutering. It has been found that some bucks with prior breeding experience, however, continue to exhibit sexual behaviors, including mounting, for up to 10 weeks postcastration.[1] Larger breeds may take up to 6 months for these negative sexual behaviors to decrease.[81] Males may also have viable sperm for a short time after neutering; therefore they should be kept separate from intact females for at least 4 to 6 weeks.

Female Reproductive and Maternal Behaviors

In the wild, matings are generally polygynandrous,* although males will attempt to monopolize particular females.[93] The estrous cycle of rabbits varies from 4 to 17 days in the absence of mating, and mating induces ovulation. Gestation lasts from 29 to 35 days, and litter sizes range from 4 to 10. Females have 3 to 5 pairs of mammary glands, which increase in size several days before kindling.

Sexual behaviors may be noted when a female is introduced into the cage of a male. Receptive females will either flatten to the floor or circle. Other behaviors that indicate sexual receptivity in the doe include lordosis

---

*A kind of polygamy in which a female pairs with several males, each of which also pairs with several different females.

and hyperactivity (except when mounted by the male). Lordosis occurs when pressure is placed over the back (such as when mounted) and the pelvis is raised in an effort to present the perineum to the male. The restless doe shows increased interest in other rabbits and rubs her chin on enclosures and objects. The vulva also becomes congested, moist, and a deeper purplish-tinged color.

Does tend to be more receptive when progesterone levels are lower.[92] A doe that is not receptive will react to the male by running away, cornering the male, biting, and vocalizing.[27] Rabbits are induced ovulators, and ovulation occurs approximately 10 to 13 hours after copulation. If the doe is stressed by overcrowding, predators, or disease, she may resorb the embryos at midterm. In this case, lactation will still occur, and she will come into estrus just as she would have if parturition had occurred normally.[66]

Female pet rabbits may be seen mounting other rabbits (both males and females) as a show of dominance. Female rabbits tend to become more aggressive, aloof, and territorial when sexually mature, even showing aggression and irritability to their owners. Ovariohysterectomy helps to quell aggressive behavior and marking tendencies, which makes for a better relationship between pet and owner.

Pseudopregnancies are common in unspayed females. Ovulation without fertilization may occur sometimes when the doe is in proximity to a male, if the vagina is mechanically stimulated, or if other females mount the doe. Many behaviors seen in gestation are exhibited during false pregnancies, including the pulling of fur from the dewlap area and the ventrum in order to make nests, mammary gland development, and lactation. Pseudopregnancy usually lasts 17 days and resolves spontaneously. It often recurs and may make the rabbit more susceptible to hydrometra or pyometra. Affected does should be spayed prophylactically.

The female's body temperature decreases during the last two thirds of pregnancy.[52] Nesting occurs from a few days to a few hours before parturition, and does will pull fur from their dewlap, abdomen, and sides to line the nest. Food intake decreases in the 48 hours prepartum.[33]

Regulation of nest building is dependent on hormones, but maintenance of maternal behavior is stimulated by the presence of the litter.[32] Kindling usually occurs in the morning hours, and uncomplicated parturition normally is accomplished within 30 minutes. It is not unusual for kits to present in anterior or breech positions. Any evidence of straining without production of kits beyond 30 minutes indicates the need for immediate veterinary intervention.

Primiparous does and those of smaller breeds usually produce smaller litters of four to five kits, whereas larger breeds may produce litters of 8 to 12 kits.[27] Rabbits are placentophagic.[63] Does usually nurse for a very short period of time (usually less than 4 minutes), in the morning or evening,[15,51,86] spending the rest of the time out of the nest. This limited nursing behavior leads many clients to think that wild rabbit does have abandoned their litters. Clients should be instructed to leave a wild rabbit nest alone, as the doe is probably nearby.

The presence of young kits stimulates milk production in the female, whereas older kits inhibit production.[64] Females are able to recognize their kits by their odors. A specific compound, dodecyl propionate, which is released by the kit's preputial glands, will stimulate the maternal anogenital licking behavior.[56] As stated previously, females are unlikely to foster kits from other litters unless they have been rubbed with the scent of the litter and the bedding[26,48] (see Sensory Behaviors). A gland in the region of the nipple produces a pheromone that attracts kits.

Intact female rabbits over the age of 2 years have an extremely high rate of neoplasia in the reproductive tract, especially uterine adenocarcinoma (Figure 1-4).[84] Clinical signs can include hematuria or serosanguineous vaginal discharge, cystic mastitis, and increased aggressiveness. Often, frank blood is most evident at the end of urination.[78] Mammary tumors are also common.

Rabbits should be spayed when they are approximately 4 to 6 months of age. A rabbit is a better surgical candidate if these surgeries are done prophylactically rather than when the rabbit is older and possibly more compromised from preexisting disease. Older intact female rabbits in good health, however, should also be considered candidates for ovariohysterectomy, because early reproductive disease may not be evident. Uterine adenocarcinoma is a relatively slow-growing neoplasm,[16] so uterine tumors may be removed through ovariohysterectomy potentially before metastasis occurs.

Neonatal and Juvenile Behaviors

Newborn kits are altricial and they are born without hair, their eyes are closed, and they require anogenital stimulation for elimination. Newborn rabbits compete vigorously for the doe's milk, so they may actually benefit from the death of littermates. They are, however, very prone to hypothermia, and because the doe spends the majority of the day away from the nest, those raised alone have lower body temperatures and are less likely to survive.[4] The kits huddle together in the nest to keep warm for the first 10 days of life, until their fur grows in.[46] In the wild, mortality rates in the first year of life have been reported to be as high as 90%.[93]

Kits have been shown to be equally attracted to the odors of placentae and colostrum, and it is believed that the fetoneonatal transitional environment affects the ability of the kits to obtain colostrum and milk

16 Exotic Pet Behavior

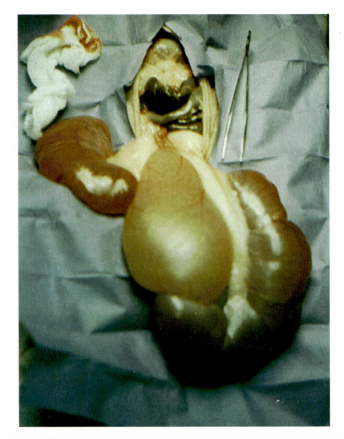

Figure 1-4
Ovariohysterectomy should be recommended in all rabbits, as reproductive pathology is common above the age of 2 years; such pathology includes severe hydrometra, as seen in this dwarf rabbit. Presenting signs included abdominal distension, anorexia, decreased fecal production, and, behaviorally, attempts to keep the cranial half of the body elevated to keep pressure of the distended uterine horns off the diaphragm in order to facilitate respiration. (Courtesy Teresa Bradley Bays.)

readily.[20] They are able to respond to pheromonal cues for nipple-search behavior and are able to recognize them even when they have been delivered by cesarean section.[44] Once nursing is established, however, it appears as though the intraoral stimulation associated with sucking is an important reinforcer to nursing even when a novel odor is applied.[45]

Experimentally, kits have been found to show a preference during the nipple-search behavior for females in early lactation.[21] They ingest more than 30% of their body weight during the daily feeding by the seventh postpartum day,[15] although milk yield decreases after lactation day 19.[33] Kits begin to leave the nest and eat solid food at approximately 3 weeks of age. They are usually weaned at approximately 42 days of age. It is less stressful on the weanlings at this time to be left in the familiar cage and to remove the doe.[13]

Eating Behaviors

In the wild, rabbits are herbivorous, selective feeders that prefer the more tender portion of plants and also consume small amounts of coarse roughage to aid in gastrointestinal motility. The dentition of rabbits allows for cutting the vegetation with the incisors and grinding it with the premolars and molars. Food is chewed thoroughly with a lateral motion of the jaws, highly organized tongue movements, and up to 120 jaw movements per minute.[19]

Domestic rabbits should eat and defecate frequently and continuously throughout the day. Because domesticated house rabbits are diurnal, they eat mostly at dawn and at dusk (crepuscular). Clients should be counseled regarding appropriate dietary items and advised to monitor what is actually eaten versus what is offered.

High-fiber diets stimulate cecocolic motility because of the "scratch factor" and the distending effect of the bulk.[49] Fiber also creates a lattice-like food ball in the stomach that allows for penetration of gastric acids.[16] Rabbits kept on low-fiber diets, on the other hand, are predisposed to hypomotility and reduced feed intake. Often a hard mass of food is created in the stomach that cannot be as easily penetrated by stomach acids and, especially in light of decreased water intake, can create obstruction. As herbivores, rabbits should be fed mostly green leafy vegetables, free-choice grass hay, and only a small amount of pellets daily.

Juvenile rabbits should get a small amount of alfalfa pellets daily, greens, and alfalfa hay. Alfalfa hay, alfalfa pellets, and other legume hays are not recommended for adult rabbits, however, as they tend to be too high in protein and calcium and may predispose the rabbit to forming cystic calculi and/or hypercalciuria, a sludge of calcium carbonate in the bladder. Also, alfalfa is also not as high in fiber as grass hays such as timothy, prairie grass, and brome. For adults, grass hay, such as timothy, prairie grass, or brome, should be offered free choice throughout the day.

A variety of fresh green, leafy vegetables should be offered twice daily, in the morning and in the early evening, the two times of the day when rabbits are most likely to be active. Recommended greens include the following: collard greens, endive, dandelion greens and flowers (no pesticides), carrots and carrot tops, mustard greens, parsley, cilantro, snow peas, romaine lettuce (not iceberg or head lettuce), red and green leaf lettuce, watercress, bok choy, clover, celery, and broccoli (mostly leaves and stems). Spinach and kale may also be offered in small amounts occasionally. Small amounts of fruit may be offered occasionally, as long as loose stools do not result, including apple, strawberries, melon, peach, and pear.

Timothy-based pellets are preferred for adults over the more readily available alfalfa pellets. Adult rabbits that get fresh grass hay and greens as recommended should not get more than $1/4$ cup of pellets per 5 lb (2.2 kg) of body weight per day. Overweight rabbits and those with chronic diarrhea or clumpy stools should have their pellet intake decreased or even eliminated. Obesity, as in other pets, has become common in pet rabbits and especially in those fed free-choice pellets, which are highly concentrated and low in fiber. These rabbits are also more likely to have chronic soft stools or diarrhea, because a low-fiber diet also decreases peristalsis, slowing gastrointestinal transit time and allowing more time for pathogenic bacteria to proliferate.

Rabbits are very social and will learn to beg food from their owners at mealtimes, often receiving table foods that are inappropriate for them. Foods that are high in carbohydrates or sugars should never be fed. Carbohydrate overload of the hindgut can increase the risk of enterotoxemia, and the carbohydrate byproduct, glucose, is used in the formation of iota toxin when *Clostridium* spp. are present. Chew sticks with honey and seeds on them, chocolate, bread, breakfast cereals, oats, crackers, cookies, corn or popcorn, pasta, potato peelings, chips, yogurt drops, and other obviously sugary table foods and treats should never be fed. For a treat, it is best to save back a portion of the rabbit's favorite leafy green vegetable or a small piece of apple or a carrot to be hand-fed at special times.

Small mammal and rodent "treat" mixes that may include seeds, dried vegetables, Canadian trapper peas, or other additives should be avoided. Rabbits will choose the favored treat items over the nutritionally complete pellets. Feeding these mixes may lead to nutritional deficiencies, obesity, and gastrointestinal problems.

Food bowls and water bottles should be cleaned daily and completely washed in hot soapy water at least once per week. Vitamins should not be added to the water, as they can alter the color and taste, making it less likely that the rabbit will drink as much water as it should. Additives in the water also encourage a bacterial slime buildup on the inside of the water bottle or bowl, making it necessary to clean it daily with hot soapy water.

Rabbits will drink 50 to 150 mL (1.6 to 5 oz) of water per kilogram per day,[16] which is more than most other mammals. This is important to realize when calculating fluid therapy for rabbits. Common dosages (mL/

kg/day) used in cats and dogs are not enough to adequately hydrate a rabbit. Polydipsia will occur if food is withheld or if renal pathology is present. Anorexia will occur with water deprivation. Water consumption may be decreased if consumption of fresh green vegetables increases. It is therefore important to question clients about water intake and how water is provided when assessing clinical signs and symptoms in rabbits.

Medical problems may be indicated by changes in food preferences, eating less, defecating smaller and less frequent stools, picking up or showing interest in a food item but not eating it, hypersalivation, or bruxism. The presence of anorexia and decreased or absent fecal output is considered an emergency for a rabbit, and immediate veterinary care should be sought (see gastrointestinal stasis in Elimination Behaviors as well as in Medical Implications of Abnormal Behaviors). Rabbit patients that are not eating on their own should be syringe-fed a supplement made for herbivores (Critical Care, Oxbow Pet Products, Murdock, NE), along with other medical support, under the direction of a veterinarian.

Dental malocclusion, abscesses, and other orofacial problems may be detected early by noting subtle changes in behavior. Food preferences may be altered because of difficulty in prehension or painful mastication. More advanced orofacial problems may be evidenced by hypersalivation, bruxism, pawing at the mouth, anorexia, decreased or total lack of grooming (increased dandruff and loose hair, unclean ears and perianal scent glands), pain on palpation of affected area, or chewing on only one side of the mouth. Rule-outs for these behavioral changes include tooth root abscesses, sharp dental spurs, viral papillomas, oral neoplasias, and facial abscesses.

Limited oral examination in an unanesthetized rabbit may be accomplished using an otoscope with a large aural cone and should be part of every routine rabbit physical examination (Figure 1-5). These so-called "chew" cones are kept separately from the aural cones. Obvious dental spurs and oral lesions may be readily seen; however, resistance to examination with an otoscope cone and increased amounts of saliva noted in the mouth (especially if both are noted unilaterally) may indicate less obvious problems that warrant further investigation with the rabbit under anesthesia.

An index finger inserted between the buccal mucosa and the upper molars can often detect sharp edges without visualization.[57] The rabbit will not appreciate this procedure, and it should be done quickly. However, if sharp points are palpated laterally on the maxillary molars, then anesthesia and molar trimming will be needed, and the extent of other dental disease can be determined when the rabbit is anesthetized.

Examination and treatment of orofacial problems is most safely and thoroughly performed with the rabbit under anesthesia, and treatment is not recommended without proper speculums and other instrumentation

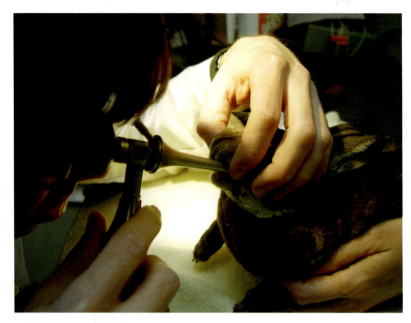

Figure 1-5
Rabbits are obligate nasal breathers and do not like to have their sensitive noses touched, so examination of the oral cavity is performed by placing the thumb and fingers around the cheeks of the rabbit and lifting the lip slightly. Talk to the rabbit quietly as you are performing the examination. (Courtesy Teresa Bradley Bays.)

that is made specifically for lagomorphs (oral instrumentation for small mammals is available through Dr. Shipp's Laboratories, Spectrum, Jorgensen Laboratories, and Sontec). The tongue should be manipulated gently using a cotton-tipped swab and never pulled outside of the rabbit's mouth. The head should be kept in a normal position and never overextended or flexed, as this may occlude the airway. The nares must be protected from accidental occlusion, which can occur when an induction mask is pressed against the nares. All surfaces of each tooth should be checked for spurs and sharp edges (especially the buccal surface, which is more difficult to visualize). Analgesics should be provided before, during, and after dental procedures, as needed.

Elimination Behaviors

Defecation is a fairly continuous process and, in healthy rabbits, is a relatively passive process whereby the rabbit assumes a sitting position with the tail down.[9] Gastrointestinal time for hard feces is 4 to 5 hours.[16] Owners should be instructed to seek veterinary consultation immediately if a rabbit is producing fewer stools, straining to eliminate, or not defecating at all.

All too frequently, the client or referring veterinarian will present a rabbit for treatment for constipation based on the fact that no stool is being produced or straining in the litter box is noted. The abdomen may be distended, or the rabbit may be assuming a strained or hunched posture. This presentation is more likely caused by anorexia and gastrointestinal stasis, which is often secondary to other medical problems.

Gastrointestinal pain may be evidenced in rabbits by anorexia, bruxism, polydipsia, pressing of the abdomen on the floor, or assumption of a hunched posture. Gastric ulcers, partial or total gastric obstruction, gastrointestinal stasis, ileus, or enteritis may cause this discomfort. It is essential to immediately address the need for analgesics and treat the gastrointestinal stasis regardless of the cause (see Medical Implications of Abnormal Behaviors).

The contents of the gastrointestinal tract can constitute up to 10% to 20% of a rabbit's body weight. The stomach contains about 15% of ingesta, and food and cecotropes should always be present in the stomach of a healthy rabbit. The small intestines contain about 12% of ingesta. The large, thin-walled cecum contains about 40% of the ingesta, with a capacity of up to 10 times that of the stomach.[16]

Rabbits are coprophagic and ingest the soft, grapelike clusters of round cecotropes (also known as cecals or night feces) directly from the anus. Coprophagy is seen about 3 to 8 hours after eating.[18] It has been suggested that coprophagy is initiated by the expanding effects of the fecal material on the colonic or rectal wall.[29] These cecals have a mucilaginous membrane that protects them from the acidic pH of the stomach so that they can pass through to the small intestines for reabsorption.

Rabbits that are obese or geriatric rabbits with arthritis or discospondylosis are often unable to reach these cecals, and the perianal area may become soiled. Also, a diet too high in protein may cause an overproduction of cecals. Often clients who may not have noticed them before will call the veterinarian distressed that their rabbit has diarrhea. In severe cases the anus may become blocked by dried fecal mats, creating perianal irritation and dermatitis. Every physical examination should include a careful inspection of the anogenital area, and clients should be counseled to check this area daily so problems may be detected early.

Wild rabbits create a latrine area in their warrens for urination and defecation. This behavior is also seen in domesticated rabbits, which tend to deposit urine and feces in the same place in their enclosures. This makes it possible to litter box train them (Box 1-3). Rabbits may litter train easily

> **BOX 1-3 Litter Box Training Suggestions for Rabbits**
>
> - Begin by confining the rabbit to a small area such as the cage, a fenced-off pen, or a bathroom. As a "denning" species, rabbits prefer not to soil in the areas in which they eat or sleep.
> - Offer several large litter boxes with absorbent compressed newspaper pellet litter or newspaper fiber litter. Do not use clay or clumping litters.
> - Place a litter box in the rabbit's cage in the area that the rabbit frequently uses for urination and defecation. It may be necessary to wire this in place so that it is not easily tipped.
> - Place a fresh supply of hay at one end of the litter box, and freshen daily. Rabbits will spend time in the box eating hay and will often defecate as they eat, thus establishing a use for the box.
> - Fresh fecal pellets defecated outside the litter box should be gathered as they are produced and placed in the litter box.
> - Fresh urine (urinated outside the box) should be wiped up with a paper towel, and the towel placed in the litter box.
> - If the owner is present at the time of defecation and micturition, the fresh urine or feces should be put immediately into the litter box, and the rabbit should then be placed in the litter box. Repeat this as often as is necessary.
> - Clean litter boxes frequently, as a dirty box may discourage use. A mixture of water and vinegar can be used to help remove urine stains.
> - Spayed and neutered rabbits are easier to litter train, as they are generally less interested in marking their territory.
> - If a rabbit spends too much time in the litter box, consider making a more appealing resting area nearby using an alternate bedding material.
> - When the rabbit is using the litter box(es) consistently in the smaller space, pen, or cage, gradually increase the amount of space to which it has access. If mistakes are made, then go back to the smaller space for a bit longer until the rabbit again uses the litter box(es) consistently.
> - Often a rabbit will choose its own place to urinate and defecate. A litter box should be placed in this area, and once the rabbit is using it consistently, it can slowly be moved to a more convenient (for you) location—but maybe not!
> - Some rabbits object to litter of any type. For these, newspapers covered with hay or straw can be placed in the litter box. These will need to be changed more frequently than if other litters are used, as they are not as absorbent.
> - Some rabbits are harder to train than others. Be patient, and never punish the rabbit.
> - Be consistent, and use a lot of praise when the litter box is used.

as adolescents, but when intact rabbits become sexually mature they will begin to mark their territory with strong-smelling urine and feces, thus disrupting their litter habits. This behavior can be quelled by castration and ovariohysterectomy, preferably by 4 to 6 months of age.

Healthy rabbits produce a large amount of urine and stool each day. Therefore litter should be spot cleaned daily and totally changed and cleaned at least once per week. Pine, cedar, and other wood shavings should be avoided, as they have been found to increase liver enzymes in rabbits and rodents, and the volatile aromatic oils may also cause respiratory and dermatologic problems. Wood chips can also harbor mites. Recycled newspaper products, either fiber or pelleted, are preferred, as they are absorptive and safe if eaten. Paper towels and newspapers are also safe to use. Straw and hay can be used as well but do not absorb urine well. Clumping, clay, or corncob litters should not be used, as they may be ingested, leading to gastrointestinal stasis or obstruction.

Urinary Behaviors

Micturition is a relatively passive process during which the tail of the rabbit is only slightly lifted. Urine excretion ranges from 10 to 35 mL/kg/day (0.3 to 1.1 oz).[16] Stranguria is evidenced by a strained posture during micturition as the tail and hind end are lifted much higher with attempts to produce urine and may be accompanied by vocalization. Stranguria may be seen with urinary tract infections, urinary calculi, and hypercalciuria and may be associated with reproductive problems in unspayed females. A rabbit with stranguria may exhibit oliguria and pollakiuria and, in a litter box trained rabbit, inappropriate urination.

The serum level of calcium reflects the dietary intake of calcium, and rabbits excrete 45% to 60% of it in the urine (as opposed to less than 2% in other mammals). Because micturition is the major route of calcium excretion in rabbits, thick urine sludge can form as calcium carbonate precipitates out and create hypercalciuria (see Medical Implications of Abnormal Behaviors).

Occasionally a rabbit's urine will be orange or brownish in color because of porphyrin pigment production. This may occur in rabbits that are taking certain antibiotics, are under stress, or have ingested certain plant pigments. The owner often mistakes this urine discoloration for hematuria. A urine dipstick test can be performed to differentiate the pigmentation from hematuria. In addition, porphyrin will fluoresce under ultraviolet light, whereas blood will not.

See Box 1-3 for litter box training suggestions.

Locomotor Behaviors and Activities

Although wild rabbits are endogenously a nocturnally active animal, domestic rabbits have readily become diurnal when stimulated by external noise, light, and feeding schedule during the daylight.[51] It has been shown that with artificial light the rabbit has a different rhythm than with natural light.[77] Healthy rabbits that are kept in groups spend much of the day together. Although wild rabbits dig burrows that serve as a primary haven, and their home ranges are restricted, observations have shown them to be active above ground—moving around, hopping, running, chasing, and playing. Hopping is the main mode of locomotion.

Rabbits tend to rest for long periods of time in the afternoons and will huddle together, mimicking the natural "safety in numbers" tendency.[10] They will either lie on their sides with feet extended or lie in sternal recumbency with the rear legs stretched back, often with their eyes open (Figure 1-6). Occasionally they will wobble or lean as the depth of sleep increases.[10] They may even lie on their backs with their feet up in the air. Snoring, twitching, thrashing, and fluttering of the eyelids or whiskers may occur and can be mistakenly described by owners as seizing. Therefore, care should be taken when evaluating these behaviors as described by the owner.

Exercise is important for maintaining both physical and mental health of rabbits. Rabbits that are continuously caged, especially in cages that are

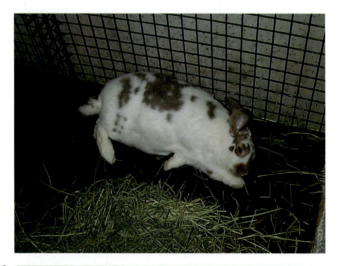

Figure 1-6
A relaxed rabbit may sleep on its side or abdomen with the rear feet extended back. Some rabbits sleep on their backs with their feet up in the air when they feel totally safe. (Courtesy Darice Heishman.)

Rabbit Behavior 25

too small, have an increased risk for obesity, pododermatitis, osteoporosis, and spinal injuries.[38] Rabbits allowed to roam freely in a room or in the home often demonstrate a happy "dance." This entails running quickly and kicking up their rear legs. Excited, joyous rabbits may even leap off the ground with all four feet (similar to a newborn lamb), often with sideways kicks and body shaking in what is fondly referred to as the "binkie." Happiness may also be expressed by a shake of the head or a sudden flop onto the side or back. Rabbits may also stand on their hind legs to use sight, hearing, and smell to evaluate their surroundings. Enclosures should be large enough to allow them to do this easily.

Rabbits will climb onto objects if they have the opportunity and will lie together and sleep on raised platforms. If they are able to move from level to level, they will often be found sitting on shelves 6 to 8 feet (1.8 to 2.4 m) above the floor (Figure 1-7). Unfortunately, the use of vertical space for laboratory rabbits has not been studied. From studies performed

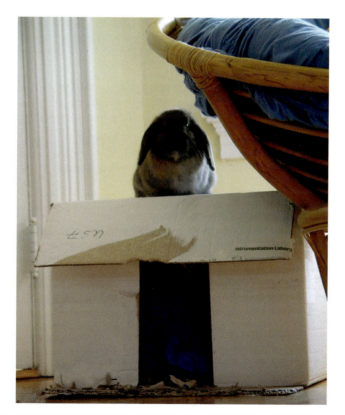

Figure 1-7
Rabbits love to perch on top of objects and up on shelves. This behavior should be encouraged if safe access can be provided. (Courtesy Jörg Mayer.)

by Love,[60] however, it was concluded that space to move around is important. Rabbits should have the minimal space required to indulge in hopping, standing up on their hind legs, and perching at higher levels; a prey species, rabbits need a safe haven when frightened.

Juvenile rabbits act much as teenagers do. They tend to be hyperactive, rambunctious, playful, and mischievous. They are intensely curious and can be active chewers and diggers. It takes up to a year for them to become more sedate and predictable, with occasional periods of activity. Many rabbits are given up by their owners because this adolescent behavior is misunderstood and not properly redirected (Box 1-4).

BOX 1-4 Modifying or Preventing Negative Behaviors in Rabbits

1. Chewing and digging are natural behaviors, and they cannot be controlled. Instead, divert the rabbit's attention, and provide areas that are rabbit safe and appropriate items to dig at or chew on.
   - Cover electric, phone, and data cords with PVC tubing or plastic aquarium tubing that has been slit on one side.
   - Eliminate dangling cords.
   - Protect baseboards and floors with grass or straw matting or thick plastic.
   - Cover flooring with cotton matting, straw, or grass mats.
   - Block or cover up any small places in which a rabbit could get trapped.
   - Provide rabbit-safe "toys," and rotate them periodically:
     - Woven straw and untreated wicker baskets
     - Toilet paper rolls, cardboard boxes (untreated), paper cups (not Styrofoam), paper towel rolls
     - Untreated wood blocks
     - Paper grocery bags and other commercial "tunnels"
     - Sturdy hard plastic toys that are made for large birds (such as macaws) and large dogs
     - An empty soda can with a rock inside
     - Plastic Slinkies and newspapers or old phone books that are positioned beneath table legs
     - Hay and straw, provided to lie in, burrow under, and eat
     - A tub, cardboard box, or paper bag filled with loose hay or straw
     - Grass and straw mats
     - Green leafy vegetable treats hidden in various areas to simulate foraging
2. Be as consistent as possible with your feeding schedule, and provide food items twice per day (early morning and early evening). Provide grass hays free choice.

> **BOX 1-4** **Modifying or Preventing Negative Behaviors in Rabbits—cont'd**
>
> 3 Be consistent with the day-night cycle to which your rabbit is exposed. Rabbits are not meant to stay up late.
> 4 Rabbits like to perch on high places such as couches, desks, and shelves. Provide places such as these that are easily and safely reachable and that do not have any dangerous (to rabbits) items on them. Encourage use of only these special places by putting bedding boxes where it is acceptable for them to perch.
> 5 Although rabbits often initiate chase games, they should not be chased, because this resembles the predator-prey situation and is stressful to the rabbit.
> 6 Remember that juvenile rabbits tend to be extremely rambunctious and mischievous and they like to dig, chew, and spray urine, especially as they approach sexual maturity. Rabbits calm as they mature, and this "stage" does not last forever.
> 7 Spaying and neutering will help to quell or eliminate urine spraying and decrease fecal marking of territory.
> 8 Aggression has multiple causes and therefore should be analyzed to try to improve the situation:
>   - Learned behavior—owner does not handle the rabbit because it is being aggressive
>   - Improper socialization
>   - Boredom
>   - Territorial aggression
>   - Previous trauma creating aversive behavior
>   - Pain or illness
> 9 As with other pets, using communication that a rabbit understands helps to curtail negative behaviors. If a rabbit nips or bites, an immediate short high-pitched scream (to mimic what another rabbit might do) may indicate to the rabbit that the behavior is unacceptable. If a rabbit is getting close to a dangerous situation or an off-limits area, the owner can stomp his or her foot to alert the rabbit of impending danger, just as another rabbit might do to signal danger or an impending predator.

Geriatric rabbits (above the age of 5 or 6 years old) tend to move more slowly and to sleep more. As in all other species, however, age does not create lethargy, decreased appetite, or weight loss—these are signs of illness that should be explored. Preventive care for geriatric rabbits should be a part of the veterinary practice's goals, including biyearly examinations and yearly blood work in an effort to manage disease as in other species.

In order to recognize abnormal locomotor behaviors, the clinician must understand how rabbits ambulate normally. Rabbits hop with their rear legs, and when they hop the entire palmar surface of each foot is used and both feet leave the ground simultaneously. When rabbits ambulate more slowly, however, just the toes of the rear feet touch the ground. Normally body weight is distributed evenly among all four limbs when the rabbit is standing quietly or sitting. When rabbits are sitting, the entire plantar surface, from the hock to the toes, touches the ground.

Behavior changes in posture and locomotion can include subtle differences such as walking rather than hopping with the rear legs. In a normal sitting posture, a rabbit will have both rear legs squarely beneath it and the back will be well rounded.[9] Rabbits with an *Encephalitozoon cuniculi* infection may exhibit mild posterior paresis and often have a flattened rather than a rounded posture over the back and hindquarters.[9] A lame rabbit may also sit unevenly with one limb extended slightly away from the body or lean slightly to one side with one limb held closer to the body. Clients and referring veterinarians often perceive that the leg held under the rabbit's body is the affected limb, when actually the rabbit may be shifting weight away from the damaged limb.

Head tilt or torticollis occurs acutely and can have multiple etiologies. Many clients mistake a cocked ear or occasional tilting of the head as torticollis, but this behavior is usually caused by otitis externa or mite infestation. True torticollis is not intermittent and may be accompanied by rolling and circling, especially in the early weeks to months of the disease process. Clients must be counseled that torticollis may be permanent despite treatment and that careful management of associated symptoms is necessary while possible causes are ruled out and treatment is begun.

Often rabbits can function and live well despite permanent torticollis, once they have been supported through the earlier stages, if given appropriate treatment and managed carefully by the owners. For instance, the eye that points downward may need to be lubricated to keep it protected from abrasion. A temporary tarsorrhaphy may even be needed in severe cases. Daily management also includes keeping cage or pen furniture in the same position and furnishing nonslick surfaces such as cotton carpets or rubber-backed carpets for better traction. Litter box sides should be lowered, and water and food should be placed so they are easily accessible. Affected rabbits should be kept with their bonded mates to decrease stress or, if possible, provided with mates if they are not already paired.

Rule-outs to be considered for locomotor and postural abnormalities and torticollis include soft-tissue trauma, fracture or dislocation, otitis interna, *E. cuniculi* infestations, neoplasia, encephalitis, septicemia, toxicities, and larval migration of *Cuterebra* organisms. Vertebral fractures or luxations can cause posterior paralysis. Rabbits that are less active, exhibit pain on palpation of the dorsal abdomen or the epaxial area, and assume abnormal postures should be radiographed to check for discospondylosis or arthritis. The potential for an idiopathic vestibular syndrome, as is seen in dogs and cats, has not been ruled out in rabbits.

After several days or weeks of supportive care, regardless of the cause of the torticollis, rabbits have often adapted sufficiently to regain their appetite. However, the longer that severe torticollis remains, the less likely is the recovery of normal or near-normal posture. Physical therapy consisting of stimulation to encourage the rabbit to turn its head to the opposite side has been amazingly successful in many cases.[57] This can be accomplished with the application of a cat laxative to the opposite leg or flank, or scratching of the flank to elicit a reflexive turning of the head in that direction.

Grooming Behaviors

Like most other small mammal species, rabbits are meticulous groomers (Figure 1-8). Mutual grooming of conspecifics and of human companions is a sign of acceptance and affection.[10] Grooming after handling or after a treatment or procedure is an excellent sign of a return to normal behavior. Rabbits that do not groom themselves completely or at all should be checked for illness or pain. Causes of lack of grooming include obesity, arthritis, discospondylosis, orofacial pathology, intense pruritus associated with parasites, and any lethargy-associated illness.

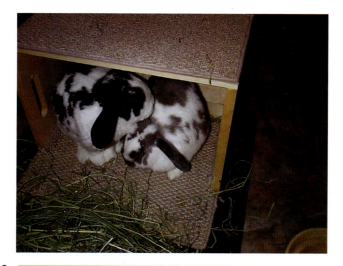

Figure 1-8
Mutual grooming is commonly seen among bonded rabbits. It is important to brush rabbits frequently so that the rabbit doing the grooming does not ingest an excess amount of hair. (Courtesy Darice Heishman.)

Because of rabbits' grooming behavior, it is normal for hair to be present in the gastrointestinal tract. If a rabbit is on an appropriate high-fiber diet and remains hydrated, this does not cause a medical problem. Shorthaired rabbits should be brushed several times per week in general and every day during periods of shedding (molting). Longhaired rabbits should be brushed daily and trimmed occasionally in order to prevent tangles and matting. During periods of molting, longhaired rabbits should be brushed up to twice daily.

Many owners of longhaired rabbits have their pets shaved on a regular basis. This should probably be done under anesthesia to decrease stress to the rabbit. Bathing rabbits for other than medical purposes should be actively discouraged, as the loose hair created after bathing will be ingested during grooming. Because rabbits are unable to vomit, this ingested hair can cause gastrointestinal obstruction.

Barbering occurs between rabbits when a dominant rabbit pulls hair from the subordinate rabbit. Rabbits may barber themselves in late gestation or in pseudopregnancy to prepare a nest or if they are on low-fiber diets, bored, or stressed. Self-barbering may also represent a stress-related dissociative behavior in rabbits.[42] Increasing access to grass hays and greens, providing safe toys to play with, decreasing overcrowding, altering light cycles and light intensity, and increasing exercise will help to quell these behaviors. Easy epilation, seborrhea, alopecia, pruritus, and a rough hair coat are indicative of parasitic infections such as lice or mites.

Rabbits use their rear feet to dig wax out of their ears and then ingest the wax. Wax buildup in one or both of the ears may indicate the presence of medical conditions that limit the movement of the rear legs. The inguinal scent glands may also remain unclean in a rabbit that is overweight or has a medical condition of the spine or pelvis such as arthritis or discospondylosis.

Rabbits have a pad of thick fur on the bottoms of their feet that protects skin and bone beneath. If the integrity of this pad is compromised by moisture, matting, and/or shaving, pressure necrosis pododermatitis may result.

Toenails are not retractable, and declawing rabbits should never be presented as an option to clients as this is a painful elective procedure. Instead owners should be taught how to cut their pet's nails and be counseled to have styptic powder available in case a toenail is cut too short. Nails should be trimmed every 2 to 3 weeks or whenever they are overlong. Overgrown nails get caught in cages, carpets, or other materials and can be pulled off, which can lead to excessive bleeding. Rabbits are exquisitely sensitive to pressure applied to the nail at a level where the nerve (and therefore the vessel) extends. When a rabbit's nails are clipped, the clippers should be applied and lightly closed around the nail. If the rabbit then retracts its foot, the clippers are likely positioned too high and should be repositioned before cutting.

Rabbits in Outdoor Enclosures

Many people still house rabbits in outdoor enclosures. This situation is not ideal, as it limits social contact with conspecifics as well as with human companions. Many hutches that are made specifically for rabbits do not provide enough space for them to move around and to stand up on their hind legs. It is also more difficult to maintain an environment that is safe and comfortable for rabbits and that protects them from predators such as other domesticated pets and wildlife.

In general, rabbits tolerate cold better than heat, but if kept outdoors it is imperative that an enclosed portion of the enclosure provide protection from wind and insulation from the cold. Rabbits are very sensitive to heat and do not tolerate temperatures above 85° F (28° C). They are able to sweat only through glands that are on the lips, and only a small portion of the heat is dissipated through the surface area of their ears, which have a large arteriovenous anastomotic system.[38] They pant ineffectively, and if they become dehydrated they will stop panting.[27] Signs of heat stress include decreased food consumption, gastrointestinal stasis, and assumption of postures that are stretched or prone.[48]

In outdoor enclosures, shade and ventilation are absolute necessities for survival, and clean, fresh water must be available at all times. Care should be taken that wild rabbits do not have access to the domestic rabbits' outdoor enclosures, as infection with *E. cuniculi* could occur via contamination of the grass and subsequent consumption by the domestic rabbit.

Behavioral Enrichment

Rabbits are very social by nature, and as stated previously (see Social and Antisocial Behaviors) tend to do better in bonded pairs or trios. When placed in a cage system that allowed access between two cages, rabbits preferred to be in the same cage with other rabbits.[47] They are intelligent and playful and often initiate play with both human and animal companions. They need attention and mental stimulation in order to thrive. Each has its own personality, but most like the attention of petting and gentle handling. They will initiate games of tag with humans, bat a ball around with the forepaws, and chase toys as they are pulled by their owners, as well as toss toys into the air and retrieve them.[10]

For rabbits kept in enclosures, wire cages are preferred over aquariums because they provide better ventilation. Since rabbits produce a lot of urine daily, ventilation is important so that ammonia levels do not build up and create an unhealthy environment. Rabbits on wire-bottomed cages should be provided with a platform made of wood or cardboard or even hay to allow them to have some time off the wire. It is important that all surfaces be smooth, with no sharp edges, to prevent injury.

Cages should have at a minimum enough space for a rabbit to complete three hops[60] and be at least tall enough for a rabbit to stand up on its hind feet. Studies have shown that rabbits kept in conventional cage systems without enrichment showed more restlessness, excessive grooming, bar-gnawing, and timidity.[37]

Periods of exercise should be provided at least daily. A rabbit-safe area can be created by eliminating the hazards of electric cords and dangerous items that can be eaten or chewed. Decorative houseplants can also be hazardous, as some of them, including dumb cane *(Dieffenbachia seguine)* and oleander *(Nerium oleander)*, are poisonous when eaten. Exercise pens can be created easily by using baby gates or standing pens. During exercise periods owners can lie on the floor with their pets and talk softly to them. A shy rabbit will generally be much more likely to approach a person who is no longer at predator height.

Wild rabbits often use burrows for shelter and safety, and domestic rabbits prefer having tunnels or a hide box to spend time in (Figure 1-9). Care must be taken to ensure that a rabbit does not spend an entire day in a hide box, however, and that whatever is provided is well ventilated. A shy rabbit that stays inside an enclosure with little ventilation and urinates and defecates where it lies can develop respiratory disease, dermatologic problems, and pododermatitis over time.

Even rabbits that are allowed to roam free in rooms or houses should be provided with a cage or box to which they can escape if they feel threatened. Studies with enriched cage systems showed that rabbits often preferred to sit on top of hide boxes[37] and therefore enclosures should be large enough to provide an elevated area on which rabbits can perch.

Grazing arks can be created by placing the top of a cage or a solid frame with wire mesh sides and top over areas of untreated lawn. Water and shade should be provided, and the rabbits should be supervised by an adult to prevent escape or predation by other domestic pets or wild animals. Rabbits like to dig shallow holes to lie in and may try to dig out of a pen if precautions are not taken to prevent escape.

The best and safest toys for rabbits are readily available and inexpensive and include straw baskets, toilet paper rolls, cardboard boxes (untreated), paper cups (not Styrofoam), paper towel rolls, and untreated wood. Paper bags and other "tunnels" can also provide entertainment and resemble burrows used in a more natural environment. Sturdy hard plastic toys that are made for large birds (such as macaws) and large dogs can also be pro-

Rabbit Behavior

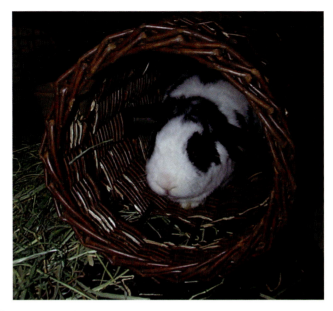

Figure 1-9
Providing tunnels and hide boxes using materials that are safe if chewed or eaten helps to simulate the natural tendencies of this denning species. (Courtesy Darice Heishman.)

vided as long as they cannot be chewed apart and do not have any sharp parts (Figure 1-10).

Small blocks of untreated wood are great for chewing on and batting around. An empty soda can with a rock inside of it will also create a distraction. Plastic Slinkies and newspapers or old phone books that are positioned beneath table legs for resistance can be pulled and chewed. Care must be taken to ensure that rabbits are not able to hurt themselves with damaged toys or toys that can be chewed apart.[87] Studies show that interaction with enrichment devices decreases over time, indicating the necessity to rotate enrichment devices to increase the success of using them.[53]

Providing hay and straw to lie in, burrow under, and eat also helps to provide daily distractions. A tub or box of loose straw or woven straw baskets, untreated wicker baskets, and sea grass and straw mats can also provide diversions. Hiding green leafy vegetable treats in various areas enriches the environment, and studies have shown that total activity time was significantly greater in rabbits that were enriched with food than in those enriched only with nonfood items.[39]

It was also shown that rabbits given loose hay were less likely to exhibit barbering of conspecifics as evidenced by alopecia on the forehead of

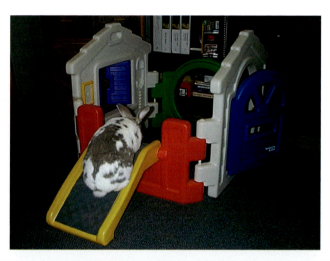

Figure 1-10
This rabbit clubhouse provides the ultimate in behavioral enrichment. Food can be hidden inside to allow foraging and to encourage exercise. (Courtesy Darice Heishman.)

cagemates.[67] Providing a variety of rabbit-safe distractions, toys, and healthy food treats will encourage exercise, decrease boredom, and help to decrease destructive behaviors and conspecific-directed abusive behaviors (see Box 1-4). Environmental enrichment therefore should be considered as important as nutrition and veterinary care.[3]

Medical Implications of Abnormal Behaviors

It is essential for veterinarians to be able to understand and recognize how behavior in rabbits can change with clinical disease and to help educate clients regarding signs of illness in rabbits. Healthy rabbits are inquisitive, alert, and always exploring and sniffing around their environment. The presence of a dull, rough coat or lifeless eyes that appear glazed and unfocused indicates serious illness in rabbits. Also, a rabbit that normally seeks attention from its mate and human companions may isolate itself and become less active when ill.

Rabbits, like other prey species, tend to mask signs of illness and pain, especially if they are frightened and in the strange surroundings of a veterinary clinic. Fortunately, today's rabbit owners are more educated than in the past and are likely to present their pets earlier for veterinary care. Veterinarians should be attentive to owners' observations concerning behavior that is abnormal for their pet rabbits.

Rabbit Behavior 35

Routine well-care visits should be scheduled for any new rabbit and then annually or semiannually thereafter. Well-care visits have the benefits of allowing a practitioner to become familiar with the pet and helping to establish a rapport with the owners in order to counsel them on updated husbandry (diet and environment) recommendations. Most important, problems may be detected earlier, possibly before they are evident to the owner. Annual blood work is recommended for rabbits 5 years old or older to check for common geriatric conditions so that they may be managed proactively.

Rabbits stress very easily and if overhandled or held for too long against an owner's chest can easily become overheated and begin to pant (Figure 1-11). If this behavior is noted it should be addressed immediately by increasing the ventilation in the room and allowing the rabbit to get down on the floor away from the handler. Temperature should be assessed early in the examination process before stress and handling falsely elevate the body temperature.[2]

The most common clinical presentation in rabbits is gastrointestinal stasis evidenced by decreased appetite, anorexia, and decreased or no fecal pellets. Clinical signs also include decreased water intake, hunched postures, tender abdomen, and bruxism. Complete obstruction will be evi-

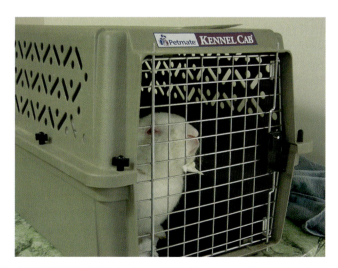

Figure 1-11
This rabbit has its head elevated and nostrils alternatively pinched or flared as it struggles to breathe. With such obvious respiratory distress, handling should be done carefully and diagnostic procedures postponed until the rabbit's condition is more stable. (Courtesy Teresa Bradley Bays.)

denced by severe depression, dehydration, abdominal distention, and hypothermia and will quickly lead to shock and death if not immediately treated.

Gastrointestinal stasis is usually secondary to other illness, stress, or pain and is often associated with high-carbohydrate, low-fiber diets, lack of exercise, and increased ingestion of hair. Once the patient's condition is stable, diagnostics should be performed in order to determine the inciting cause while the gastrointestinal tract function is supported with fluids, antigas products, analgesics, motility stimulants, and antibiotics if deemed appropriate. Gastrointestinal motility will be enhanced and supported by syringe-feeding the rabbit several times per day. Oxbow Pet Products (Murdock, NE) has a formulation (Critical Care) that is nutritionally complete for herbivores and comes in several flavors that are palatable to rabbits. This product has greatly increased the success rate of treatment of gastrointestinal stasis in herbivores.

Because rabbits are unable to vomit, they should not be fasted before surgery except for gastrointestinal surgery, at which time a 6- to 12-hour fast may help to reduce gastrointestinal contents.[14] Because of the weight of the gastrointestinal contents, the rabbit's head and thorax should be elevated when the animal is anesthetized to decrease pressure on the diaphragm.[14] Subcuticular sutures using synthetic absorbable suture material are recommended for skin closure, as rabbits are less likely to chew at the incision than with skin sutures. Rabbits are obligate nasal breathers, so maintaining the patency of the nares is important at all times.

Dacryocystitis is a common problem in rabbits and will cause epiphora. The nasolacrimal duct is very small and narrows at the proximal maxillae and at the base of the upper incisors. Teeth, ears, eyes, and nasolacrimal ducts should be examined if epiphora or ocular discharge is present. Cytology and culture and sensitivity should be performed on ocular and aural discharges, and skull radiographs taken if the condition persists. Upper respiratory infection can be overlooked if a fastidious rabbit licks or grooms away the nasal discharge. Dried residue on the medial aspect of the forepaws, however, may indicate the presence of a discharge.

Prominent causes of morbidity and mortality in female rabbits are reproductive disorders including uterine adenocarcinoma and other neoplasias, as well as cystic ovaries, ovarian neoplasias, hydrometra, pyometra, and metritis. Often hematuria or a serosanguineous discharge from the vulva will be noted (see other clinical signs under Female Reproductive Behaviors). Reproductive disorders in rabbits may also be accompanied by behavioral changes including increased aggression, nesting behaviors, pulling hair from the abdomen or dewlap, polydipsia, polyuria, and inappropriate urination. Hydrometra, pyometra, or abdominal neoplasia that causes distention of the abdomen may cause the rabbit to rest with its head and forelimbs elevated in order to relieve the pressure of abdominal contents on the diaphragm, making it easier to breathe.

It is medically prudent to promote routine, prophylactic spaying of rabbits as part of a preventive health care regimen. The risk for reproductive neoplasia far outweighs the risks of surgery and anesthesia, and the procedure eliminates the need to perform the same surgery in a more severely compromised patient later in life.

Pregnancy toxemia may be seen in late gestation in obese rabbits that are exposed to stress and environmental changes that may cause them to eat less. Does become weak, depressed, and ataxic and may be dyspneic with an acetone odor to the breath. They will become anorexic and may succumb to seizures, coma, and death. Ovariohysterectomy and supportive care are recommended, but the prognosis is grave.

Obesity has become a common problem among pet rabbits, often because of excessive food and treats, inappropriate food items, and too little exercise. Obesity can lead to many medical problems including difficulty grooming, especially in the perianal area, inability to reach and consume cecotropes, and, as in other species, elevated heart rates, hypertension, and cardiac hypertrophy. Obesity and inactivity can also be associated with hypercalciuria and cystitis,[38] probably because of urinary retention. Obese rabbits that become stressed and anorexic are also more likely to develop hepatic lipidosis.

E. cuniculi is transmitted from rabbit to rabbit through the urine and can affect the renal and central nervous systems of rabbits. Although many rabbits are asymptomatic, others may have urinary incontinence and posterior paresis,[16] as well as nystagmus, rolling, and seizures, often after a stressful period in a rabbit's life.[25] A stiff-gaited posture and walking rather than hopping with the rear feet may be all that is clinically evident.[9] Torticollis may also be seen and should be considered a symptom of *E. cuniculi* infection if otitis media has been ruled out (see Locomotor Behaviors and Activities).

Renal failure can be a common presentation in very young rabbits and as rabbits get older. Clinical signs in older rabbits may include lethargy, depression, anorexia, polyuria, polydipsia, and urine scalding. If diagnosed early, rabbits may respond to supportive care and subcutaneous fluids. Grass hay and greens should be increased, and the amount of pellets offered should be decreased. Synthetic erythropoietin can be administered if anemia is present in rabbits with chronic renal failure.

Polyuria, polydipsia, inappropriate urination, perineal urine scalding, hematuria, stranguria, pollakiuria, hunched posture, and bruxism may be evidence of urinary tract infection or disease. Urolithiasis and hypercalciuria (see Urinary Behaviors) may be seen, often in obese rabbits fed high-calcium diets including alfalfa hay and pellets as well as those receiving vitamin and mineral supplementation. Urolithiasis is more common in sedentary, obese, or geriatric rabbits.[13] A diet similar to that used for renal failure is recommended, as is increasing exercise and avoiding highly mineralized water sources.

Urine scalding and urinary incontinence may also be seen in older obese rabbits with discospondylosis or osteoarthritis and secondary to *E. cuniculi* infection. Weight loss is recommended; however, surgery may become necessary to remove excess skinfolds in rabbits with chronic urine scalding.

Many texts list the use of marginal ear veins for venipuncture. Perivascular necrosis can occur, especially in breeds with smaller ears and veins. The lateral saphenous vein is superficial, is easily accessible, and is my preferred site for venipuncture.

Rabbits and the Hospital Environment

A fearful rabbit flattens its body in a crouched position with the feet tucked beneath it and the head extended, often with eyes bulging and ears flat against the head.[10] Stress-related catecholamine release, as seen in rabbits that are frightened, causes increases in heart rate and respiratory rate, renal ischemia, and decreased body temperature.[27,50] This catecholamine release will also interfere with anesthesia and recovery from surgery.

It is therefore important to decrease stress as much as possible during hospitalization in order to increase the success of a medical or surgical patient. Teach clients to place open pet taxis or carriers containing a small amount of hay out in the open at home between visits. When rabbits have ready access to these, they will be less frightened when confined to the carrier for transport. Rabbits should also be prepared for the veterinary visit by occasionally acclimating them by driving them around in the pet taxi or carrier.

In the examination room, provide a towel or cloth mat for the rabbit to sit on in order to provide traction and to decrease stress. Timidity in the hospital environment might create a more quiet rabbit, but the eyes of a healthy rabbit should be bright and the posture should remain normal. With calming the rabbit will begin to groom, exhibit curiosity by sniffing the environment, and eat if offered appropriate food items. Approach the rabbit patient slowly, and handle it gently. Quietly talk to the rabbit patient about what you are doing as you perform your examination.

A rabbit should be lifted up gently but firmly by scooping the rear end with one hand as the rabbit is grasped behind the front legs with the other hand. If the rear legs are not well supported, the rabbit can break its own

Rabbit Behavior 39

back by kicking. Rabbits can be held like a football against the handler's chest with the head tucked into the elbow and the scruff held gently but firmly if necessary.

Rabbits often try to twist and kick or thump as they are released into a cage, which can lead to spinal injury or injury to the handler. They should therefore be placed backward into a cage or a pet taxi. If a rabbit is struggling, the handler should try to cover the rabbit's eyes and place the rabbit down on a secure surface. A frightened or angry rabbit will go to a back corner of the cage and face outward with the head tilted slightly downward, eyes glaring and ears laid back. A rabbit in this posture should be picked up slowly and carefully, as it may lunge at, scratch, or bite the handler when approached.

For examination of the ventrum, temperature taking, and nail trimming, the rabbit can be placed in the **C** position with the back against the handler's chest, the rear end cupped with one hand, and the front legs supported with the other hand (Figure 1-12). In this position the feet are

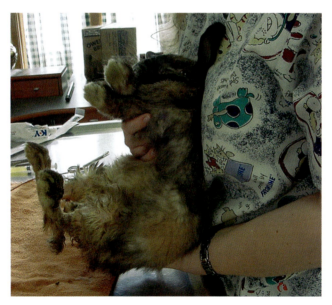

Figure 1-12

Holding rabbits in the **C** position, in which the rump is cupped with one hand and the other hand is placed below the front legs, allows for nail trims, examination, and procedures of the ventrum and perigenital area. The feet are never restrained in this position. If the rabbit struggles, the curve of the **C** can be altered until the rabbit is more comfortable. (Courtesy Teresa Bradley Bays.)

never restrained, and the **C** position is gently altered if the rabbit struggles, until it feels comfortable and more secure.

It is very important to ask the owner whether a rabbit is accustomed to drinking from a sipper bottle or a bowl and to provide this when it is hospitalized. Pathology and pain of the oral cavity should be taken into consideration when choosing food items and in deciding on whether an impaired rabbit is given a water bottle or water bowl. For example, impaired rabbits may eat better if provided with a gruel (such as Oxbow's Critical Care; see Eating Behaviors) or a blended mush of greens to eat, and may be able to obtain water more easily from a bowl than from a sipper bottle.

Preferred food items should be available, especially if a rabbit is not eating well. Even preferred treats that are not necessarily good for rabbits can be fed on a short-term basis in order to encourage rabbits to eat and then changed back to a better diet once eating resumes. A rabbit that has undergone surgery (except for gastrointestinal surgery) should be eating and defecating within a very short time of anesthetic recovery. If this does not occur, supportive care with warmed subcutaneous fluids, additional analgesics, and syringe-feeding with Critical Care (see gastrointestinal stasis under Medical Implications of Abnormal Behaviors) should be instituted.

Hospitalized rabbits should be kept in a quiet area away from predator species. Provide plenty of greens and grass hay for hospitalized rabbits in order to provide them with familiar items and to encourage them to eat despite the stress. Allowing bonded mates or rabbit companions to stay together during hospitalization and boarding is very important to decrease stress and to increase the success of treatment.[10,48] Allowing them to be together while hospitalized will also help to eliminate changes in their social hierarchy when they return home, as they will both (or all) have a similar smell that might otherwise alienate them from one another. Efforts to return the rabbit to its home environment as soon as possible should be made in order to limit stress. A litter box should be provided when the rabbit is hospitalized, containing rabbit-safe litter including pelleted or fiber-type recycled newspaper products, as many rabbits will not urinate or defecate outside of a litter box.[14]

Rabbits naturally burrow, so providing a nest box or hide box for a long-term stay in the hospital or boarding may provide some additional security and therefore decrease stress. These can be made out of wood, cardboard, or plastic. As stated previously, it is important that such boxes are well ventilated, and care should be taken that a shyer rabbit is not spending all of its time in the box and lying constantly in urine and feces.

Pain Management Considerations

Veterinarians who treat rabbits must be especially aware of the need for pain management in the primary treatment of these patients. It has been shown that small mammals have the same or similar neurologic components to perceive pain as those found in domestic species as well as in humans and that antinociceptive mechanisms to modulate pain are present.[91] Therefore rabbits display appropriate behavior in response to stimuli that are known to be painful in other species. Pain management in rabbits and other prey species should be addressed immediately *before* diagnostic procedures and other treatments are performed.[11]

The physiologic "stress response" to pain in rabbits and other small mammals includes vasoconstriction, increased heart rate and stroke volume, and decreased gastrointestinal and urinary tone.[95] Endocrine responses lead to a catabolic state with decreased kidney function.[95] Also, nociceptive stimulation of the brain enhances reflex sympathetic responses, which create increased blood viscosity, prolonged clotting time, fibrinolysis, and platelet aggregation.[95]

Clinically, as in all species, the response to pain in rabbits can include immune suppression, impaired wound healing, decreased food and water intake,[83] and secondary medical problems including gastric ulcers, gastrointestinal stasis, decreased peripheral circulation and body temperature, shock, and even death. In general, a higher rate of anesthetic mortality is associated with surgery in exotic species, and one must wonder if this is related to the inadequate use of preoperative and postoperative analgesics.[83]

Physiologic changes that accompany pain can create secondary medical problems, may inhibit response to treatment, and may even precipitate death in the patient. These detrimental responses make it necessary for practitioners to reevaluate the need for analgesia in rabbits that are experiencing trauma, disease, surgery, or other invasive procedures in which pain is a known component. As with all species, a return to normal behavior indicates a positive response to analgesic treatment. Specifically for rabbits, this includes eating and drinking, defecating, sleeping, playing, stretching, and grooming. Any disease, trauma, or process that has pain as a known component in other species should be considered painful in these species as well and treated accordingly.[11]

Behaviors Associated with Pain

Becoming familiar with normal behaviors of each species that a veterinary practitioner treats is the first step needed in order to recognize pain behaviors as early as possible. Identification of pain behaviors in rabbits and other prey species, however, is made more complicated because they exhibit less overt pain-associated behaviors in order to decrease their chances of being caught by predators.[58] Immobility is a common behavior displayed by all prey species that are presented for examination, making it even more difficult to determine if pain is present.[31] This would especially be true for rabbits that are excessively nervous or not well socialized. Also, anxiety has been associated with a lowered threshold of pain perception.[62] It is therefore imperative that attempts be made to decrease the rabbit patient's anxiety in the hospital environment by keeping it in a quiet environment away from dogs, cats, and excessive noise. Practitioners should remember that rabbit owners may be the most attuned to normal behavior for their pets, and therefore we should never discount an owner's assessment of pain and anxiety in a pet. See Box 1-5 for clinical signs associated with pain in rabbits.

Hypnosis

Some handlers have the ability to use hypnosis as a method of restraint whereby the rabbit is placed on its back with the neck stretched out, sometimes with the rear legs restrained. The ventrum of the rabbit is then rubbed gently while the handler speaks softly in a monotone voice. The breathing rate is said to decrease, and the eyes stay open with the pupils constricted.

Although this technique *might* be useful for noninvasive, nonpainful procedures, it should *never* be used as a method of restraint for castration or other surgical procedures in this prey species. Anesthetics and analgesics are imperative; this is a classic case of "just because you can, doesn't mean you should."

Euthanasia and Adoption

Humane euthanasia is a difficult task with any species, but euthanizing prey species is made more difficult by the fact that restraint is frightening to them. Rabbits that are compromised and suffering can be gently and humanely euthanized by anesthetizing them first with injectable or gas anesthetics, followed by an intracardiac or intravenous injection of euthanasia solution.

Like cats and dogs, exotic species are more frequently being taken to shelters and rescue groups when owners tire of the responsibility of caring for them as pets. Rabbits are no exception, and like dogs and cats are often euthanized if space becomes limited in shelters. It is imperative that we as practitioners guide our clients toward adoption of these pets. Rabbits

BOX 1-5 Clinical Signs Associated with Pain in Rabbits*

- Production of fewer, smaller, or no fecal pellets
- Half-closed or dull, unfocused eyes
- Holding the head in an elevated and extended position
- Aggression in a normally docile animal
- Pressing abdomen on the floor
- Chewing at affected site
- Immobility, lethargy, or reluctance to move
- Decreased interest in the environment
- Isolation
- Overgrooming or lack of grooming
- Hair pulling at affected site
- Vocalization (squeal usually indicates fear in rabbits)
- Stretching with back arched
- Stinting/splinting on palpation
- Hunched posture
- Teeth grinding (bruxism)
- Tucked appearance to abdomen
- Strained facial expression with bulging eyes
- Squinting of the eyes
- Increased frequency and depth of respiration
- Rapid shallow breathing
- Abdominal breathing
- Lameness, ataxia or stiff movements
- Anorexia
- Polyuria and polydipsia (especially with gastrointestinal pain)
- Piloerection
- Porphyrin secretion (stress)
- Self-mutilation
- Absence of normal behaviors

*All of the clinical signs listed can be associated with any disease process in rabbits. If pain is a known component of the existing disease process or procedure, then analgesics should be used preemptively, but especially if these signs or behaviors are noted.

can be adopted from shelters and also through rescue groups such as local chapters of the National House Rabbit Society (www.rabbit.org).

Veterinarians should also counsel owners not to continue to breed rabbits just for the sake of allowing their children to "experience nature" or to provide pet stores with additional rabbits that may be purchased as

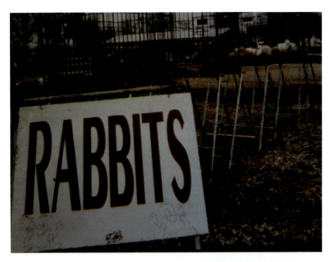

Figure 1-13
Rabbits, as well as other exotic pets, are often purchased as impulse buys without thought or knowledge of how much attention and care they will need. This photo was taken on Easter day on a roadside in Missouri and shows an all-too-common occurrence. (Courtesy Teresa Bradley Bays.)

impulse buys such as those purchased for Easter presents (Figure 1-13). In addition, pet store employees should be schooled regarding the husbandry and care of rabbits so that potential buyers have a full understanding of what it takes to be a rabbit owner.

Acknowledgments

I wish to acknowledge Thomas Donnelly, BVSc, Diplomate ACLAM, for his guidance with this chapter.

References

1. Agmo A: Sexual behavior following castration in experienced and inexperienced male rabbits, *Z Tierpsychol* 40(4):390-395; *Anesth* 21:73-77, 1976.
2. Antinoff N: Physical examination and preventative care of rabbits. In *Veterinary Clinics of North America, Exotic Animal Practice—Physical examination and preventative medicine*, Philadelphia, Saunders, 1999.
3. Bausman V: Environmental enrichment for laboratory rodents and rabbits: requirements of rodents, rabbits, and research, *ILAR J* 46(2):162-170, 2005.
4. Bautista A, Drummond H, Martinez-Gomez M, et al: Thermal benefit of sibling presence in the newborn rabbit, *Dev Psychobiol* 43(3):208-215, 2003.
5. Bell DJ: Social olfaction in lagomorphs, *Symp Zool Soc London* 45:141-164, 1980.

6. Bell DJ: The behavior of rabbits: implications for their laboratory management. In *Standards in laboratory management, Part 2*. Proceedings of Universities Federation for Animal Welfare Symposium. Edinburgh, 1984, Churchill Livingstone.
7. Bigler L, Oester H: Raising pairs of young non-reproducing female rabbits in cages, *Berl Munch Tierarztl Wochenschr* 107(6):202-205,1994.
8. Bilko A, Altbacker V: Regular handling early in the nursing period eliminates fear responses toward human beings in wild and domestic rabbits, *Dev Psychobiol* 36(1):78-87, 2000.
9. Bradley TA: Rabbits: medical implications of selected abnormal behaviors, *Exotic DVM Magazine* 2(4):27-31, 2000.
10. Bradley TA: Rabbits: understanding normal behavior, *Exotic DVM Magazine* 2(1):19-24, 2000.
11. Bradley TA: Pain management considerations and pain-associated behaviors in reptiles and amphibians. Proceedings of the Association of Reptilian and Amphibian Veterinarians and American Association of Zoo Veterinarians, Orlando, Fla., September 2001.
12. Brooks DL: Rabbits, hares, and pikas (lagomorpha). In Fowler ME, editor: *Zoo and wild animal medicine,* ed 2, Philadelphia, 1986, Saunders.
13. Brooks DL: Nutrition and gastrointestinal physiology. In Quesenberry KE, Carpenter JW, editors: *Ferrets, rabbits, and rodents: clinical medicine and surgery,* ed 2, St Louis, 2003, Saunders.
14. Brown SA: Clinical techniques in rabbits, *Semin Avian Exot Pet Med* 2(6):86-95, 1997.
15. Caba M, Rovirosa MJ, Silver R: Suckling and genital stroking induces Fos expression in hypothalamic oxytocinergic neurons of rabbit pups, *Brain Res Dev* 143(2):119-128, 2003.
16. Carpenter JW: Lagomorpha (pikas, rabbits, and hares). In Fowler ME, Miller RE, editors: *Zoo and wild animal medicine,* ed 5, Philadelphia, 2003, Saunders.
17. Chawan CB, Rao DR: Influence of type of housing on the performance of growing rabbits, *J Appl Rabbit Res* 3:24-25, 1987.
18. Cheeke PR: *Rabbit feeding and nutrition,* Orlando, 1987, Academic Press.
19. Cortopassi D, Muhl ZF: Videofluorographic analysis of tongue movement in the rabbit (*Oryctolagus cuniculus*), *J Morphol* 204:139-146,1990.
20. Coureaud G, Schaal B, Hudson R, et al: Transnatal olfactory continuity in the rabbit: behavioral evidence and short-term consequences of its disruption, *Dev Psychobiol* 40(4);372-390, 2002.
21. Coureaud G, Schaal B, Langlois D, et al: Orientation of newborn rabbits to odours of lactating females; relative effectiveness of surface and milk cues, *Anim Behav* 61(1):153-162, 2001.
22. Cowan DP: Group living in the European rabbit *(Oryctolagus cuniculus):* mutual benefit or resource localization, *J Anim Ecol* 56:779-795, 1987.
23. Cruise LJ, Brewer NR: Anatomy. In Manning PJ, Ringler DH, Newcomer CE, editors: *The biology of the laboratory rabbit,* ed 2, San Diego, 1994, Academic Press.
24. Davis H, Gibson JA: Can rabbits tell humans apart? Discrimination of individuals and its implications for animal research, *Comp Med* 50:483-485, 2000.
25. Deeb BJ: Neurological and musculoskeletal diseases. In Quesenberry KE, Carpenter JW, editors: *Ferrets, rabbits, and rodents: clinical medicine and surgery,* ed 2, St Louis, 2003, Saunders.

26. Donnelly TM: Basic anatomy, physiology, and husbandry. In Hillyer EV, Quesenberry KE, editors: *Ferrets, rabbits, and rodents: clinical medicine and surgery*, St Louis, 1997, Saunders.
27. Donnelly TM: Basic anatomy, physiology, and husbandry. In Quesenberry KE, Carpenter JW, editors: *Ferrets, rabbits, and rodents: clinical medicine and surgery*, ed 2, St Louis, 2003, Saunders.
28. Drescher B: Housing of rabbits with respect to animal welfare, *J Appl Rabbit Res* 15:678-683, 1992.
29. Ebino KY, Shutoh Y, Takahashi KW: Coprophagy in rabbits: autoingestion of hard feces, *Jikken Dobutsu* 42(4):611-613, 1993.
30. Eisermann K: Longterm heartrate responses to social stress in wild European rabbits: predominant effect of rank position, *Physiol Behav* 52:33-36, 1992.
31. Flecknell PA: Advances in the assessment and alleviation of pain in laboratory and domestic animals, *J Vet Anesth* 21:98-105, 1994.
32. Gonzalez-Mariscal G: 2001. Neuroendocrinology of maternal behavior in the rabbit, *Horm Behav* 40(2):125-132.
33. Gonzalez-Mariscal G, Diaz-Sanchez V, Melo AI, et al: Maternal behavior in New Zealand white rabbits: quantification of somatic events, motor patterns, and steroid plasma levels, *Physiol Behav* 55:1081-1089, 1994.
34. Gonzalez-Mariscal G, Melo AI, Zavala A, et al: Variations in chin-marking behavior of New Zealand female rabbits throughout the whole reproductive cycle, *Physiol Behav* 48:361-365, 1990.
35. Gonzalez-Mariscal G, Melo AI, Zavala A, et al: Chin-marking behavior in male and female New Zealand rabbit: onset, development, and activation by steroids, *Physiol Behav* 52:889-893, 1992.
36. Grizmek B, editor: *Grizmek's encyclopedia of mammals*, New York, 1990, McGraw Hill.
37. Hansen LT, Berthelsen H: The effect of environmental enrichment on the behavior of caged rabbits (*Orytolagus cuniculus*), *Appl Anim Behav Sci* 68(2):163-178, 2000.
38. Harcourt-Brown F: *Textbook of rabbit medicine*, Oxford, UK, 2002, Reed Educational and Professional Publishing, Alden Press.
39. Harris LD, Custer LB, Soranaka ET, et al: Evaluation of objects and food for environmental enrichment of NZW rabbits, *Contemp Top Lab Anim Sci* 40(1):27-30, 2001.
40. Hayes RA, Richardson BJ, Claus SC, et al: Semiochemicals and social signaling in the wild European rabbit in Australia: II. Variations in chemical composition of chin gland secretion across sampling sites, *J Chem Ecol* 28(12):2613-2625, 2002.
41. Hayes RA, Richardson BJ, Wyllie SG: To fix or not to fix: the role of 2-phenoxyethanol in rabbit, *Oryctolagus cuniculus*, chin gland secretion, *J Chem Ecol* 29(5):1051-1064, 2003.
42. Hess L: Dermatologic diseases. In Quesenberry KE, Carpenter JW, editors: *Ferrets, rabbits, and rodents: clinical medicine and surgery*, St Louis, 2003, Saunders.
43. Hesterman ER, Goodrich BS, Mykytowycz R: Behavioral and cardiac responses of the rabbit to *Oryctolagus cuniculus* to chemical fractions from the anal gland, *J Chem Ecol* 2:25-37, 1976.
44. Hudson R: Do newborn rabbits learn the odor stimuli releasing nipple-search behavior? *Dev Psychobiol* 18(6):575-585, 1985.
45. Hudson R, Labra-Cardero D, Mendoza-Soylovna A: Suckling, not milk, is important for the rapid learning of nipple-search odors in rabbits, *Dev Psychobiol* 41(3):226-235, 2002.

46. Hull J, Hull D: Behavioral thermoregulation in newborn rabbits, *J Comp Physiol Psychol* 96(1):143-147, 1982.
47. Huls WL, Brooks DL, Bean-Knudsen D: Response of adult New Zealand white rabbits to enrichment objects and paired housing, *Lab Anim Sci* 41(6):609-612, 1991.
48. Jenkins JR: Rabbit behavior. In *Veterinary Clinics of North America, Exotic Animal Practice—Behavior 2001*, Philadelphia, 2001, Saunders.
49. Jenkins JR: Gastrointestinal diseases. In Quesenberry KE, Carpenter JW, editors: *Ferrets, rabbits, and rodents: clinical medicine and surgery*, ed 2, St Louis, 2003, Saunders.
50. Jenkins JR, Brown SA: *A practitioner's guide to rabbits and ferrets*, Lakewood, Colo., 1993, American Animal Hospital Association (AAHA).
51. Jilge B: The rabbit: a diurnal or nocturnal animal? *J Exp Anim Sci* 34(5-6):170-183, 1991.
52. Jilge B, Kuhnt B, Landerer W, et al: Circadian temperature rhythms in rabbit pups and in their does, *Lab Anim* 35(4):364-373, 2001.
53. Johnson CA, Pallozzi WA, Geiger L, et al: The effect of an environmental enrichment device on individual caged rabbits in a safety assessment facility, *Contemp Top Lab Anim Sci* 42(5):27-30, 2003.
54. Lehmann M: Interference of a restricted environment—as found in battery cages—with normal behavior of young fattening rabbits. In Auxila T, editor: *Rabbit production systems including welfare*, Luxembourg, Official Publications of the European Communities, 1987.
55. Lehmann M: Social behavior of young domestic rabbits under semi-natural conditions, *Appl Anim Behav Sci* 32:269-292, 1991.
56. Levy F, Keller M, Poindron P: Olfactory regulation of maternal behavior in mammals, *Horm Behav* 46(3):284-302, 2004.
57. Lightfoot T: Personal communication, 2005.
58. Livingston A: Physiological basis for pain perception in animals, *J Vet Anaesth* 21:15-20,1994.
59. Lockley RM: Social structure and stress in the rabbit warren, *J Anim Ecol* 30:385-423, 1961
60. Love JA: Group housing: meeting physical and social needs of the laboratory rabbit, *Lab Anim Sci* 44:5-11, 1994.
61. Maertens L, DeGroote G: Influence of the number of fryer rabbits per cage on their performances, *J Appl Rabbit Res* 7(4):151-155, 1984.
62. Mathews KA: Pain assessment and general approach to management. In Mathews KA, editor: *Veterinary Clinics of North America, Small Animal Practice—Management of pain*, Philadelphia, 2000, Saunders.
63. Melo AI, Gonzalez-Mariscal G: Placentophagia in rabbits: incidence across the reproductive cycle, *Dev Psychobiol* 43(1):37-43, 2003.
64. Mena F, Clapp C, Martinez de la Escalera G: Age-related stimulatory and inhibitory effects of suckling regulated lactation in rabbits, *Physiol Behav* 48:307-310, 1990.
65. Metz JHM: Behavioral problems of rabbits in cages. In Auxila T, editor: *Rabbit production systems including welfare*, Luxembourg, 1987, Official Publications of the European Communities.
66. Mohamed MMA, Szendro ZS: Studies on nursing and milk production of does and milk intake and suckling behavior of their kits, *J Appl Rabbit Res* 15:708-716, 1992.
67. Mulder A, Nieuwenkamp AE, van der Palen JG, et al: Supplementary hay reduces fur chewing in rabbits. *Tijdschr Diergeneeskd* 117(22):655-658, 1992.

68. Myers K: The rabbit in Australia. In den Boer PJ, Gradwell GR, editors: *Dynamics of populations.* Proceedings of the Advanced Study Institute on Dynamics of Numbers in Populations, Oosterbeek, the Netherlands, September 7-18, 1970. Wageningen, the Netherlands, 1970, Centre for Agricultural Publishing and Documentation (PUDOC).
69. Myers K, Parer I, Richardson BJ: Leporidae. In Walton DW, Richardson BJ, editors: *Fauna of Australia. Mammalia, vol 1B,* Canberra, Australian Government Publishing Service, 1989.
70. Myers K, Parker BS: A study of the biology of the wild rabbit in climatically different regions in Eastern Australia. VI. Changes in numbers and distribution related to climate and land systems in semiarid North-western New South Wales, *Aust Wildl Res* 2:11-32, 1975.
71. Mykytowycz R: Social behavior of an experimental colony of wild rabbits, *Oryctolagus cuniculus.* I. Establishment of the colony, *CSIRO Wildl Res* 3:7-25, 1958.
72. Mykytowycz R: Social behavior of an experimental colony of wild rabbits, *Oryctolagus cuniculus.* II. First breeding season, *CSIRO Wildl Res* 4:1-13, 1959.
73. Mykytowycz R: Territorial marking by rabbits, *Sci Am* 218:116-126, 1968.
74. Mykytowycz R: The role of skin glands in mammalian communication, *Adv Chemoreception* 1:327-360, 1970.
75. Mykytowycz R: Reproduction of mammals in relation to environmental odors, *J Reprod Fertil* 19(suppl):431-444, 1973.
76. Mykytowycz R, Fullagar PJ: Effect of social environment on reproduction in the rabbit *Oryctolagus cuniculus, J Reprod Fertil* 19(suppl):503-522, 1973.
77. Nelissen M: On the diurnal rhythm of activity of *Oryctolagus cuniculus* (Linne, 1758), *Acta Zool Pathol Antverp* (61):3-18, 1975.
78. Pare JA: Disorders of the reproductive and urinary systems. In Quesenberry KE, Carpenter JW, editors: *Ferrets, rabbits, and rodents: clinical medicine and surgery,* ed 2, St Louis, 2003, Saunders.
79. Parer I: The population ecology of the wild rabbit (*Oryctolagus cuniculus*) in a Mediterranean-type climate in New South Wales, *Aust Wildl Res* 4:171-205, 1977.
80. Pongracz P, Altbacker V, Fenes D: Human handling might interfere with conspecific recognition in the European rabbit *(Oryctolagus cuniculus), Dev Psychobiol* 39(1):53-62, 2001.
81. Richardson R: Behavior. *Rabbits—health, husbandry and diseases,* Oxford, UK, 2000, Blackwell.
82. Roberts S: Group-living and consortships in two populations of the European rabbit (*Oryctolagus cuniculus*), *J Mammol* 69:28-38, 1987.
83. Robertson SA: Analgesia and analgesic techniques. In Heard DJ, editor: *Veterinary Clinics of North America, Exotic Animal Practice—Analgesia and anesthesia,* Philadelphia, 2001, Saunders.
84. Saito K, Nakanishi M, Hasegawa A: Uterine disorders diagnosed by ventrotomy in 47 rabbits, *J Vet Med Sci* 64(6):495-497, 2002.
85. Sandford JC: Notes on the history of the rabbit, *J Appl Rabbit Res* 15:1-28, 1992.
86. Seitz K, Hoy S, Lange K: Effect of various factors on the suckling behavior of domestic rabbits, *Berl Munch Tierarztl Wochenschr* 111(2):48-52, 1998.
87. Shomer NH, Peikert S, Terwilliger G: Enrichment-toy trauma in a New Zealand White rabbit, *Contemp Top Lab Anim Sci* 40(1):31-32, 2001.
88. Southern HN: Sexual and aggressive behavior in the wild rabbit, *Behaviour* 1:173-194, 1948.

89. Southern HN: The ecology and population dynamics of the wild rabbit (*Oryctolagus cuniculus*), *Ann Appl Biol* 27:509-526, 1940.
90. Stodart E, Myers K: A comparison of behavior, reproduction and mortality of wild and domestic rabbits in confined populations, *CSIRO Wildl Res* 9:144-159, 1964.
91. Stoskopf MK: Pain and analgesia in birds, reptiles, fish and amphibians, *Invest Ophthalmol Vet Sci* 35:755-780, 1994.
92. Stoufflet I, Caillol M: Relation between circulating sex steroid concentrations and sexual behavior during pregnancy and post partum in the domestic rabbit, *J Reprod Fertil* 82(1):209-218, 1988.
93. Tislerics A: *Oryctolagus cuniculus.* Animal Diversity Web. 2000. Available at: http://animaldiversity.ummz.umich.edu/site/accounts/information/Oryctolagus_cuniculus.html. Accessed May 15, 2005.
94. Whary M, Peper R, Borkowski G, et al: The effects of group housing on the research use of the laboratory rabbit, *Lab Anim* 27:330-341, 1993.
95. Wright EM, Woodson JF: Clinical assessment of pain in laboratory animals. In Rollin BE, Kesel ML, editors: *The experimental animal in biologic research*, Boca Raton, Fla., 1990, CRC Press.

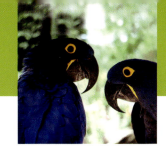

CHAPTER 2

TERESA LIGHTFOOT
CARINA L. NACEWICZ

Psittacine Behavior

Introduction

Members of the order Psittaciformes are the most commonly kept pet birds worldwide. The bond between humans and psittacines is centuries old. The existence of over 300 species of Psittaciformes and their wide variations in behavior emphasizes that we have knowledge of a mere fraction of the significant behavioral parameters of these birds. Despite this paucity of information, the keeping and breeding of psittacines in captivity is likely to continue to expand. With the decimation of habitats worldwide, captive reproduction of many species has become the route to ensure survival of these species.

Ornithologists, ethologists, aviculturists, and veterinarians must combine their knowledge and experience and incorporate theories and discoveries by allied professions in their own work in order to ensure not only survival but optimal quality of life of these captive psittacine species.

For a compelling and inclusive treatise on the need for a cohesive approach to avian behavior, along with more than 1400 references regarding individual studies, the reader is strongly encouraged to read Kavanau's *Behavior and Evolution*.[20]

Wild Bird Behavior

As stated in the introduction, although thousands of articles have been published on various aspects of psittacine behavior in the wild, what is unknown still far exceeds what is known. The development of ethograms for most parrot species has not been accomplished. An ethogram is a systematic behavioral inventory consisting of (1) a detailed list of all behavioral elements that occur in a given context and (2) guidelines for definition of and discrimination among those elements. The nature of the observations required, specifically tracking individual birds for prolonged periods of time, is daunting. Detailed chronologic records would need to be obtained relating to parent and sibling interactions, interactions with conspecifics of various ages and relationships, play behavior in juvenile birds, and the development and maintenance of pair bonds. This research, if and when accomplished, would identify various wild behaviors but not necessarily elucidate their functions.

Intriguing discoveries have been made in the past two centuries. Some of these are useful for directing future research. Others may be more immediately applicable in improving the environment of the current captive psittacine population, encouraging breeding, and improving physical and mental development.

Many studies are intrinsically fascinating but have no direct application or concrete interpretation at this time.[3,4,19,20] Disagreements among researchers about general theories and terminology complicate the documentation and advancement of psittacine ethology. Studies of captive populations of psittacines have yielded fascinating data, but the captive environmental context may alter the results from what would occur in nature.

Species Differences

Nomadic psittacines (such as many Australian species), which by definition migrate in order to find sufficient food and water, have evolutionarily developed significant differences in their social and individual behaviors when compared with birds in tropical climates (such as South American macaws and Amazons), where food supplies are more consistently present within a localized area. For example, nomadic species (budgerigars, lovebirds) tend to be colony breeders. This adaptive survival mechanism serves them well. The larger number of individuals in these flocks provides protection from predators and increases the efficiency of foraging. Socialization, therefore, tends to be less pair specific, and fewer confrontational dominance displays occur. Not surprisingly, these large-flock nomadic birds learn more readily from conspecifics—for example to consume new food items—than do South American species.[29]

Although generalizations regarding psittacines are taken from representative studies, significant variations may exist among species or individuals and according to the breeding status of the birds.

Time Allocation and Behaviors

The percentage of waking hours spent performing the following major categories of behaviors has been averaged from the sources cited (Box 2-1). These were quantified when birds were *not* at nest, although some studies

> **BOX 2-1 Time Allocation and Behaviors**
>
> - Grooming (self-preening and allopreening)
>   20%-66%
> - Foraging for food
>   40%-60%
> - Vocalizing
>   2%-5%
> - Social interactions
>   10%-40%
>
> References 7, 13, 20, 43.

did involve degrees of courtship or territoriality that may indicate peri-breeding behavior.

Senses

Vision and hearing are the predominant senses in most birds. Tactile sensation is also well developed but used in a closer and more limited fashion. Smell and taste are less significant than are these senses in many mammals.

Vocalization

The range of vocalization in birds is extensive, and they can discriminate and identify individual songs and cries in order to interpret conveyed information. Evidence from studies conducted in disparate disciplines indicates that the left and right hemispheres of the brain in avian species have asymmetric functions; specifically, as in humans, the left brain is markedly dominant in the learning and reproduction of vocal communication (i.e., "song") in birds.[31]

Unrelated newly hatched budgerigars *(Melopsittacus undulates)* produce comparable vocalizations. However, by 3 weeks of age their cries have been shaped to mimic those of their parents.[4] Mutual vocal recognition of chicks and parents is universal. Parents equidistant from their own young and those of conspecifics will react frantically to distress calls by their offspring while ignoring the calls of others. Likewise, cockatiel *(Nymphicus hollandicus)* chicks in the nest will respond to the song of a parent bird outside their field of vision but not to that of other adult cockatiels.

Amazons in contiguous regions of Central America have been determined to have regional dialects. Individual birds in adjacent areas can vocalize and recognize both dialects.[31]

Extensive studies of avian neurology and neuroanatomy have shown it to be unlikely that birds that are not conspecifics can fully "understand" vocalizations of other species, although mimicry is obviously within the ability of many birds. The strength, duration, and timing of song in conspecific birds located in temperate climates vary significantly from birds in tropical climates. The potential significance of these differences is still controversial.[20,31,40]

Body Language

Posturing is used to display various messages to conspecifics. Territoriality and breeding behavioral displays, including filoerection, voluntary pupillary constriction and dilation, fanning of tail feathers, spreading of the wings, and beak lunging are all noted in captivity as well as in nature. It is likely that, in addition to recognizing these overt behaviors, humans do not fully recognize more subtle body language displays and the messages they are intended to convey (Figures 2-1 and 2-2).

Foraging Behaviors

Natural foraging habits of birds have several ramifications in captivity:
- Species that forage in flocks (often nomadic, arid-dwelling species such as cockatiels and lovebirds) tend to have more intense social interactions with conspecifics and to be colony breeders.
- Flock foragers (both psittacine and nonpsittacine) also tend to learn new food choices and feeding behaviors readily from conspecifics, unlike species that forage singly.
- Adult birds (as most adult animals) are conservative in their selection of foods while foraging. This is logical for survival, to minimize the ingestion of both toxic and less-nutritious foods. However, this makes conversion to improved diets as adults a greater challenge in captivity.
- Foraging consumes a great deal of energy on a daily basis. Foraging "deficiency" decreases constructive physical and emotional energy outlets, which may lead to health and behavioral problems in captivity.

Intraspecies Contact and Species Variations

Cockatiels engage in extensive head preening as part of their pair-bonded and parent-offspring interactions. However, this preening can take on an aggressive component. Adult birds (usually males) will "preen" the female's head to get her to move from the nest box. This preening can turn into pecking if the preening hint is not taken.[20] Most veterinarians have noted

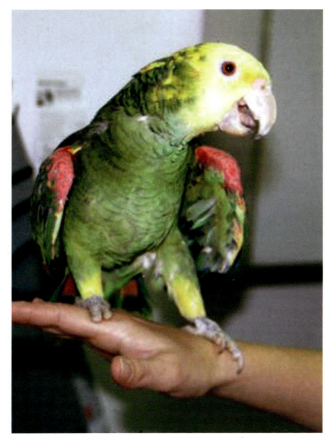

Figure 2-1
Note the partially open beak and the posture, with the body leaning away from the handler, indicating nervousness or fear. (Courtesy Teresa Lightfoot.)

the tendency of some parent cockatiels to overpreen, pluck, or damage the heads of baby cockatiels in the nest.

Cockatiels are also notorious for becoming irritable if their head is being preened and the preener stops. What role in dominance or pair-bonding this demand for preening plays is either not known or not recorded.

Conversely, adult cockatiels tend to avoid body contact with conspecifics, startling readily if they accidentally touch another bird. This contact avoidance is present in most psittacine species.[30]

Compare this with Peach-faced Lovebirds (*Agapornis roseicollis*), which tend to enjoy "huddling" not only as young in the nest but also as adults.

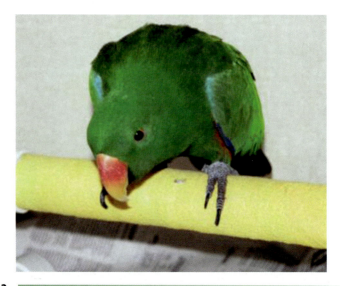

Figure 2-2
This pensive posture and a tendency to observe items or situations for prolonged periods of time have given *Eclectus* the undeserved reputation for being dull-witted. (Courtesy Teresa Lightfoot.)

In lovebirds, extensive body contact may be seen at all ages. Lovebirds are much less aggressive with their preening; males will often (when the female is in the nest box) preen the female all over her body without becoming aggressive.[20]

Tremendous variation appears to exist among species regarding the timing and extent of grooming and allogrooming. This makes it difficult to identify in captive psittacines when allogrooming may begin to be abnormal or excessive. (See Feather Destruction.)

Parenting

Although the exact conditions of chick development in the wild are unknown in most species, many critical developmental factors can be assumed from watching captive-raised birds and from knowledge of development in other species. The visual, tactile, and auditory development of birds in nature is greatly influenced by interaction with parents and siblings. The ontogenetic comparisons of development in parrots seem to correlate more closely with those of the great apes than they do with those of dogs and cats.[39] The importance of weaning and fledging in wild psittacine development may contribute to the plateaus in learning that occur in captive-tested psittacines.[31]

Captive Psittacine Development

The typical psittacine breeding facility has advanced in recent decades to meet many of the physiologic needs of neonatal birds, including regulation of temperature, humidity, and improved nutrition in the form of formulated hand-feeding diets. The acclimation of our birds to physical contact and handling has been part of the hand-raising process and generally produces a bird with more attachment to and positive interaction with people, at least initially. However, the emotional and social development of these birds is undoubtedly affected by the lack of conspecific interactions comparable to those that would occur in nature. Unacceptable and exaggerated behaviors such as feather destruction, excessive screaming, and biting have manifested in a large percentage of our current population of hand-raised pet psittacines. These behaviors are generally not noted in wild-caught pet psittacines or those captive-bred but allowed to be raised by the parents. These behavioral abnormalities have been postulated to be similar to the "orphanage syndrome" or relative attachment disorder described in human children deprived of affection and stability in their early months and years of life. Such behavioral abnormalities in children (and also those in human-raised psittacines) often do not manifest until later in life.[22,23,50]

Allowing the parents to incubate and raise their chicks creates potential financial and emotional liability for psittacine breeders. Broken eggs, abused or neglected chicks, and accidental injury can all occur when chicks are left in the nest. However, little doubt exists that this is the ideal environment for emotional and social development. There also are physical advantages to development within the nest box, as a study conducted on Dusky Pionus parrots *(Pionus fuscus)* demonstrated. Between 16 and 45 days of age, when bone growth is rapid and the skeletal structure still weak, chicks housed separately in incubators stumbled about, apparently in search of sibling or parental contact. Clutches maintained together huddled closely and moved little, and this huddling aided in supporting the appendicular skeleton.[15] Additional studies have shown increased bony deformation and osteodystrophy in chicks housed individually in incubators. Fortunately, increasing numbers of breeders are now allowing the parents to incubate, hatch, and raise the chicks through fledging.

Human interaction with the chicks can begin either in the nest box (known as *co-parenting*) or after the chicks have fledged. In this way, young birds become acclimated to human handling by brief daily interactions while still benefiting from parental and sibling interaction. Ongoing work at the University of California, Davis has shown the benefit, at least in Orange-winged Amazons *(Amazona amazonica)*, of handling the young on a regular basis while still allowing parent rearing of the chicks. In some species and individuals, interaction with humans may increase the risk of abuse or neglect by the parents, so this technique will not be applicable in all situations.

If it is necessary to hand-raise a psittacine chick, every attempt should be made to meet the physiologic and psychologic needs of that individual. Lack of concrete data regarding the exact nature of these needs leaves us with a duty to replicate the environment and interactions provided in the wild. This includes body pressure; warmth and contact; a dark, safe, secure nest box area; feeding on demand; the ability to incrementally explore the nest environment; and visualization of the outside world without physical exposure. Phoebe Linden has labeled these aspects of neonatal and juvenile psittacine developmental care, along with specific feeding techniques and materials, as *Abundance Weaning*.[22-25] Readers are urged to review this material in order to properly understand and inform their clients of the necessity for initial and ongoing developmental enrichment.[24]

Socialization

As stated previously, there likely is a window of time in early development during which exposure of psittacines to various species (conspecifics, other birds, humans, other household pets) and objects results in acceptance of these, or minimally in a reduction of fear and avoidance. Lack of exposure to conspecifics during this time may prohibit normal development and the potential for successful pair-bonding.[41] Substitution of the human caregiver for the parent, sibling, and/or mate occurs in many captive psittacines.

Psittacine owners usually seek a strong emotional and physical "bond" with their bird, which removal from the nest and hand-feeding provide. However, the oxymoron that results is that many of the behavioral and medical problems of pet psittacines stem from this abnormal bonding relationship.

The same phenomenon is documented with captive-raised birds of prey.[18,30] Intensive socialization during hand-raising of falcons and hawks creates a bird that is less readily disturbed by the presence of civilization (humans, vehicles, hunting dogs, and so on). This imprinting on people is also used to encourage mating with humans who have been equipped with semen collection devices (hats or other designs) for later use in artificial insemination of pure and hybrid falconry birds. However, removing the fear of humans increases the potential that the normal territoriality of mature raptors may be violently directed at any humans invading this territory. Again, as in psittacines, certain species seem to be more prone to territorial aggression.[18]

Stimulation

Stimulation is similar to socialization but does not require an individual (person or animal) to interact with; it instead connotes experiences or situations. Generally, the more numerous and varied the stimuli to which a bird is exposed at a relatively young age, the less likely it is to develop fears of these objects, noises, or phenomena (Figure 2-3). The ability to retreat from overstimulation via a hide box should be provided, especially for the young but also for adults.

In addition to preventing fears, this mental stimulation is challenging for the bird as it attempts to determine the nature and function of the events or objects. A simple example is placing the bird's cage where the bird can see outdoors (preferably through a screened window) and observe the sky, trees, other birds, and squirrels; hear traffic noise; and feel barometric pressure changes. This is much preferable to leaving the television or radio on for the bird.

Consequences of Inactivity

The absence of normal stressors in a safe, clean, stable captive environment is often the main cause of problem behaviors such as feather destructive behavior or stereotypy. In fact, these "problem" behaviors are typically displaced and/or exaggerated normal behaviors. A common presentation to veterinarians is the bird owned by a loving, attentive, conscientious

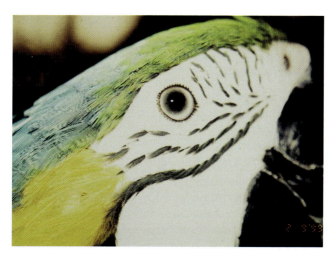

Figure 2-3
The innate curiosity and high energy level of young macaws require stimulation and socialization to prevent the development of inappropriate behaviors. (Courtesy Teresa Lightfoot.)

owner who provides a clean and stable environment, constant access to sufficient food and water, and multiple toys. These owners are particularly distressed when their bird initiates feather destructive behavior, and they believe that the bird must be lacking some comfort or necessity. In fact, the opposite is often true. These birds are secure and all their needs are met without the expenditure of any physical or mental energy. They therefore have no mental or physical stimuli—no need to forage for food, guard against predators, seek shelter, attract or keep a mate, locate nesting areas, or provide for offspring. It follows that, of the natural behaviors remaining, one such as preening may then assume a dominant role and be accelerated to an abnormal degree. There likely is also a similarity to the phenomenon seen in people with autism—a need for stimuli, albeit negative stimuli, in an environment devoid of any natural challenges often results in hair pulling or self-mutilation.

Toys

Depending on the individual bird, toys may be useful displacers for mental and physical excess energies.[27] Varieties of toys are available, and these can serve multiple purposes. Objects such as old telephone books provide an outlet for the need to chew and mechanically dispel excess energy. Puzzle toys (with a food treat or other object that is revealed and obtained after manipulation) provide both physical and mental stimulation (Figure 2-4). However, the ability and desire to interact with toys is not universal and may be learned to some degree. Seldom will the instillation of toys into the environment substitute for human interaction and training.

Behavior Modification

Much of the remainder of this chapter discusses various aspects of behavior and its manipulation in captivity. The following applicable generalities bear mentioning here.

Exaggeration of Normal Behaviors

The most common objectionable behaviors in captive psittacines will likely stem from exaggeration or expansion of normal behaviors. This must be understood in order to have reasonable expectations of reducing, not necessarily eliminating, these behaviors. For example, some degree of vocalization is an innate behavior in psittacines in the morning and late afternoon. Preening is also a normal behavior, occupying a large percentage of time in any situation (wild or captive birds). The critical function of feather maintenance in psittacines, and therefore the need and ability

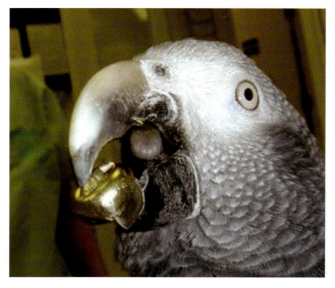

Figure 2-4
This photo illustrates the necessity to choose bird safe toys to avoid injury. This African Grey was presented with a metal bell caught on its mandibular beak. (Courtesy Dan Johnson.)

to preen, must be considered when mechanical barriers to feather destructive behavior are considered.

Positive Reinforcement for the Owner

Owners of psittacines often have lives, jobs, and families in addition to their pet bird. This can make compliance with frequent or complex training sessions difficult if not impossible. Besides the need to tailor any recommendations for interactions with the bird to a reasonable schedule, the veterinarian should consider motivation and long-term commitment. Some people cannot or will not consistently devote time to their birds. Others will, if the potential for improvement and the inherent value (e.g., bonding, enrichment, safety) of such interactions is adequately explained. This commitment can be greatly enhanced if both the owner and the bird derive enjoyment from the process. Discovering tricks, treats, and interactions that the bird enjoys is crucial to successful behavior modification. Similarly, the most devoted owners are often created when their bird learns some behavior that is rewarding to the owner (e.g., wave goodbye, play eagle, sing part of "Dixie"). The mutual excitement between bird and owner that this engenders greatly increases the likelihood that that owner will continue to work with the bird. The reinforcement received by the bird also increases the odds of continued performance of these behaviors as well as the acquisition of new ones.

Initiation

An initial period when the bird is in the hands of an avian trainer—be this a parrot behavioral consultant, a veterinarian, or another individual—may allow the implementation of some basic behavioral modification. Particularly with adult birds, a new environment or new person to interact with is often a prerequisite, being enough of a change to interrupt a chronic pattern and stimulate a willingness to learn, explore, and exhibit new behaviors. Learning to step on command and to allow the person holding the bird to place a thumb over a foot to prevent flight are two basic training exercises that expedite further learning. These are also very important for safety during an unforeseen event.

Never Punish

At no time is physical punishment ever an acceptable or productive training method for birds. Although punishment is already generally discouraged by behaviorists and trainers for any type of pet, this is particularly true for birds. There are multiple reasons for this. First and foremost, most normal interactions with conspecifics are not physical beyond general grooming. Birds communicate and interact using vocalization, display, access to resources, location in the environment, and even space occupation to intimidate or establish dominance; therefore these are the inherent training tools used to shape behavior. The rare occasion of physical violence usually involves either a particularly dominant individual or a life-changing event (e.g., a territorial dispute); this type of interaction would normally breed avoidance or resentment, not the type of continued harmonious and intimate relationship that an owner is trying to foster. Even if desired, it would be impossible for a human to replicate the typical negative physical interaction because of anatomic differences: whereas humans interact primarily with their hands, birds interact with their beaks, for example, darting the head in close to provide a carefully placed warning nip. They do not interact with, nor seem to comprehend despite their intelligence, any gestures or acts made with hands and arms that are not for mere display.

Often, the types of behaviors that punishment is used to suppress (screaming, biting) are at their core a normal behavior that cannot be absolutely suppressed without risking emotional health. Sadly, extremely intelligent psittacines that are "acting up" because of boredom will be positively reinforced by the mere attention that punishments convey, no matter how aversive the reaction.

Identifying and Creating the Proper Human-Psittacine Relationship

Establishing, or even defining, a healthy relationship between bird owner and captive psittacine is challenging. The degree of interaction desired by owners often either is not normal for a given species in the wild or is encountered only between parent and offspring or mated pairs. Excessive or improper bonding (malimprinting) can have negative physical and behavioral outcomes in captivity.

For example, the inherent dependence in a relationship in which an Umbrella Cockatoo *(Cacatua alba)* perceives the owner as its parent may result in prolonged or incomplete weaning. In addition to the emotional stunting that may accompany this relationship, the constant crying for food can be both an annoyance and a precipitating factor in the production of cloacal prolapse (see Cockatoo Prolapse Syndrome later in the chapter).

As the parrot matures, it may transfer its affection to another person in the household. This often occurs following the absence of the previous "bonded" individual, who was perceived as the parent figure. It should not be surprising that the developing parrot seeks a companion, if not a mate, other than its perceived surrogate parent. Ideally, the mate would be a conspecific of the opposite gender. However, the need for a companion, and possibly the increased security and advantages provided, is apparently stronger than the requirement for a member of the opposite gender. In nature and in large aviary populations in which there exists a disproportionate number of one gender, homosexual pair bonding is commonly encountered. (Author note: No studies were located that attempted to determine whether a predisposition to homosexual pair-bonding exists when sufficient numbers of both genders are available.)

During maturation, the transference of affection from the original person who has raised and nurtured the bird to another may occur. This can be very traumatic for the individual to whom the bird was originally bonded. In certain situations, there may be no other person to whom the bird can or desires to transfer the bond; in such cases the relationship remains with the same individual but changes in character.

In nature, most parrots practice "perennial monogamy" or long-term, year-round pair-bonding to the same individual.[45] Pair-bonded Glossy Black Cockatoos *(Calyptorhynchus lathami)*, for example, are found to be higher on the dominance hierarchy than any given individual and also to be very closely ranked in the dominance scheme relative to their mates. Much has been written regarding the reasons for the endurance of the pair bond throughout the nonbreeding season. Continued care of juvenile offspring and ease of mate location during subsequent breeding seasons are involved in some species. However, studies of wild cockatoos, lorikeets, and White-fronted Amazons *(Amazona albifrons)* have shown that the primary advantage seems to be the dominance conferred by a mated pair acting in unison—usually to supplant other conspecifics from a preferred food tree, therefore ensuring optimal nutrition throughout the year.

In captivity the mated-pair relationship may induce behaviors such as territoriality, mate or nest protection, aggression, and ovulation or egg laying when a bird perceives its owner as its mate (Figure 2-5). However, if this perceived relationship can be maintained as a prolonged nonbreeding season alliance, some or most of the negative aspects may be avoided. This is what most veterinarians and behaviorists, intentionally or not, are recommending when they advise clients on frequency and type of interaction allowed with the pet bird, the caveat being to avoid all behavior that can be construed as sexual (petting, feeding by mouth).

Is this the best solution to the relationship between owner and captive pet psittacine? Are we even wise to look for natural equivalent relationships for which to strive with our captive-raised pet psittacines? The answer may vary among species, individual birds, and owners. Long-term relationships between bird and owner that appear psychologically healthy are commonly encountered. This would connote both a mutual enjoyment regardless of the amount of physical contact and an absence of serious unacceptable behaviors (possessiveness, separation anxiety, copulatory behavior, biting, screaming, and so on, by bird or human).

Obviously, this area requires more study and the acknowledgment that what is desired by the owner may not be within the comfort zone or ability of an individual captive psittacine.

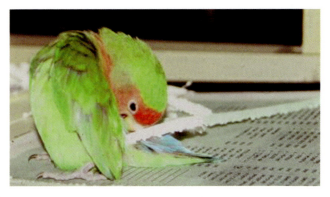

Figure 2-5
Note the behavior of placing strips of paper under the wings, practiced by lovebirds during nest construction. Aggressive and defensive behavior with humans may drastically increase during breeding season. (Courtesy Teresa Lightfoot.)

Husbandry Considerations

Caging

Many factors are involved in the selection of appropriate caging for pet psittacines.

Size

The size of the cage depends in part on the species and the relative amount of time the bird will spend in its cage. Minimally, the bird should (1) be able to spread its wings in all directions without contacting the cage sides and (2) have sufficient clearance that the tail does not contact either the floor or other objects while the bird is perched. It is preferred to provide a cage that is one size larger than what is advertised for that species. Obviously, toxic materials such as galvanized wire (e.g., in caging, dishes, toy parts, or clasps) should be avoided.

Perches

Ideally, perches of various diameters and textures will be available to the caged pet psittacine. Also, because most birds will develop a favorite location to perch, these will need to be rotated or changed. The less active and the heavier a bird is, the more critical this is for the prevention of pododermatitis.

The use of appropriate concrete perches, located such that the bird must stand on the perch and walk a few steps to access a desirable toy or food treat, can accomplish toenail maintenance without the need for manual trimming. This works most effectively on birds weighing between 200 and 1000 g. Smaller birds do not seem to place enough force on the nail to effect smoothing, and very large birds may develop irritations on the feet from the rough surface. The introduction of these perches has reduced the need for nail trimming dramatically, thereby reducing stress in birds that have not had adequate training to allow grooming to be accomplished without objection. These concrete perches are also used by birds to rub their beaks, removing both excess food and keratin and thus eliminating a majority of the cosmetic beak trims requested.

Soft wood branches can serve as disposable perches of variable diameters and as an outlet for chewing. However, crashing to the bottom of the cage can occur when these perches are chewed through.

Bathing

Bathing is critical for both physical and mental well-being. Species and individual variations may dictate in which form this is provided. Many birds enjoy being in the shower with their owners. Many birds also enjoy natural rainfall while in their cage placed outdoors. Before the rain, the perception of a barometric pressure change often sends these birds, particularly South American species, into postural displays in anticipation of the rain. Allowing the bird to dry outside or on a lanai when the weather is suitable encourages normal preening. Some people use blow dryers on their birds. This is potentially drying to the skin and may remove some of the natural grooming instincts. However, it is desirable if no other way exists to assure that the bird stays warm while it dries naturally.

Nutrition

This subject is intimately involved in both the physical and emotional health of pet birds. It must be recognized that a bird, as any animal, will be at its emotional best when its nutritional needs are met.

In many species the presence of certain foods serves as a trigger for breeding behavior. Sprouts, fresh greens, and high-fat nuts can all potentially serve as stimuli for increased breeding activity. This may be detrimental in a pet bird, in which ovulation may cause physical problems and excessive sexual agitation is not compatible with human coexistence. The importance of diet in stimulating reproductive activity varies with the species, other environmental factors, and the degree to which these foods are an innate or absolute trigger (as opposed to one that may be diminished through constant exposure).

Photoperiod

The day and night lengths, respectively, to which pet psittacines are exposed can affect their general health (e.g., obtaining sufficient rest) and their reproductive cycling or lack thereof. Particularly with regard to behavior disorders, it is important to remember that overall emotional health is dependent on adequate sleep. A dark, quiet area without disruptions should be reliably provided for an adequate duration at a consistent time. It is often surprising to new owners how quickly a developing problematic behavior can be eliminated by this simple correction.

Generally, increasing day length is a sign of incipient spring and summer, with the concurrent food availability and warm ambient temperature conducive to breeding and raising young. Although many other factors will affect reproduction, the maintenance of a 12-hour light and 12-hour darkness routine will prevent some birds from becoming sexually active.[19]

Grooming: Nail, Beak, and Wing Trimming

The trimming of toenails in young and middle-aged birds is done almost exclusively for the comfort of the owners and to the detriment of the bird's physical (and therefore emotional) stability. Sharp, needlelike points are normal on psittacine nails and enable them to have a secure hold on various-sized branches during adverse weather conditions such as rain and wind. However, most owners will not tolerate multiple puncture wounds on their hands and arms in order to allow a pet parrot to have optimal perching stability. Therefore dulling of the nails is often performed in the veterinary office. Owners generally need to be educated about the bird's need for some degree of sharpness to assure a secure grip. They may also need to be shown that the nails they consider long are often normal for the individual. The exceptions most commonly are geriatric birds, birds with poor nutritional history, or those with decreased hepatic function. In these cases the nails tend to curl prematurely and often must be trimmed to allow the bird to perch comfortably and securely. Concrete perches, mentioned previously in regard to toenail maintenance, do not usually work on nails that have very acute curvatures

Wing trimming is another subject with implications beyond a mere grooming procedure. The removal of the ability to fly and the compromised balance that occur when symmetrical wing flapping is disrupted are major impediments to full function in captive psittacines. It is rightfully argued, however, that the dangers of being full-flighted in captivity may outweigh this handicap. If wing trimming is elected by the owner (to prevent escape or injury or to assist in training), several factors need to be considered.

- Wing trimming should initially be done gradually when possible, allowing the bird time to acclimate not only to reduced flying ability but also to needed balance and wing-exercise adaptations.[23,35,44,47] This may thus involve taking only a feather or two from each wing over a period of weeks.
- In the interest of balance, it is ideal to avoid performing wing trimming and nail trimming concurrently. Encourage owners to stagger the procedures over time. If it is necessary to perform both, each should be done to a lesser extent.
- The wing trim severity will depend on several factors: the size of the bird (which is inversely proportional to the number of feathers that need to be clipped); the purpose of the trim (e.g., prevention of accidental escape or injury indoors versus the bird that, despite advice to the contrary, will be on the owner's shoulders as they walk down beaches

or city streets); the household situation with regard to other pets and children; and the disposition of the bird (e.g., dominant, independent, insecure, fearful).
- The trim should result in the retention of the ability to glide gently to the floor from a height (rather than fall like a stone). If this function is not retained, the bird risks severe injury from fall-related crashes (not to mention possible permanent injuries to mental and emotional stability).
- Numerous variations exist with regard to which feathers are trimmed and to what length. It is wise to start by asking owners if they have a particular trim to which their bird is accustomed or that they prefer (usually because of brightly colored primaries). If not otherwise indicated, it is most efficient for reducing flight to start with the most distal primaries. Attention should be paid to the remaining shaft after trimming: a sharp or pointy calamus that irritates the skin of the body can initiate feather destructive behavior.
- Contrary to the insistence of some, blood feathers can and should be trimmed (rather than leaving such feathers exposed and vulnerable by having trimmed the remainder of feathers on the wing). Blood feathers can be cut only beyond the vessel-containing portion of the feather shaft, which varies as the feather matures and the vessel recedes. It is recommended to provide additional protection by trimming the adjacent feathers to the same length, thereby creating a guard on either side of the blood feather.

Disease Considerations

Neurologic Disease

This section addresses selected neurologic signs and associated diseases. Additional information may be obtained from the references.

Sudden Blindness

In one author's experience, sudden blindness is most commonly attributable to cataracts or retinal detachment (Figure 2-6). Intracranial tumors, primarily pituitary, are the second most frequent cause. Additional causes include toxicity or severe metabolic disease, but in these cases clinical illness is usually obvious to the owner and the veterinary practitioner. When sudden blindness occurs in the absence of other functional disease conditions, birds may exhibit a variety of reactions. Some become lethargic and unreactive to stimuli. Others become hyperesthetic, which may be interpreted by the owner as either aggression or seizure activity.

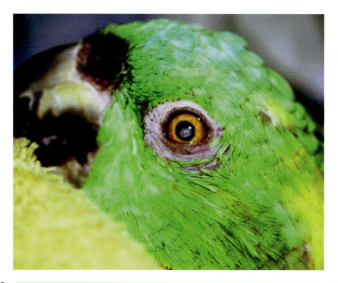

Figure 2-6
Mature cataract in a >30-year-old Amazon. As in dogs, gradual onset of cataracts is often well tolerated, but acute onset can be disorienting and result in severely altered behavior. (Courtesy Teresa Lightfoot.)

Although gradual onset of cataracts and acclimation is more common in birds, the practitioner should be aware of the potential for sudden blindness and its presentations.

Hepatic Encephalopathy

Several cases of hepatic encephalopathy have been reported anecdotally in the literature, with at least one case documented by the author of this chapter. A 1-year-old African Grey *(Psittacus erithacus)* was presented with weight loss, ataxia, and marigold-colored urates. Chemistries demonstrated bile acids over 899 µmol/L (reference range 20 to 100), aspartate aminotransferase (AST) >1200 U/L (reference 40 to 340), alanine aminotransferase (ALT) 35 U/L (reference 0 to 11), and lactate dehydrogenase (LDH) 954 U/L (reference 55 to 340). A hepatic biopsy revealed bile duct stasis and fibrosis, with cellular infiltrate suggestive of a previous infection. The bird responded clinically to ursodiol, antibiotics, and supportive care. Over the subsequent 2 years, two episodes of severe ataxia recurred during separate attempts to discontinue the ursodiol, both times accompanied by recurrent elevations in bile acids, AST, ALT and LDH.

Heavy Metal Toxicity

The incidence of lead poisoning in birds (and other species) was significantly higher several decades ago than it is today. Variable numbers of birds with lead toxicity were noted to have pronounced neurologic signs (other than the moderate to severe depression normally accompanying any heavy metal toxicity). Hyperexcitability, seizures, and functional blindness have been noted with lead poisoning.[16]

Egg Yolk Stroke

In ovulatory female birds, proteins for production of the egg yolk are made in the liver and transported to the infundibulum across the celomic cavity. This yolk protein may be absorbed into the bloodstream, creating arterial occlusion and subsequent neurologic impairment. Common clinical presentations of this condition include a recently laying hen with an acute onset of ataxia or an inability to right herself or ambulate, although often she still retains muscular strength. These birds are often panicked by their condition and may demonstrate what is interpreted by the owner as a prolonged seizure, vocalizing loudly and flapping frantically. Self-induced trauma is common. Preliminary evidence suggests that, in addition to supportive care, intravenous hyaluronidase may be a viable therapy for this condition (as could other enzymatic proteinases theoretically be, including trypsin or chymotrypsin derivatives).[22]

Pituitary Adenoma

This neoplasm has been historically documented in budgerigars and cockatiels. Anecdotal reports and occasional literature citations note its occurrence in other species as well, including Amazons and African Greys. This tumor may be a manifestation of whichever pituitary hormone is being produced in excess. The most common example of this is the polyuric-polydipsic (PU/PD) bird, in which the adenoma causes an increase in ACTH production, elevating corticosterone.[16,22,23,50] Alternate presentations include seizures, opisthotonus, and unilateral exophthalmus created by retrobulbar space-occupying lesions.

Miscellaneous Neuropathies

Birds demonstrate numerous neurologic presentations for which causes have yet to be identified. Several of these are expected to prove to be degenerative neuropathies. Spongiform encephalopathy, lysosomal storage disease, and avian vacuolar myelinopathy[32] are infrequent but are documented neurologic conditions in birds. Clinical signs of these degenerative conditions include depression, ataxia, head tremors, nystagmus, strabismus, and functional blindness. It is likely that these and other degenerative conditions exist to a greater degree than is documented because of inadequate necropsies and histopathology submission after neurologic disease fatalities.

Pain-Associated Behaviors

As with any prey species, vocal demonstrations of pain are rare, being counterproductive to survival in the wild. Still, when a localized injury (e.g., swollen tarsometatarsal joint, fracture of the tibiotarsal bone, or bruised carpometacarpus) is palpated, vocalization and a withdrawal response are often elicited.

More difficult to identify is diffuse or chronic pain. Conditions known to be invariably painful, such as advanced bilateral articular gout or severe bilateral pododermatitis, should be aggressively treated with antiinflammatories and analgesics. These two particular conditions, because of the poor prognosis and the extreme pain caused by the constant need to bear weight on the affected surfaces, are situations in which euthanasia should be strongly considered as the humane course of action.

With clinically ill birds it can be difficult to distinguish among lethargy, depression, debilitation, fear, and pain. Reluctance to move, excessive muscle fasciculations, and anorexia all may reflect one or more of these conditions. Unless contraindicated by a known metabolic impairment, a trial of both a synthetic opioid (such as butorphanol) and a nonsteroidal antiinflammatory drug (NSAID) (such as meloxicam) can assist in differentiation among potential causes of such clinical manifestations. If improvement is (subjectively) noted, continuation of analgesic medications should be considered.

Captive Behavior and Training

Much anecdotal information is available on parrot behavior and training. Recently, principles of behavioral analysis and modification as applied to psittacines have been published. Many parrot behavioral consultants have come to use methods that parallel those described in the following sections through their own experience, extrapolation from other species, and common sense.

Behavior Analysis

Dr. Susan Friedman discusses in detail behavior analysis in birds and its application to learning and/or manipulating captive behaviors.[13] The fact that the principles she describes are often those used by bird trainers in the demanding venue of commercial bird shows attests to the efficacy of these techniques. Many behaviorists and veterinarians successfully employ some of these techniques, albeit often without knowledge of the underlying principles of behavioral science. The extensive description and explanation of behavioral analysis and operant conditioning in her referenced works[13] provides a matrix for understanding why these techniques, which have been subjectively employed, are effective.

Because behavioral science is a field in which most veterinarians are not well versed, practitioners may have difficulty conveying this information to their clients in a usable form. In addition, many clients anthropomorphize their bird's behavior, and not all owners are amenable to applying or able to apply these training techniques to their pet psittacines. Despite these difficulties, the innate value of this information and the advantage its application confers are quite remarkable. A synopsis and examples of behavior analysis and modification techniques are provided in the following paragraphs.

Accurate identification and modification of behavior require that the conditions under which a behavior occurs be defined. Because behaviors are learned (or are present innately) for a functional reason, identification of the applicable circumstances (both those preceding the behavior and the consequences that follow) will elucidate the reason for or function of the specific behavior. This will then allow manipulation of that behavior—whether for the purpose of reinforcement (as in associating it with a command, which can then be rewarded in the appropriate context), distraction, desensitization, or extinguishing (eliminating any rewards, such as with biting or excessive screaming).

Modification Techniques

Reinforcing Desired Behaviors

An example of reinforcement of desired behaviors is a bird that will step onto the owner's hand at some times, but at other times will run away or lunge as if to bite. Analyze the circumstances under which the bird most readily steps onto the hand: Is it when the bird is lower than the owner, when the owner is not wearing a brightly flowered shirt, when the bird is not on top of or inside its cage? Next, what are the results of stepping onto the hand? Does the bird get returned to its cage, which would be perceived as negative reinforcement? Or is it taken somewhere for positive interaction? Altering both the circumstances related to the behavior and the consequences of the behavior can reinforce that behavior.

Substituting Acceptable Behaviors or Teaching New Behaviors

The primary requirement for use of this technique is that the person working with the bird remain constantly aware of positive reinforcers for that bird—that is, what the bird considers worth obtaining (e.g., attention, food treat, petting). The following example, using one author's more than

20-year-old imported Yellow-naped Amazon (*Amazona ochrocephala*), named Cookie, illustrates the main points.

> "When I return to home or hospital where Cookie is currently residing, she says 'Hello', 'Cookie pretty girl!' 'Want to play?' and other slightly loud, excited greetings. I meet this with a somewhat softer but pleasant and happy response. I am usually still out of her sight, because (as is typical) she has become aware of my presence through either conversations with employees, the sound of my car door, the clearing of my throat, and so on.
>
> "I reply to her initial flock greeting call, as this is needed reassurance. However, her tendency is to escalate the volume and frequency of her phrases to a point that is not tolerable. After one or two well-modulated responses, I lower my voice in reply. If she becomes even louder, I don't respond at all. When she responds more quietly, I quickly respond in kind and move closer, continuing as she continues to speak quietly until I eventually remove her from her cage for at least a few moments of interaction. Cookie receives what she desires from her behavior of talking more softly: my vocal response, proximity, and interaction. This results in a quiet greeting and handling that is devoid of the raucous voice for which these birds are known. Any breakdown in this process, which does happen, is caused by my lack of attention or compliance."

Extinction of Undesirable Behaviors

Once the reinforcers—intentional or inadvertent—have been identified for an undesirable behavior, these reinforcers can be eliminated. When the behavior no longer achieves its desired consequence (e.g., if the bird yells but the owner no longer yells back), the behavior loses its function and will be diminished or extinguished unless it holds some other inherent value or reward.

Use of the technique of behavior analysis and shaping is inherent in the training of psittacines for complicated tricks and feats performed at bird shows. Although the reinforcers for these tricks may vary, and no doubt the quantity of time spent in training is significant, the intelligence and aptitude for some of these tricks are present in many of our pet psittacines. However, our knowledge and time constraints, as well as our roles as owners, generally preclude the degree of training seen in these professionally handled birds. For example, professional bird trainers have been called to task for using food deprivation as a reinforcer for learning a behavior. We all agree that starvation or severe food deprivation is inhumane. However, the delay of a meal or food treat until a task is completed is often used by people with their own children. Common sense and compassion make this a reasonable and effective reinforcer in the right hands. (Note the references to the work by Dr. Irene Pepperberg with African Greys at the end of this chapter. Within her text, the determination and use of rewards is incidentally but usefully discussed.)

The previous section is intended as a brief overview of operant conditioning; the reader is encouraged to review "The Natural Science of Behavior" by Susan Friedman, in *Clinical Avian Medicine*, Harrison and Lightfoot (editors), Spix Publishing (in press), and Steve Martin's article "Name that Article!" in the 2002 AAV Proceedings.

The benefits of this type of training include the displacement of undesirable behaviors (e.g., screaming, sexual behavior with the owner), the production of new enjoyable and acceptable behaviors, and the prevention of stereotypic behaviors that can occur when parrots are deprived of sufficient stimulation.

(Note: The relationship between stereotypic behaviors in birds and various psychologic conditions in people is an active area of research in the sciences of behavior, psychology, and neurophysiology. The references cited in the previous paragraphs will give the reader an introduction to these various disciplines and potential ramifications of parallels between avian stereotypy and human schizophrenia, obsessive-compulsive disorder [OCD], and autism.)

Problem Behaviors or Syndromes

Dominance

The existence of dominant and submissive individuals among parrots is well documented, but its significance in pet psittacines is subject to debate.* Dominance usually correlates with increased exploratory behavior in young individuals and increased aggression in adults. Some studies, such as that done on cockatiels by the University of Georgia's Department of Applied Behavioral Science, have demonstrated that dominance (at least in this species and situation) is specific to both the circumstances and the individuals involved.[40] This study took seven cockatiels and established their dominance hierarchy by observation. These birds were then moved to different locations within the same enclosure, and the less dominant members were treated with testosterone. The hierarchy remained the same. When the testosterone-treated individuals were then removed and placed in a new enclosure with new males, these formerly submissive, exogenously androgenized birds became dominant. However, when their original male counterparts were subsequently introduced into this new enclosure, they again assumed submissive roles.

The conclusions reached by this study reinforce what has been observed in other domesticated species, such as our canine and feline companions,

---

*References 8,10,20,28,34,35,38,40.

Psittacine Behavior

where it has long been observed that (1) the most seemingly unlikely individual of a pair may turn out to be dominant and (2) even the most established relationships can be upset by illness or aging changes in the dominant member. It is important to recognize that this is indeed the case in order to establish realistic hope for changing relationships between individuals in an established environment (e.g., between bird and owner).

Although dominance carries a negative connotation for many people, it should also be appreciated for its value as an evolutionary technique. In some avian species, dominance is necessary for successful copulation and reproduction; for example, in Harris' Hawks *(Parabuteo unicinctus)*,[19] only the dominant female will mate. In nature, dominance is a trait that enhances survival by attempting to control social interactions—the selection and maintenance of a preferred mate, nest selection, and access to high-quality food sources and territory.

With the pet psittacine owner, the idea of dominance creates mixed feelings. Compassionate owners do not want to dominate their birds, preferring a more harmonious relationship with their pet. Conversely, owners well versed in the behavior of domesticated species, such as dogs, may find it difficult not to draw parallels between avian flock and canine pack social interactions.

Following are two behaviors that have been accepted as displays of dominance in pet birds, which are redefined to more appropriately describe the actual captive behaviors.

Height Dominance

In the wild, dominance has not been demonstrated to be related to the height of a perching position within a tree. Depending on the species, the favored location may be related to food source, temperature, protection from the elements, or proximity to other flock members or nesting sites.

However, there is no doubt that captive parrots show a greater willingness to step up onto a proffered hand when at ground level than when they are on the top of a cage or curtain rod. Birds at a low height are nervous and anxious to be elevated. Birds at considerable height feel more self-assured and less inclined to step up onto a hand. Intraspecies dominance does not seem to play a part in this basic survival perception. Perhaps this effect should be more loosely termed "height advantage."

Many experienced avian veterinarians, incidentally or purposefully, use height advantage in the animal hospital. When coupled with experience and a steady demeanor, it can allow the veterinarian to move the bird to different locations within the hospital and to initiate restraint for other procedures. It is often amazing to owners who can no longer handle their birds that the veterinarian or staff person is so readily accepted by their pet. Two different reasons may motivate this behavior in birds, which may also vary by individual. Firstly, if the bird has learned that people are basically good and safe, the newly proffered, confident hand may appear to provide the safest location in a strange environment. Alternatively, the disorientation afforded by new surroundings, new sights and other sensations, and a different voice and manner may distract, surprise, or preoccupy the bird so that it finds itself perched on a hand without conscious stepping. This phenomenon can be seen in young children, where a tantrum may stop after a few words from an unfamiliar adult, while the pleading, threatening, and cajoling of the parents have no effect. Regardless of the true impetus behind this behavior, it is useful in the animal hospital but of limited value to the owners once they return home.

Innate or True Dominant Behavior

Most birds, when confronted with a confident, experienced bird handler, will accept minor instruction and interaction such as stepping up quite readily. This obviously varies by species and individual. Occasional birds, however, are tractable and compliant until they perceive a threat or a challenge. These birds will attack when one becomes firm or disciplinary. Increased assertiveness from a human will increase their fury and determination, as the human involved accelerates his or her attempts to force compliance. This phenomenon is not well described or understood and seems to occur somewhat disproportionately in male cockatoos.[50] Such individuals may be those that would have innately demonstrated increased exploratory behavior and aggression in the wild, being destined to be more dominant within the flock.[31,50]

The following two examples demonstrate the distinction between this form of innate or true dominance and a learned behavior strengthened by positive reinforcement.

Example 1: "True" or innate dominance

A 9-year-old male Umbrella Cockatoo is being fostered by an experienced psittacine behaviorist. This male will occasionally chase visitors or family members off of furniture in the home with ferocious attacks. For over 7 years, the male had been extremely tractable and affectionate with one author while at the animal hospital, allowing physical examination, venipuncture, and wing trims without restraint. However, on one occasion after a physical examination, the author absentmindedly reprimanded him with a loud, stern "No!" when he attempted to grab the pen with which she was writing. This cockatoo then launched himself with a raucous scream, crest erect, feet and beak on the attack, at her face. After a moment, she spoke softly to him, and he stepped up to cuddle as though nothing had occurred.

Psittacine Behavior

Example 2: Learned dominant or aggressive behavior

A 7-year-old male caique will readily interact physically and vocally with multiple individuals. He will step up on command, provided that the command is given sweetly and with eye contact. However, an aggressive, irritated, or distracted command to step up will be met with a severe bite.

The first of these two examples, the male cockatoo, seems to have its problem behavior stem from dominance and aggression. This is a difficult situation, and extreme caution must be used when working with these birds to prevent serious injury to the owner or handler.

The second example is easily explained and corrected by employing the behavior analysis model. The caique will step up readily when it is stepping onto an attentive, pleasant hand, a situation already promising a positive experience for this social bird that enjoys attention. If the person is either surly or distracted, biting may accomplish one of two results that are preferable to stepping up: (1) the person may leave the bird alone, or (2) the person may yell, which is reinforcement for many birds.

Biting

Severe or repeated use of the beak for biting is not a common defense mechanism for wild parrots. The beak is used aggressively in nature usually only for lunging displays, although if actually caught by a predator the beak is a bird's most effective weapon. Therefore it has been assumed that the reason parrots bite in captivity is a learned behavior, eliciting the response they desire (such as being left alone in the cage or, conversely, not being returned to the cage). Another reason may be the dramatic effect that it creates, as was illustrated in the previous section by the case of the caique that would bite when someone was distracted or aggressive in approaching. In addition, if a bird is truly afraid of people, being forced to step up would be equivalent to being forced into physical contact with a predator; biting then may serve the purpose of defense against that predator. In this case, biting is not the major problem but the result of a fear of humans.[49] Extensive conditioning and training would be recommended to address fear-induced biting.

Birds that bite in order to be left alone or obtain a response must have these reinforcers removed. This certainly can be difficult for an inexperienced owner, who may be afraid of the bite itself or may not have confidence that the biting behavior will indeed extinguish itself if the owner perseveres. This is one of the primary reasons that involving a behaviorist is recommended.

In cases of biting, working in a neutral location (bathrooms are often ideal) and on the floor will change the bird's perceived territory, making them much more compliant. This essentially employs the same phenomenon that occurs in the veterinary hospital, allowing us to look so accomplished in the eyes of many owners. As with most behaviors that owners desire to change, a simple outline of behavior modification is typically not sufficient. Even when the theory of behavioral analysis, including reinforcement and its consequences, is understood, identifying the significant parameters for a particular behavior can be difficult and often requires experience. Consultation with a parrot behaviorist may be essential to determine the significant aspects of a situation in which a bite is precipitated, as well as what the bird derives from biting (reinforcers) that must be removed in order to eliminate the behavior. Even with specific parameters and their expected modifications well understood, exhibiting the proper response in the face of an inherent emotional reaction (e.g., to biting or incessant screaming) can be difficult for many owners.

In general, the following steps will be involved in decreasing biting behaviors (although again, various other factors may be involved and should be identified):

- Move the bird to a neutral location, such as a small bathroom.
- Use praise when the bird is perched on the hand or arm without biting. Use positive eye contact as well.
- If the bird attempts to bite, use the wobble or earthquake method (rapidly drop the perching hand a short distance, forcing the bird to forego biting in order to regain balance).
- If the bird does manage to bite, do not reward it by letting it go or yelling a dramatic "Ouch!" It is likely that either or both of these results are what the bird is seeking to achieve. Again, use the earthquake technique, concurrently placing the thumb over the foot if needed to prevent escape.
- Laddering is an effective technique for desensitizing birds that inappropriately bite advancing hands; however, because of the potential that several bites will occur during training, this should not be attempted by children or those sensitive to the discomfort or pain of being bitten.
- Gloves or towels may be used by some to decrease the likelihood and/or severity of biting, but they may also cause a fearful response in some birds.

Phobias or Neuroses

As was discussed earlier, severe behavioral problems are developing in an alarming percentage of our hand-raised psittacines. A strong correlation to the relative attachment disorder described in children exists and may account for this phenomenon. The use of the terms "neurosis" and "phobia" are controversial in their application to birds, and the general term "anxiety disorder" may be more appropriate. What seems most pertinent is the similarity of these exaggerated manifestations of fear of an object, event, or situation, to human psychologic disorders. The parallels that exist to certain documented emotional disorders in humans provide hope that their corresponding treatment approaches could be equally effective.

Whether fear reactions in birds constitute the equivalent of a neurosis or phobia is beyond our ability to determine. However, an increased incidence of birds that are easily startled or consistently fearful in situations in which they were previously comfortable is noted in captive hand-raised psittacines. The connection between hand-raising and the prevalence of this behavior is a fact, but causation is difficult to prove.

Cockatoo Prolapse Syndrome

This syndrome is extremely common in adult Umbrella and Moluccan *(Cacatua moluccensis)* Cockatoos (Figure 2-7). The exact cause has not been conclusively proved, but several characteristics have been shown to be

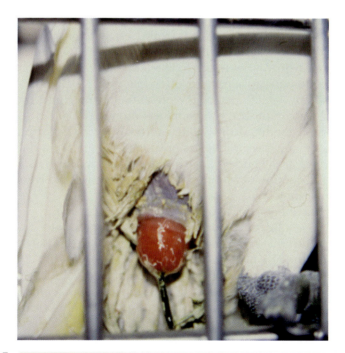

Figure 2-7
Cloacal prolapse in an Umbrella Cockatoo. See text for the multifactorial causes. (Courtesy Teresa Lightfoot.)

involved in all or most of these cases. These birds will generally be characterized by one or more of the following descriptions:
- Were hand-raised
- Experienced delayed weaning, and/or exhibited continued begging for food
- Are psychologically attached to at least one person
- Demonstrate either child-parent or mate-mate relationships with their owners, although these signs may not be obvious to the humans at which they are directed
- Tend to hold the stool in their vent for prolonged periods (e.g., overnight) rather than defecating in the cage

These factors contribute in the following manner:
- Prolonged begging (whining) for food will cause straining and dilation of the vent.
- Displaced sexual attraction to the "human" mate will cause vent straining and movement.
- Retention of stool in the vent for prolonged periods will stretch and dilate the cloaca.

All of these factors added together may account for the high incidence of prolapse in these birds.

If this problem is detected and treated early, surgical correction combined with behavioral modification may correct it. Secondary infection from irritated cloacal tissue and fecal retention is common, with *Clostridia* species or gram-negative bacteria often involved. A fetid odor to the feces often develops, which may be the presenting complaint. Surgical correction can be accomplished by several techniques.

Behavioral modification is often difficult for owners to accomplish, because in many ways it involves breaking the tight bond that they have with the bird. If the bird still perceives its owner as either its parent or its mate, it will continue to strain, and the problem will likely recur eventually, despite surgery.

The types of behavior to avoid include the following:
- Stroking the bird, especially on the back (i.e., petting)
- Feeding the bird warm foods, or food by hand or mouth
- Cuddling the bird close to the body

Cockatoos that are independent of humans do not have this medical problem. If an owner is serious about trying to change a bird's behavioral patterns, the aid of a parrot behavioral consultant will likely be necessary. A recent study suggests that improvement may also be achieved with oral clomipramine (further described under Psychotropic Medications), although the study's author attributes its effectiveness to increased urethral or cloacal muscle tone from the drug's anticholinergic properties rather than its psychologic or emotional effects.[51]

Feather Destruction

The constellation of clinical manifestations grouped under this label and the extensive variety of attributed causes warrant its independent discussion. Some general points regarding this behavioral abnormality should be noted before attempting diagnostics or therapeutics.
- Normal preening, shredding of feathers, plucking out of feathers, and some cases of self-mutilation are all on a continuum of intensity of grooming behavior.
- Purely behavioral feather plucking does occur, induced by one or more stressors. The normal preening activity becomes increased in duration, forcefulness, or both by psychologic factors (see Behavioral Contribution later in this section).
- Purely medical causes of feather plucking also occur, and a thorough medical diagnostic workup may then lead to proper therapeutics and elimination of the behavior.
- Nutritional deficiencies often create less-than-optimal organ system function, with subsequent amino acid deficiencies in the feathers, vitamin A deficiency in the skin, and resultant itchiness and irritability.
- Plucking can be caused or exacerbated by lack of exposure to sunlight, insufficient humidity, or inadequate ventilation.
- Feather picking can also be caused by such environmental factors as tobacco smoke, aerosols, low-level zinc toxicity, hand creams transferred to the bird's feathers, and numerous others.
- Any of the preceding conditions (bullet points 2 to 6) can lead to feather follicle irritation and secondary folliculitis. In certain cases (as occurs with other companion animals, although for different reasons), the inciting cause may be transient and already gone by presentation; however, if subsequent infections are not diagnosed and resolved, the irritation will persist or worsen.
- More often than not, multiple causes are involved in feather plucking.
- Importantly, once the plucking has become habitual, correction of the underlying problems may or may not stop the plucking.

Associated Medical Conditions
- Endoparasites: Particularly giardiasis in cockatiels, but occasionally also seen with tapeworms or roundworms in larger species.
- Ectoparasites: An uncommon but potential source of pruritus and feather destructive behavior. The red mite *(Dermanyssus gallinae)* may be the most common ectoparasite involved in actual feather plucking.
- Hepatic disease: Regardless of the nature of the hepatopathy, pruritus associated with liver dysfunction may cause plucking.

- Coelomic cavity granuloma or mass.
- Folliculitis or dermatitis: These conditions can be primary or secondary to excessive plucking and/or mutilation. Bacteria, virus, fungus, or yeast may be involved. Note that severe primary bacterial folliculitis may require prolonged antibiotic therapy. The skin in these birds is usually grossly abnormal in affected areas. Biopsy and culture are necessary for proper diagnosis and selection of antimicrobials. Severe fungal infection (often with *Aspergillus* species but occasionally with a yeast or saprophytic fungus) is usually secondary and localized; it may be invasive and refractory to treatment because of the destruction of skin and underlying musculature by both the infection and self-trauma.
- Allergies: Although it is difficult to confirm, a change in environment or diet may lead to a decrease in allergen exposure, decreased plucking, and a tentative diagnosis of allergy based on this response.
- Endocrine abnormalities: The most common endocrinopathy in birds is hypothyroidism. However, hypothyroidism is still overdiagnosed in birds. Established normal values for avian thyroid levels are lacking. Nevertheless, some obese birds that demonstrate a lack of weight loss following a rigid diet, accompanied by poor-quality feathers and infrequent molts, may be thyroid deficient. The plucking exhibited by these birds is often an attempt to rid themselves of old, damaged feathers.
- Heavy metal toxicity (notably zinc): Barbering and feather plucking from zinc ingestion has been theorized. Many of these cases will not have radiographic evidence of heavy metal and require a blood zinc analysis for documentation of elevated zinc levels.

Environmental and Nutritional Factors

Environmental and nutritional factors may be more common contributors to feather destructive behavior than the classic medical conditions listed in the previous section.
- Basic seed and table food diets often create multiple nutritional deficiencies. These deficiencies cause abnormal skin and feather development, resulting in plucking behavior, as well as a myriad of other medical problems that may occur later in life.
- The dyes and preservatives that are added to seeds and most pelleted diets may be detrimental to birds. This seems to be most common in species such as African Greys, Eclectus, and some cockatoos.
- The relatively low humidity in most households also has a drying effect on the skin.
- Being deprived of natural sunlight, fresh air, humidity, and the normal light-dark cycle has negative physiologic and psychologic effects on birds.

Behavioral Contribution

Many times, although treatment of medical and environmental factors may reduce the severity of feather plucking, a strong behavioral component is also involved. It is common to treat for the abovementioned problems and note an initial improvement, only to have a recurrence of the condition at a later date. The psychologic factors that can lead to plucking are numerous, but it is important to remember that these cases represent displaced behavior in response to some psychologic stressor. The analogy of fingernail biting in people is apt and often allows the client to relate to the problem—a person may begin to bite the fingernails while undergoing a very stressful time in their lives and once the stress has been relieved, the habit may still remain. This analogy also explains the persistence of plucking even when the apparent causes have been remedied—the habit itself has become self-rewarding (Figure 2-8).

It is noteworthy that feather destructive behavior does *not* occur in the wild. Wild birds are occupied with finding food, maintaining their positions in the flock, seeking out and finding a mate, avoiding predators, breeding, and raising young. Therefore often the best-loved birds, with all their apparent needs met, will be the purely behavioral pluckers. The owners find comfort in this explanation, because they often feel that they have been somehow negligent or their bird would not be bald!

Psychologic conditions that may cause feather plucking in birds vary, and situations that cause plucking in one bird may cause the cessation of

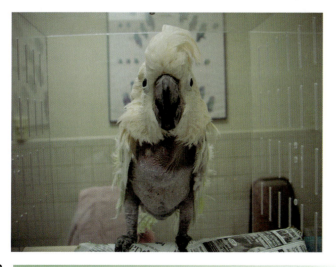

Figure 2-8
The localization of feather loss to the chest suggests a self-trauma, as opposed to cagemate trauma or generalized feather disease. (Courtesy Jörg Mayer.)

plucking in another. Overstimulation (e.g., a house full of active children) may initiate plucking in a nervous bird. A second bird that was plucking from boredom may feel both stimulated and slightly threatened by the presence of this increased activity in the home, and it may stop plucking in order to pay attention to the environment. This capitalizes on the bird's basic instinct to guard itself against potential predators. Birds that are reaching sexual maturity may begin to pluck as an outlet for their increased energy and agitation. Owners of these birds often report that their birds are showing more cage territoriality, more aggression toward one or more family members, and possible sexual behavior toward a perceived human mate or inanimate objects.

A thorough understanding of the environment of the bird and the behavioral changes that have accompanied the onset of plucking will allow the veterinarian to make the appropriate suggestions for environmental manipulation. Tremendous variation in the initiating factors and subsequent recommendations to remedy these problems exists. It is extremely helpful to have a questionnaire for the owner that covers multiple aspects—the bird's origins, husbandry (diet, caging, environment, humidity, schedule, and so on), and behavioral interactions.[36,37] Requesting that the owner fill out the form in advance of a discussion will often preclude the need for prolonged diatribes on areas not applicable to that individual bird. The owners can often identify concerns or potential exacerbating factors in the course of answering a well-designed questionnaire.

The ongoing services of a parrot behavioral consultant are often needed for the specific identification of problem situations, appropriate initial corrections, ongoing owner support, and modification of the behavioral plan as needed.

Medical Modification of Behavior

When the anamnesis points to a psychologic basis for plucking, the veterinarian and owner may elect to combine environmental manipulation and training with either hormonal or psychotropic medications. Similarly, the idea long advocated by behaviorists is that the most efficient use of pharmacotherapy is to potentiate behavioral modification techniques (i.e., using medications concurrently to reinforce behavioral training). Although this would seem particularly true for psittacines exhibiting feather destructive behavior (both purely behavioral cases and those persisting once other inciting factors have been resolved), it is arguably applicable to any chronic behavior patterns that an owner wishes to change.

Following are partial lists of these drugs, their indications, contraindications, and potential usefulness. None of these drugs is ideal for producing long-term positive results, and side effects are possible with several of these medications. (Note: All doses are oral [PO] unless otherwise indicated.)

Psychotropic Medications

Diazepam: For birds that appear anxious (notably, that pluck or destroy feathers when left alone—that is, separation anxiety), diazepam may be helpful. In addition to being anxiolytic, it may be advantageous for its appetite stimulant, anticonvulsant, or hypnotic properties. Initial treatment at 0.5 to 1 mg/kg PO q8h may be successful in decreasing feather destructive behavior, separation anxiety, and "phobic" reactions. Dosages as high as 2.5 to 4 mg/kg q6-12h PO have also been reported for these same indications. Diazepam also greatly decreases stress during the application of an Elizabethan collar, and in this situation is often administered intramuscularly (IM) while the bird is under inhalation anesthesia or before collar application.

Haloperidol (Haldol): Numerous reports document that this dopamine-blocking antipsychotic is reasonably efficacious, notably in cockatoos. Serious side effects, including anorexia, hepatic dysfunction, and central nervous system (CNS) signs, have been reported in various species of psittacines. Occasional adverse reactions including severe excitation or depression and gastric upset have also been reported. Suggested doses are 0.15 mg/kg every 24 hours for larger birds and 0.2 mg/kg every 12 hours for smaller species.[5,6,15]

Fluoxetine (Prozac): Reports of the usefulness of selective serotonin reuptake inhibitors (SSRIs) have varied widely. A dose of 2 mg/kg every 12 hours for fluoxetine is reported empirically. However, because an initial loading period of several weeks is necessary for the manifestation of therapeutic effects in humans, owner compliance is often poor. Preparing the client for the prolonged interval before an observable improvement may aid in its successful use.

Amitriptyline (Elavil): Tricyclic antidepressants (TCAs) have sedative, antihistamine, anticholinergic, and some serotonin reuptake inhibition properties. The antihistamine portion may cause a sedative effect. As with fluoxetine and other SSRIs, an initial loading period is necessary for an observable response. Barring side effects of the anticholinergic properties, it may be worth a more prolonged course of this medication to determine its usefulness in birds. Dosages published for amitriptyline are 1 to 2 mg/kg every 12 to 24 hr.[5]

Clomipramine (Clomicalm): This relatively new TCA is unique in that it is thought to act primarily through serotonin reuptake inhibition. In humans it is used for a variety of disorders including depression, anxiety,

---

*References 9,11,12,17,26,33,38.

and obsessive-compulsive disorder (OCD)*; it is also licensed for obsessive-compulsive conditions in dogs. Empiric dosages used in birds are most commonly reported as 0.25 to 0.5 mg/kg daily, but a recent study involving cloacal prolapse in cockatoos used a dose of 3 mg/kg every 12 hours.[51] Some avian behaviorists advocate dosages in the range of 3 to 5 mg/kg/day.[39] Potential side effects relate to the anticholinergic effects of TCAs and include seizures, arrhythmias, and cardiovascular collapse; for similar reasons, TCAs should be avoided with decreased gastrointestinal motility, urinary retention, cardiac arrhythmias, or increased intraocular pressure.[21] Clomipramine should also be used with caution in patients with liver disease.

Because of the stress of restraint for oral administration, mixing the medication into a readily acceptable soft food vehicle (e.g., yogurt, mashed potatoes) may greatly increase client and patient compliance. Use of these medications in the drinking water is a potential alternate route. Empirically, some positive responses have been noted with drinking water administration. However, potency, efficacy, toxicity, and palatability of most of these medications in water have yet to be determined.

Research evaluating treatment success and elucidating pathways involved in human psychologic disorders provides insight that may be applicable to our companion psittacines. Obvious parallels exist between OCD in humans and feather destructive behavior, and self-mutilation disorders exist in people as well as birds. Psychiatry today recognizes anxiety and depression as a continuum of manifestations of frustration or feelings of emotional helplessness, varying in whether these perceptions are externalized (anxiety) or internalized (depression); in fact, the same drugs are now used to treat both conditions.

One new meta-analysis evaluating treatment for OCD has shown cognitive behavioral therapy to be the most successful single therapy, being superior to medication alone and not showing a significantly improved response when combined with drug therapy (in this case, clomipramine).[12] However, many other studies show significant improvement with drug therapy alone, with or without behavioral therapy.[9,11] SSRIs and clomipramine, grouped as "serotonergic antidepressants," are considered the most effective medications for OCD and have also been effective in decreasing self-injurious behavior in intellectually disabled humans.[9,11,12,17] Still, similar to the situation encountered in psittacines, meta-analysis also suggests that regardless of the type of appropriate treatment (including behavioral therapy), the effect is usually partial, and moderate levels of symptoms persist.[9,11]

New information on the pathways involved in chronic stress and the development of depression suggest that these same drugs should be useful in modulating desired behavioral changes, particularly at the onset of therapy. Investigations of chronic stress (both physical and psychosocial) and subsequent behavioral effects have been insightful.[1,6,14] Results reveal effects on gene transcription via several pathways. Retraction of dendrites and an impairment of neurogenesis in the hippocampus mediated by the described changes in gene transcription were found with chronic stress. This implies both a morphologic and a neurochemical basis for disease that decreases the underlying neural plasticity necessary for normal brain functioning (particularly learning and emotional association).[1,14] Upregulation of mediators controlling cortisol production may have behavioral effects in the brain even before their release is appreciable in the bloodstream.[6] It is interesting to note that the behavioral changes and most of the neural gene transcription alterations produced by chronic stress were prevented by clomipramine treatment.[6]

Very few objective investigations have studied the effectiveness of pharmacotherapy for feather destructive behavior. A study of clomipramine in feather-picking cockatoos showed significant improvement at both 3 and 6 weeks of treatment.[39] Although analogies to human disorders and insights from research hold promise of effectiveness, caution is warranted. Neonatal treatment with clomipramine is so reliable in producing depression that it is used as an animal model.[2] Other studies show that OCD-like alterations in decision making can be produced by chronic dopamine agonism, reinforcing the potential applicability of dopamine blockers such as haloperidol.[42] Finally, significant juvenile hyporesponsiveness to psychotropic manipulations has been demonstrated in people.[42]

Hormonal Medications

Medroxyprogesterone acetate (Depo-Provera): This drug was used for many years as a deterrent to sexual behavior, including feather plucking. Unfortunately the side effects ranged from weight gain, PU and PD, and lethargy to more severe conditions such as hepatopathy, diabetes mellitus, and death. The response of each bird to a given dose varies. This medication is not recommended for use in routine feather plucking. When the risks are determined to be acceptable to the veterinarian and the owner, the dosage range is between 5 and 25 mg/kg intramuscularly. The lowest possible effective dose should be used, and all efforts to modify the bird's behavior should be made in conjunction with this therapy so that the injection need not be repeated.[2,5]

Human chorionic gonadotropin (hCG): This drug has met with low to moderate success, mainly in female birds. The predominantly luteinizing hormone (LH) activity of hCG stimulates the production and release of endogenous progesterone in females. When successful, the female bird tends to pluck much less and be less aggressive without experiencing the side effects identified with Depo-Provera. In male birds, testosterone as well as progesterone is produced in response to LH, making the success rate much lower. An exception seems to be Eclectus males, in which the response to hCG has been equal to that of females of other species. This correlates with the lower levels of testosterone and higher levels of progesterone found normally in the limited number of Eclectus males that have been tested. Dosage protocols are exclusively empirical at this point in time. A commonly used regimen is the administration of 500 to 1000 units/kg intramuscularly.[6] Generally, if no response is seen within 3 days, the dose is repeated. If no response is noted after this second injection, it is our experience that repeated or increased doses are unlikely to be effective. The injection, if successful in reducing plucking, will initially need to be repeated after 4 to 6 weeks. The major drawback of this medication is that with repeated use, the interval between injections must be decreased; presumably, this increased resistance represents the development of hCG antibodies.[6] After 3 years of treatment with hCG, some birds need injections as frequently as every 10 days. Although repeated serum chemistries have shown no adverse effects, this frequency is inconvenient for the owner, and long-term use at this interval has not been studied.

GnRH agonist (Depo-Lupron, leuprolide acetate)[12]: This medication functions to increase the release of LH and follicle-stimulating hormone (FSH). Its efficacy is probably based on the bird's response to LH. The role of FSH in birds is not well understood. The disadvantage to this medication is that it is extremely expensive. The advantage is that there does not appear to be antibody production to GnRH. In my experience, birds that respond to hCG initially but subsequently develop a tolerance often respond to Depo-Lupron. Dosages are empirical, and current subjective administration is cited at 800 µg/kg every 4 weeks.

Acupuncture: In addition to the traditional medical therapies, acupuncture has been used with some reported success. In one author's experience, the birds that have responded favorably were usually of the genus *Cacatua*. This has been reported by other avian veterinarians as well.

Essential fatty acids: Omega fatty acids have been used as a dietary supplement to treat feather plucking with some success. Whether this is because of the antiprostaglandin effect or a true fatty acid deficiency is not certain. The canine product DermCaps can be punctured with a needle, and the contents added by the drop to the bird's food.

An ideal medical treatment is not likely to be found for feather plucking in captive birds. Manipulation of the environment, ensuring quality nutrition, and psychologic adaptations suited to the species and temperament of the bird offer the best hope for reducing this syndrome. The maintenance of a nondomestic species in a domesticated environment requires that we use all available resources to ensure the highest quality of life for our avian patients.

Psittacine Behavior in the Animal Hospital

Generalizations will be given to provide the practitioner a starting point when dealing with a given species, but as in all things, exceptions are common. Observation of the bird and interpretation of the owner's statements regarding temperament can either reinforce or be contrary to general species behavioral assumptions. These generalizations apply primarily to birds raised under current production methods (i.e., without the benefit of Abundance Weaning and the associated socialization during development).

Home-Court Advantage

The unfamiliar environment of the animal hospital dampens or eliminates most birds' territorial behavior, especially if they are not in their cage or on their owner. When taking a bird from the owner, have the owner place the bird on the examination room table or floor, then move yourself between the bird and the owner. If the bird is hand-tamed, it will get on your hand to get out of the lower "prey" position. Maintain the bird at chest level, where many will be comfortable with their inferior but not dangerously low height. Most birds that are not truly phobic will respond to a calm, dominant, and fearless individual. Firm assertive and distracting techniques can get the bird onto your hand and up to a level of comfort before the bird realizes it is no longer perching on an inanimate object. Observation of the bird's posture and body language at this point will indicate what adjustments in height or attention (eye contact or lack of) need to be made.[43,46] Some birds do best with the owner absent; although they may have a close relationship, it is usually the owner that has been well trained by the bird to respond to its desires and moods. Simulated earthquakes, the use of eye contact, and voice modulation all may aid in control of the biting bird.[46] The key for many is a lack of reaction to attempted or actual bites. It should not change one's motions, behavior or expectations of the bird if it bites or attempts to bite. This rapidly removes the reward obtained by biting. Exceptions and variations occur, and undoubtedly there is much more to this aspect of psychology than pure dominance; regardless, the technique is highly effective.

Aggressive Amazons and Other Psittacines in the Animal Hospital

In the unfamiliar environment of the animal hospital, you may be able to get the aggressive bird (whether this perceived aggressiveness is a result of fear or territoriality), of which the owner has become fearful, momentarily hand-tamed. Especially after restraint, when the bird is tired, "submissive," and stressed to the extent that sitting on your hand is a viable option, you can proudly walk up to the owner with the bird perched on your arm, having "tamed" the untamable. If the owner is seated and you then hand the bird down to the owner, it will likely refuse to step and may even attempt to bite the owner. You are at a superior height and represent stability and safety. However, your goal is to help the owner of a biting, territorial Amazon (or other species) regain a positive relationship with the pet bird—not to demonstrate your (somewhat artificial) prowess. After handling a bird presented with aggression and biting behavior, the veterinarian should return the bird to the owner in a manner that allows the owner to see the potential for the bird to become an enjoyable, interactive pet. This is best accomplished by releasing the bird onto the floor or examination table while the owner is standing and you are sitting. Most birds will readily step onto the owner's hand to be rescued from this compromising position. The owner then feels good about the bird, himself or herself, and what you have taught. (Note that with older African Greys or with fearful owners of aggressive Amazons, your own hand or a towel may need to be placed between the perching bird and the owner's hand to further ensure that the owner will not be bitten.)

At this time, warn the owner that returning the bird to the same cage and same routine at home will usually reinstate the old negative behaviors. The owner should be encouraged to place the bird in a new location on returning home, such as the bathroom. The location, elevation, and orientation of the cage, and even the cage itself, should be changed if at all possible. However, these measures will only be transiently effective, the temporary goal being to give owners hope that the bird may once again become an enjoyable and joyful pet. This may be the positive incentive needed to convince them to solicit the services of a professional behavior consultant or commit to regular training sessions. Be certain to provide the clients with the telephone numbers and e-mail addresses of these consultants, as well as literature and Internet references about proper training, before they leave your office.[48] Many veterinarians and/or technicians are becoming more proficient with behavioral training and offer individual consultations or classes through their hospitals.

Conures (Sun, Jenday, Gold-capped, Blue-crown, Mitred, other *Aratinga* Species)

These are fast, often territorial birds. Attempting to take them from the owner's shoulder almost ensures either a flight to the floor, a "ring around the client," or a bite for the owner or the veterinarian. If the bird is towel trained, use this to your advantage. The owners of "towel-happy" birds tend to be more knowledgable about their bird's behavior and do not appreciate it if you ignore all their work by grabbing the bird out of the towel, screaming. One author had two wonderful Sun Conure patients that loved traveling while secure in their towel. The physical examination could be accomplished while they remained in the towel with their vision obscured. It was only when the towel was briefly removed from their faces for the examination of the head that they became indignant. Out of the towel they were little piranhas and desperately wanted retribution for years of annual venipuncture.

Umbrella Cockatoos (Cacatua alba)

Cockatoos tend to adjust quickly to new people when separated from their owners, and prefer to be cuddled and coddled rather than to step up onto a new hand. Axillary and crest rubbing are often loved, and a soft clucking sound or soothing voice as you approach the bird, with your fingers moving in a "you-are-about-to-get-a-really-good-massage" motion will convince most of these birds to accept your attentions (Figure 2-9). Umbrellas also tend to be forgiving after restraint and venipuncture; the same person that performed these procedures can then make apologies and comfort the bird. Allow the owner to be the last one to console the cockatoo, making both the owner and the bird feel better.

One can avoid initiating a startle reflex by demonstrating equipment in advance of its use (this same technique is needed with African Greys). The bird then has time to recognize it as a nonthreatening object. For example, stethoscopes and penlights should not be whipped out in front of the bird, but displayed first at a distance. Rubbing these objects against your face and talking in a soothing voice will demonstrate the nonthreatening nature of these items and often facilitate their acceptance.

Despite (or because of) their inclination for extensive interaction with humans, cockatoos are far from exempt from behavioral problems. Umbrella Cockatoos may exhibit screaming, feather picking, phobic behaviors, or chronic cloacal prolapse. A small percentage of Umbrella Cockatoos are very nervous in the hospital environment—startling and thrashing when stimulated, much like the "phobic" African Grey. These birds are rapidly identifiable by their behavior.

Another faction of cockatoos has been labeled as "super male." Whether these birds actually differ in genetic or hormonal makeup from other male cockatoos, and whether they would be destined to be one of the more superior males in the flock, is unknown. These birds' behaviors tend to be unpredictable. A male cockatoo with the "super-male" temperament may be docile and affectionate until he perceives a threat or challenge. A violent attack can follow the perception of this threat or challenge. (See the earlier section on true dominance.)

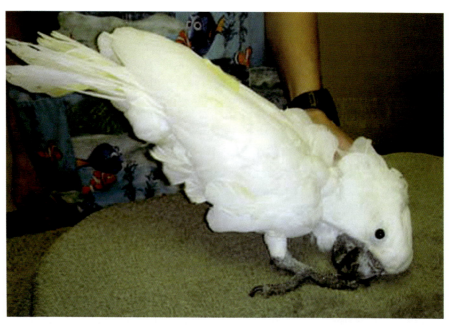

Figure 2-9
The head-down position of this Umbrella Cockatoo *(Cacatua alba)* can be a submissive gesture of a nervous or insecure cockatoo (note that the neck is being rubbed by a person in the background). This is in contrast to a truly fearful or frightened cockatoo, which will display agitated wing flapping in an attempt to remove itself from the source of its fear. The head-down, back-elevated position demonstrated in this photo can also be an invitation for petting or sexual contact. (Courtesy Dan Johnson.)

In addition to species tendencies, unsuitable or inappropriate behavioral expectations, and learned reactions to previous experiences, hormonal components are involved in some of these syndromes in cockatoos. Sadly with cockatoos, because of their incredible screaming ability and less pronounced (as compared with African Greys) talking ability, disheartened owners are likely to rid themselves of cockatoos that become problematic pets. African Greys, if their behavior becomes less desirable, are often relegated to life in a cage, being considered still somewhat "valuable" to less-perceptive owners because of the entertainment value of their talking ability.

Macaws (Ara spp.)

The inquisitive nature and athleticism of these species necessitate considerable effort on the part of the owner to assure proper development. These birds, if not extensively socialized when young, tend to become attached to one owner and to range from nervous to severely neurotic while at the animal hospital. They are also one of the species more likely to be totally acclimated to the owner's shoulder. Because of their long beak reach and ability to elevate with flapping of even clipped wings, they are one of the more difficult species to keep off of your shoulder. My personal opinion is that, in the typical tame but inadequately socialized (and therefore very nervous) in-hospital blue and gold macaw *(Ara ararauna)* discretion may be the better part of valor. If one is transporting the macaw from the owner (who did not bring the bird in a cage, of course) to the back for restraint and venipuncture, the clinician has three choices: (1) restrain the bird in the examination room and carry it to the back; (2) place the bird (most likely with appreciable commotion) in a hospital-owned carrier and transport it to the back; or (3) transport the macaw on one's arm or shoulder, allowing the owner to avoid involvement in or observation of the restraint. The first two options usually result in stress to both the owner and the bird. If the owner does not wish to be present, it is often easiest to allow the macaw to retain its position on your shoulder for the brief duration of a walk directly to your destination; a predetermined path that naturally excludes access to other rooms, the reception area, lunging dogs, or the outdoors is essential. Most macaws will be sufficiently "prey" minded to have all their attention diverted to watching their surroundings and not your ear during this time.

Wild caught or untrained macaws should be restrained firmly and as briefly as possible. They will vocalize almost constantly; the handlers, to avoid hearing damage, should wear earplugs. Many "older" practitioners lost hearing from working with imported macaws (before the 1980s). Attempts to calm these wild or unsocialized macaws during restraint are generally unsuccessful.

Eclectus (Eclectus spp.)

The generalization that male Eclectus tend to be more docile than females is supported by the fact that this is one of the few psittacine species where the female consistently attacks and injures the male. Studies performed at one of our hospitals from 1996 to 1998 (researching the use of chorionic gonadotropin) suggested, as an incidental finding, that the cause of this may be that male Eclectus have the lowest testosterone levels of any male psittacine species tested.[22] Female Eclectus had the second highest level of testosterone of all females we tested (female African Greys having the highest). However, the number of Eclectus used in our study was not large enough to be conclusive for quantification of testosterone in that species.

Generalizations are also made regarding the intelligence of this species. Eclectus tend to stare intently, as though frozen, at objects and situations.

This makes them appear dull. Actually, they seem to be quite intelligent and can develop extensive vocabularies. They are generally not overly nervous if properly socialized. Eclectus also appear to be one species in which underlying nutritional problems and disease are important factors in many abnormal behavioral manifestations, such as feather destruction and toe tapping.

African Greys (Psitticus erithacus)

Entire books can (and have) been written on behavior and African Grey Parrots. Their intelligence, cognition, and communicative skills have been studied and quantified (Figure 2-10). (See the section on intelligence and communication at the end of this chapter.) This section will address specific species traits that are applicable to the African Grey as a patient in the avian hospital.

These birds are exceedingly intelligent and therefore seem to more frequently suffer from excessive fears and related behavioral problems. When they are restrained, talking softly and holding absolutely still will usually calm these birds and temporarily stop their growling. However, the growling will begin again once movement is resumed. Still, momentarily halting your movement and soothing the bird will give it a respite from stress, and it is recommended that this be done at intervals when prolonged restraint is necessary.[5] Telling the client in advance that the growling will stop will often impress them with your knowledge. After all, their main concern is that the bird not be hurt, so the more knowledgable one appears, the less nervous the owner will be. Great care should be taken to soothe African Greys at the end of the procedures and to return them to the owner or carrier *only after* you have reestablished a degree of stability to their psyches.

Dremmel sanders, stethoscopes, and other potentially frightening instruments should be demonstrated to both the bird and owner before their use. The owner is less worried when he or she sees you apply the Dremmel sander lightly to your own face or hand. African Greys seem to respond especially well to this technique. It should be noted that a small percentage of birds will seize in response to the application of the Dremmel sander to the beak. A disproportionate number of these birds have been Congo African Greys.

African Greys have an astounding ability to accurately reproduce sounds and are notorious for mimicking a "smoker's cough." Flatulence is also readily learned. Although flatulence may occur in parrots, it is rare and is usually seen in association with severe obesity or cloacal obstructive disease, such as papillomatosis or cloacal prolapse accompanied by marked difficulty in passing stool and abnormal feces. Flatulent noises in the absence of these clinical signs are generally mimicry. We have developed

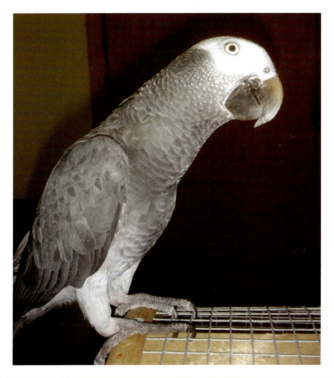

Figure 2-10
This photo of a Congo African Grey demonstrates the tilted head posture that is assumed when psittacines use their mononuclear vision to carefully assess a person, object, or event. (Courtesy Dan Johnson.)

no subtle approach for explaining this to owners, and welcome any suggestions.

Miscellaneous Species

Caiques are small, colorful, playful South American parrots. These birds will hop instead of walking when they are feeling playful or hurrying. This hopping behavior is delightful and surprising when first observed. Their talking ability is limited, but their whistling mimicry is often outstanding.

Pionus spp. may produce a rapid sniffing sound when nervous. This should not be mistaken for a respiratory condition. They are the less boisterous "cousins" of the Amazon, and a favored pet bird of many.

Senegals are often very playful, and may sleep on their backs (as do many young birds) even into adulthood.

Many species of psittacine may imitate a human sneeze. Differentiation from a true physiologic sneeze includes observation of the bird for movement of the head and/or discharge that is produced when sneezing.

Intelligence, Cognition, and Communication in Parrots

In large part because of decades of study by Dr. Irene Pepperberg, as summarized in *The Alex Studies: Cognitive and Communicative Abilities of Grey Parrots* and other works by this author,[31] a great deal of information regarding the learning abilities of parrots has been documented. The behavioral vernacular is daunting, as are the neuroanatomic structures and their associated nomenclature. Originally, the absence of an anatomic region equivalent in structure and function to the mammalian neocortex was thought to preclude learning and advanced (noninstinctual) cognitive behavior in birds. Recent studies have since concluded that there not only exists an avian anatomic structure homologous to the mammalian neostriatum (the palaeostriatum augmentatum), but that there also exists another structure homologous to the mammalian globus pallidus (the avian palaeostriatum primitivum).[6-8] These conclusions have prompted the formation of a consortium to revise the nomenclature of avian neuroanatomy.

No attempt will be made here to explore this extensive and developing subject. However, a synopsis of documented learning-related behaviors is presented, along with related explanations or hypotheses for the evolutionary advantages of these abilities. Much of this information is taken from references provided by Dr. Pepperberg or directly from her work. It is impossible to do justice to the depth, detail, intricacies of experimental design, and exacting elimination of confounding variables that characterize her studies. In attempting to summarize such a wide range of observations and hypotheses, there will admittedly be significant omissions. The reader is strongly encouraged to review this material in its entirety.

Social and Cognitive Similarities to Great Apes

Much research and subsequent hypotheses have centered on the development of intelligence, communication skills, and social interaction in great apes. Many reasons for the emergence of these characteristics have been postulated, including (1) their complex social structure and resultant need for communication among conspecifics; (2) their longevity, with adaptation to new information over time therefore representing a significant survival advantage; and (3) the inherent and immediate survival advantages conferred by such abilities (to interpret, learn, cooperate, and convey information).

Any or all of these parameters may also apply to development of these same traits in parrots and are likely examples of convergent evolution. However, studies in parrots, unlike those in nonhuman primates, are aided by these birds' vocal ability, which allows researchers to more readily quantify and qualify cognition in them.

Perireferential Communication and Categoric Class Formation

Again, the most extensive and relevant work comes from Dr. Irene Pepperberg's studies with Alex and several other African Grey Parrots. This work has determined that an African Grey Parrot can not only learn and convey a simple association—for example, the color that the word "red" represents—but can also extend the concept of "red" to a characteristic that can be shared by objects: a red ball, a red food pellet, or a red dress. From this, it can be inferred that there exists an understanding of "redness" as a quality and the ability to discern and compare qualities among objects (i.e., what is the same and what is different). In addition, although this ability has already been demonstrated in the laboratory setting, other studies indicate that this type of learning and discrimination is greatly enhanced when the categories are defined by qualities whose recognition is important to the survival of a species. Therefore, parrots' categoric class formation abilities may far exceed what can be demonstrated by the types of challenges encountered in the artificial environment of a laboratory.

Sentinel Behavior

Intelligence and categoric discrimination are both needed in order for a species to exhibit sentinel behavior, with individuals being able to produce and heed appropriate warnings. For instance, a sentinel parrot must be able to differentiate between what is potentially dangerous (e.g., a predator) and what is benign. Discrimination, learning, and recollection are capacities critical to providing proper sentinel information to the flock. These birds must interpret and screen information from their natural environment in order to avoid initiating or transmitting erroneous alarm calls. The ability to learn and differentiate "normal" from "alarming" is a complex and advanced function. The specificity of information that different avian species can, through vocalization, relay to conspecifics is still largely unknown, but this sentinel behavior has been observed in numerous species of macaws, Amazons, and cockatoos.

The significance of the innate intelligence of parrots is not of only academic or even applied scientific interest. The consideration of parrots as highly sentient beings should motivate our profession and others involved in avian stewardship to maximize our commitments to providing these creatures with an optimal quality of life, both physically and emotionally.

References

1. Alfonso J, Pollevick GD, Van Der Hart MG, et al: Identification of genes regulated by chronic psychosocial stress and antidepressant treatment in the hippocampus, *Eur J Neurosci* 3:659-666, 2004.
2. Bonilla-Jaime H, Retana-Marquez S, Vazquez-Palacios G, et al: Corticosterone and testosterone levels after chronic stress in an animal model of depression, *Neuropsychobiology* 48(2):55-58, 2003.
3. Brauth SE, Tang ZY, Liang W, Roberts TF: Contact call-driven zenk mRNA expression in the brain of the budgerigar *(Melopsittacus undulatus), Brain Res Mol Brain Res* 117(1):97-103, 2003.
4. Brittan-Powell EF, Dooling RJ, Larsen ON, et al: Mechanisms of vocal production in budgerigars *(Melopsittacus undulatus), J Acoust Soc Am* 101(1):578-589, 1997.
5. Buitenhuis AJ, Rodenburg TB, Van Hierden TM, et al: Mapping quantitative trait loci affecting feather pecking behavior and stress response in laying hens, *Poult Sci* 82(8):1215-1222, 2003.
6. Cordner AP, Herwood MB, Helmreich DL: Antidepressants blunt the effects of inescapable stress on male mating behavior and decrease the corticotrophin-releasing hormone mRNA expression in the hypothalamic paraventricular nucleus of the Syrian hamster *(Mesocricetus auratus), J Neuroendocrinol* 16(7):628-636, 2004.
7. Davis C: Basic considerations for avian behavior modification. *Semin Avian Exot Pet Med* (8)4:183-195, 1999.
8. Diamond J, Bond AB: *Kea, bird of paradox. The evolution and behavior of a New Zealand parrot,* Davis, Calif., 1999, University of California Press.
9. Eddy KT, Dutra L, Bradley R, et al: A multidimensional meta-analysis of psychotherapy and pharmacotherapy for obsessive-compulsive disorder, *Clin Psychol Rev* 24(8):1011-1030, 2004.
10. Emery NJ, Dally JM, Clayton NS: Western scrub-jays *(Aphelocoma californica)* use cognitive strategies to protect their caches from thieving conspecifics, *Anim Cogn* 7(1):37-43, 2004.
11. Foa EB, Liebowitz MR, Kozak MJ, et al: Randomized, placebo-controlled trial of exposure and ritual prevention, clomipramine, and their combination in the treatment of obsessive-compulsive disorder, *Am J Psychiatry* 162(1):151-161, 2005.
12. Fineberg NA, TM Gale: Evidence-based pharmacotherapy of obsessive-compulsive disorder, *Int J Neuropsychopharmacol* 8(1):107-129, 2005.
13. Friedman SG: The natural science of behavior. In Harrison GJ, Lightfoot TL, editors: *Clinical avian medicine,* 2006, Lake Worth, Fla., Spix Press.
14. Fuchs E: Examining novel concepts of the pathophysiology of depression: the chronic psychosocial stress paradigm in tree shrews, *Behav Pharmacol* 15(5-6):315-325, 2004.

15. Garner JP, Meehan CL, Mench JA: Stereotypies in caged parrots, schizophrenia and autism: evidence for a common mechanism, *Behav Brain Res* 145(1-2):125-134, 2003.
16. Harcourt-Brown N: Development of the skeleton and feathers of Dusky parrots *(Pionus fuscus)* in relation to their behaviour, *Vet Rec* 154(2):42-48, 2004.
17. Janowsky DS, Shetty M, Barnhill J, et al: Serotonergic antidepressant effects on aggressive, self-injurious and destructive/disruptive behaviors in intellectually disabled adults: a retrospective, open-label, naturalistic trial, *Int J Neuropsychopharmacol* 8(1):37-48, 2005.
18. Jones M: Behavior of raptors, *Vet Clin North Am Exot Anim Pract* 4:625, 2002.
19. Jurkevich A, Grossmann R: Vasotocin and reproductive functions of the domestic chicken, *Domest Anim Endocrinol* 25(1):93-99, 2003.
20. Kavanau JL: *Behavior and evolution: lovebirds, cockatiels and budgerigars*, Los Angeles, 1987, Science Software Systems.
21. King JN, Steffan J, Heath SE, et al: Determination of the dosage of clomipramine for the treatment of urine spraying in cats, *J Am Vet Med Assoc* 225(6):881-887, 2004.
22. Lightfoot TL: Avian behavior. In Proceedings of the Annual Conference of the Association of Avian Veterinarians, Monterey, Calif., 2000.
23. Linden PG: *Abundantly avian: the compiled works of Phoebe Linden*, Santa Barbara, Calif., 1999, Santa Barbara Bird Farm.
24. Linden PG: Behavioral development of the companion psittacine bird. In Proceedings of the Annual Conference of the AAV, Wesley Chapel, Fla., 1998.
25. Linden PG: Teaching psittacine birds to learn, *Semin Avian Exot Pet Med* (8)4:154-164, 1999.
26. Masi G: Pharmacotherapy of pervasive developmental disorders in children and adolescents, *CNS Drugs* 18(14):1031-1052, 2004.
27. Meehan CL, Garner JP, Mench JA: Environmental enrichment and development of cage stereotypy in Orange-winged Amazon parrots *(Amazona amazonica)*, *Dev Psychobiol* 44(4):209-218, 2004.
28. Moore BR: The evolution of learning, *Annu Rev Psychol*, 12(2):23-29, 2003.
29. Mottley K, Heyes C: Budgerigars *(Melopsittacus undulatus)* copy virtual demonstrators in a two-action test, *J Comp Psychol* 117(4):363-370, 2003.
30. Park F: Behavior and behavioral problems of Australian raptors in captivity, *Semin Avian Exot Pet Med* 12(4):232-241, 2003.
31. Pepperberg IM: *The Alex studies: cognitive and communicative abilities of Grey Parrots*, Cambridge, 2000, Harvard University Press.
32. Platt SR: Evaluating and treating the nervous system. In Harrison GJ, Lightfoot TL, editors: *Clinical avian medicine*, Palm Beach, Fla., 2006, Spix.
33. Plumb D: *Veterinary drug handbook*, ed 4, Ames, Iowa, 2002, Iowa State Press.
34. Rich, GA: Syndromes and conditions of parrotlets, Pionus Parrots, Poicephalus, and Mynah Birds, *Semin Avian Exot Pet Med* 12(3):144-148, 2003.
35. Ritchie BW, Harrison GJ, Harrison LR, editors: *Avian medicine: principles and application*, Lake Worth, Fla., 1994, Wingers Publishing.
36. Rosenthal KL, Morris DO, Mauldin EA, et al: Cytologic, histologic, and microbiologic characterization of the feather pulp and follicles of feather-picking psittacine birds: a preliminary study, *J Avian Med Surg* 18(3):137-143, 2004.
37. Seibert, LM: Animal behavior case of the month, *J Am Vet Med Assoc* 224(9):1433-1435, 2004.

38. Seibert LM, Crowell-Davis SL: Gender effects on aggression, dominance rank, and affiliative behaviors in a flock of captive adult cockatiels *(Nymphicus hollandicus)*, *Appl Anim Behav Sci* 71(2):155-170, 2001.
39. Seibert LM, Crowell-Davis SL, Wilson GH, et al: Placebo-controlled clomipramine trial for the treatment of feather picking disorder in cockatoos, *J Am Anim Hosp Assoc* 40(4):261-269, 2004.
40. Sibley DA: *The Sibley guide to bird life and behavior,* New York, 2001, Chantilleer Press.
41. Styles D: Captive psittacine behavioral reproductive husbandry and management: socialization, aggression control, and pairing techniques. Proceedings of the Annual Conference of the Association of Avian Veterinarians Monterey, Calif., 2001.
42. Ulloa RE, Nicolini H, Fernandez-Guasti A: Age differences in an animal model of obsessive-compulsive disorder. Participation of dopamine: dopamine in an animal model of OCD, *Pharmacol Biochem Behav* 78(4):661-666, 2004.
43. Welle KR: Avian obedience training. In Proceedings of the Annual Conference of the Association of Avian Veterinarians, Minneapolis, Minn., 1997.
44. Welle KR: Psittacine behavior. In Proceedings of the Annual Conference of the Association of Avian Veterinarians, Wesley Chapel, Fla., 1998.
45. Wiley RH, Steadman L, Chadwick L, Wollerman L: Social inertia in white-throated sparrows results from recognition of opponents, *Animal Behav* 57(2):453-463, 1999.
46. Wilson L: Biting and screaming behavior in parrots, *Veterinary Clin North Am Exot Anim Pract* 4[3]:641-650, 2001.
47. Wilson L: Considerations on companion parrot behavior and avian veterinarians, *J Avian Med Surg* 14[4]:273-276, 2000.
48. Wilson L: Restraint in the animal hospital, *Vet Clin North Am Exot Anim Pract* 3(4):633-640, 2001.
49. Wilson L: Screaming and biting in the psittacine pet bird, *Vet Clin North Am Exot Anim Pract,* 3(4):641-650, 2001.
50. Wilson L, Lightfoot T, Linden P: Concepts in behavior, section II: early psittacine behavior. In Harrison GJ, Lightfoot TL, editors: *Clinical avian medicine,* Palm Beach, Fla., 2006, Spix.
51. Zantop DW: Clomipramine hydrochloride for prolapsing cloaca, *Exotic DVM Magazine* 6(5):20, 2004.

Additional Reading

Blanchard S, editor: *Companion Parrot Quarterly* (formerly *Pet Bird Report*). Information available at: www.companionparrot.com.

Brown SD, Dooling RJ: Perception of conspecific faces by budgerigars *(Melopsittacus undulatus)*: II. Synthetic models, *Comp Psychol* 107(1):48-60, 1993.

Courtney J: The juvenile food-begging calls and related behaviour in the Australian 'Rose-tailed' Parrots *Alisterus, Aprosmictus* and *Polytelis;* and a comparison with the Eclectus Parrot *Eclectus roratus* and Pesquet's Parrot Vale via Glen Innes, NSW *Psittrichas fulgidus, Aust Bird Watcher* 17: 42-59, 1997.

Davis CS: Parrot psychology and behavior problems, *Vet Clin North Am Small Anim Pract* 21(6):1281-1288, 1991.

Harris LJ: Footedness in parrots: three centuries of research, theory, and mere surmise, *Can J Psychol* 43(3):369-396, 1989.

Pearn SM, Bennett AT, Cuthill IC: Ultraviolet vision, fluorescence and mate choice in a parrot, the budgerigar *Melopsittacus undulatus, Proc R Soc Lond B Biol Sci* 268(1482):2273-2279, 2001.
Pepperberg IM, Wilcox SE: Evidence for a form of mutual exclusivity during label acquisition by grey parrots *(Psittacus erithacus)? J Comp Psychol* 114(3):219-231, 2000.
Wanker R, Apcin J, Jennerjahn B, Waibel, B: Discrimination of different social companions in spectacled parrotlets *(Forpus conspicillatus):* evidence for individual voice recognition, *Behav Ecol Sociobiol* 43(3):197-202, 1998.

The following journals contain insightful information in multiple articles within the specified dates.

Auk, 1952-1985
Bulletin of the British Ornithologists' Club, 1956-1972
Condor, 1959-1985 (information available at: http://gw.roottech.com/condor)
Emu, 1980-1985
Ibis, 1964-1976
Journal of Ornithology, 1922-1964
Living Bird, 1962-1974
PsittaScene (magazine of the World Parrot Trust), 1989-2002 (information available at: www.worldparrottrust.org)
Proceedings of the International Ornithological Congress, 1962-1976
Wilson Bulletin, 1902-2001

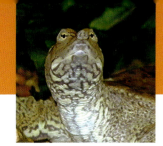

CHAPTER 3

JÖRG MAYER
TERESA BRADLEY BAYS

Reptile Behavior

Introduction

Reptiles are becoming more and more popular as pets and as research animals. With so many reptile species being presented to the practitioner, it is difficult to stay abreast of the knowledge necessary to provide appropriate care and to counsel and educate clients. Recognition of normal and abnormal behavior could alert the caretaker and the veterinary practitioner to a medical problem at an earlier stage, making treatment more likely successful.

Although more literature about the care and handling of reptiles in captivity is being published, the amount of literature available regarding behavioral studies and observations is overwhelming. This should not be surprising, considering that the green anole *(Anolis carolinensis)* lizard has been the subject of behavioral and ecologic study for more than 100 years.[83] Most of the existing literature in reptilian ethology, however, has been used to study reproductive behavior and the neural and muscular morphology that is involved. Also, direct comparison and conclusions drawn from behavioral observation in other species are of limited value because of the significant differences in the biology of reptiles versus other classes.[29] Conclusions about the uniformity of an observed behavior pattern between reptile species also have to be made with reservations. Despite the large amount of literature available on reptile behavior, little of this knowledge is adequately reflected in the resources primarily aimed at the veterinary market.

As with other species, close cooperation and exchange of information between the owner and the clinician must be part of the examination. Without this anamnesis an adequate evaluation of the behavioral issues is impossible. A significant percentage of health problems in reptiles is related to errors in management, especially environment and diet. Despite the best intentions, it appears that many reptiles in captivity do not reach adulthood, often dying of medical complications secondary to inadequate husbandry. For example, garter snakes, which are commonly used for scientific laboratory studies or kept as pets, often become ill and die young in captivity.[56] Fortunately, as our knowledge base increases and as reptile owners and clinicians become more educated, these statistics are improving.

This chapter was prepared to help to increase that knowledge base. The common postures and behaviors in reptiles, both in natural habitats and in captivity, and the clinical interpretation of these behaviors are described. It is an impossible task to include all of the behavioral aspects of all species of reptiles in this single chapter. We have attempted to focus on the relevant points of normal and abnormal behavior exhibited by popular reptiles in order to familiarize the clinician and other reptile caretakers with this complex topic.

Developmental Aspects of Behavior

To appreciate the complex discussion of behavior, we need to keep in mind the developmental nature of reptiles. The concept of ontogeny is relatively new to herpetologic research, and limited data on how behavior changes with the age of an individual reptile are available. One can roughly classify five stages of development in the life of a reptile[32]:

- Stage I is the prebirth or embryonic stage, with an emphasis on development and genetics.
- Stage II is the hatchling or juvenile stage, in which a high growth rate is characteristic and an increased level of fight-or-flight reactions can be observed, as well as intraspecific competition, mainly for food.
- Stage III is the stage of sexual maturity or young adulthood and involves a shift from growth to sexual maturity and associated behavior.
- Stage IV is adulthood, when continued growth is minimal or nonexistent and reproductive activity is increasing (e.g., large clutch size).
- Stage V is characterized by the older reptile, in which metabolic processes slow and the animal may need support for basic physiologic processes.

An excellent summary of the ontogeny of the green iguana *(Iguana iguana)* can be found in *Biology, Husbandry and Medicine of the Green Iguana*.[4] Without doubt, the behavioral patterns of individual reptiles undergo development during the different life stages, and some of the ontogenic stages are primarily based on changes in behavior. The knowledge of these different stages and their associated behavioral patterns is especially significant in managing a reproductive colony.

The ontogeny of antipredator responses in natricine snakes has been examined. Neonates were given a standardized defensive behavior test at

1 and/or 20 days of age. Another example of ontogenic shifts in antipredator responses has been seen in an Australian scincid lizard *(Eulamprus heatwolei)*. In this species it was noted that juveniles avoided predator odors, whereas adults showed no avoidance behaviors toward predator odors, suggesting an age-specific shift in predator avoidance behaviors. The likely cause is that the increased size serves as a deterrent to many predators.[62]

It has been noted in male green iguanas that femoral gland pore size and amount of secretions correlated with age and the maintenance of dominance relationships.[3] Pore size was positively correlated with the frequency of headbob displays and plasma levels of testosterone during the breeding season in individuals older than 12 months of age.

Food preferences change with age. Change in nutritional needs according to age is well established in the canine and feline dietary market, and new products are now available for the senior ferret. More research is needed regarding the dietary preferences and needs of reptiles with respect to age. The bearded dragon *(Pogona vitticeps)*, for instance, is known to be significantly more insectivorous during the juvenile stages of life and is more herbivorous during the advanced stages of life. Behavior as influenced by sexual hormones is another prime example of developmental changes and is discussed later in this chapter.

As with most behavioral patterns described for a certain species of reptile, however, conclusions about the uniformity of an observed pattern among different species have been made with reservations. Although the concept of ontogenicity is not a novel idea in other species, especially in human medicine (e.g., pediatric versus geriatric medicine), it appears to be a relatively new facet of reptilian medicine. Some of the published data regarding behavioral changes with age appear to be of academic value, but clinically significant changes in behavior exist and the clinician should be aware of these.

Environmental Aspects of Behavior

The environmental influences in the life of a poikilotherm also play a significant role in the development of behavioral manifestations. The association of gender determination in reptiles with incubation temperature is well documented but not well understood. For example, it has been reported that incubation temperature significantly affects the hormonal environment of the embryo of a snapping turtle *(Chelydra serpentina)* with temperature-dependent sex determination.[43] Environmental factors such as incubation humidity, oxygen, carbon dioxide concentration, and other microclimatic factors all influence the development of the young reptile.

Not only do environmental factors play a key role in the development of both embryonic and hatched reptiles, it appears that the development of basic behavioral patterns later in life is also significantly influenced by the development of the embryonic animal. For instance, during a study of antipredator behavior of hatchling snakes, results suggest that hatchlings incubated at medium temperatures are generally less vulnerable to predators than hatchlings incubated at higher or lower temperatures.[17] These data suggest that the development of behavior is strongly influenced by early morphologic developmental factors.

Incubation temperature during embryonic development has been found to significantly alter of adult aggressiveness and attractiveness in leopard geckos *(Eublepharis macularis)*; adult female geckos from a male-biased incubation temperature (32° C; 90° F) were more aggressive and the females less attractive than the geckos arising from female-biased incubation temperatures (26°, 30°, and 34° C; 79°, 86°, and 93° F).[49] In addition, the authors noted that postnatal hormones played a role in the sociosexual behaviors of adult geckos as well.

A later paper also suggests that male-typical behaviors in the adult leopard gecko are permanently affected by both embryonic temperature and gonadal sex during development,[30] and a still-later report suggests that developmental temperatures may primarily affect the level of circulating hormones in adulthood in geckos that are gonadally intact.[108] In the red-sided garter snake *(Thamnophis sirtalis parietalis)*, research data suggest that sex steroid hormones act to organize central nervous system mechanisms influencing courtship behavior such that temperature, and not hormonal fluctuations, activate sexual behavior in the adult.[28] The truth for most behavioral patterns might be somewhere in between; observation of certain species supports the impression that environmental and internal factors act together in the development of these complex behavioral patterns.

Without a doubt the environment is crucial in the morphologic development and the survival of reptile hatchlings. It is only reasonable that these factors will have a similar and significant influence on behavior. Although the environmental temperature strongly influences the developing animal, more and more data suggest that other influences such as humidity can have significant developmental impact. A good example of continued dependence on correct environmental factors is discussed in a recently published report regarding the influence of environmental humidity on pyramidal growth of carapaces in the African spurred tortoise *(Geochelone sulcata)*.[131] The authors concluded that the major contributing factor of this abnormality is inadequate humidity.

The influence and importance of the ultraviolet (UV) spectrum on behavior has long been established. Research is being done on the UV spectrum in reptiles and how it affects behavior. The two most important fractions of the UV spectrum are the long wave (UV-A) and the midwave (UV-B) fractions. The UV-A spectrum has been suggested to influence agonistic, reproductive, and signaling behaviors in some species of lizards.[55] In a study of courtship behavior in the agamid lizard *(Ctenophorus ornatus)* with reflectance spectrometry, which extends into the UV spectrum, it was suggested that the function of visual display in this species of lizard appears to be intersexual signaling, possibly resulting in the males' choice of females.[76]

The role of the midwave fraction (UV-B) of the UV spectrum in the synthesis of active vitamin D_3 will not be discussed here. However, it has been shown that panther chameleons *(Chamaeleo [Furcifer] pardalis)* will actively change their exposure to UV light depending on the dietary intake of vitamin D_3.[44] If the dietary levels of the vitamin are high, the animals limit their exposure to the UV light source, and alternately they increase the exposure if dietary levels are low (see Eating Behaviors). It has also been documented that some reptiles become more aggressive when exposed to unfiltered natural sunlight,[51,91] although normal behavior is usually resumed when the reptile is returned to its enclosure.

Without the proper environment, many reptiles cannot successfully reproduce, and pathologic conditions such as egg binding or preovulatory follicular stasis may result. In addition to climatic conditions, other environmental clues are sometimes needed by the reptile in order to display certain behaviors. A prime example of this is the need for a proper moist or sandy substrate for some females in order to induce egg-laying behavior.

In addition to general environmental factors influencing reptiles, data also exist that outline the impact of geographic location on morphologic and behavioral development. One of the most obvious connections between behavior and local microhabitat was documented in populations of Japanese natricine snakes *(Rhabdophis tigrinus)* deprived of their natural diet, which consists mainly of toads. With an artificial diet, these snakes lacked secretions of the nuchal gland that are used to deter predators. Without the secretory defense, these snakes more frequently exhibited a flight response when threatened.[95]

Environmental pollution has also been documented to have a profound impact on the developing reptile, and detrimental changes in behavioral patterns have been noted. High environmental concentrations of lead have been shown to affect the righting reflex of reptiles as well as having other detrimental effects.[18] Aside from environmental pollution, which can be measured and assessed fairly easily, other factors of human impact on nature and consequently on reptilian behavior are more difficult to measure. However, some of these behavioral consequences have been documented. For example, the effect of artificial light sources, referred to as *photo-pollution*, near beaches used by sea turtles has a detrimental effect on the nest site selection and interferes with the water location capability of the hatchlings.[124]

Social and Antisocial Behaviors

For proper management of reptiles in captivity it is of absolute importance to know the social structure of the reptile species, because an inadequate setup will trigger stress responses in the animals and immunosuppression can follow (Box 3-1). Additional evidence that an elevated social status may provide advantages was noted in a study of response to stress in the

---

BOX 3-1 — **How Behavior Relates to Captivity**

The following examples of how behavior relates to captivity may seem rudimentary to the practitioner, but many clients need to be educated and counseled in order to avoid harmful practices.
- Regardless of species, it is inappropriate to provide excessive numbers of prey items or to leave them in the enclosure with an uninterested reptile for lengthy periods of time. This allows the prey species (be they mice, rats, or crickets) to potentially cause damage to the reptile.
- Social or antisocial behavior of a given species must be taken into consideration when deciding whether to cage conspecifics or members of different species together (Figure 3-1).
- Reptile species that are naturally gregarious such as leopard geckos *(Eublepharus macularis)* and bearded dragons *(Pogona vitticeps)* thrive better when kept in groups, especially when a single male is kept with multiple females.
- Mirrors and other reflective surfaces should be avoided in enclosures, as a reptile's reflection may be perceived as a dominant conspecific and create undue stress or may be perceived as competition and therefore may be attacked, causing injury as the reptile strikes the surface.
- Keeping male reptiles in cages that allow for visualization of other males may prove to be socially stressful to them. Therefore it is best to avoid a setup in which direct visual contact can be established.
- The presence of other domestic pets can be perceived as threatening to captive reptiles, and attempts to minimize or eliminate visual contact are recommended.
- Providing a temperature gradient (horizontally as well as vertically) in an appropriately sized enclosure allows reptiles to thermoregulate as they move around the enclosure.

Reptile Behavior

BOX 3-1   How Behavior Relates to Captivity–cont'd

- Providing appropriate space and hiding places for reptiles may alleviate some of the stress associated with captivity.
- Feeding tendencies must be considered when placing reptiles together. For instance, it would not be appropriate to put a carnivorous species in with an herbivorous species and create a predator-prey situation.
- Obesity is a common consequence of captivity for several reasons, including lack of exercise and inappropriate or high-calorie food. Often the owner's fascination for seeing prey consumed leads to overfeeding.

(Continued)

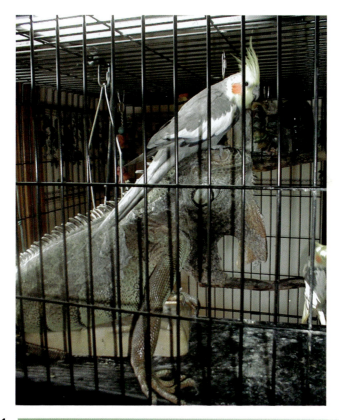

Figure 3-1

Housing multiple species is not recommended unless enough room is provided so that each has its own microenvironment. One has to wonder how stressful this is to the iguana, although the owner perceived that this iguana was content. (Courtesy Teresa Bradley Bays.)

BOX 3-1   How Behavior Relates to Captivity—cont'd

- We strongly discourage the feeding of live prey vertebrates to reptiles for both medical and ethical reasons.
- Providing a substrate that is not easily ingested (or is safe if ingested) is important in species that often flick their tongues in order to investigate their environment or those that get substrate mixed in with food items. When in doubt, newspaper is a safe substrate to recommend, with the additional benefit of allowing observation of urine and feces.
- Attempts to escape may be made and actually cause self-trauma in species maintained under certain conditions. These conditions include housing in improper environments (e.g., sharp wire edges), enclosure walls that are transparent or provide a reflection of the reptile, or situations in which interspecies or intraspecies aggression, overcrowding, or other social stressor is present.
- Under-tank heaters may be inappropriate for burrowing reptile species that may expose themselves directly to the heat and be more likely to develop thermal burns.
- Overhandling of shy species can lead to stress, anorexia, and ill health. Species such as chameleons and ball pythons may not be the best pet choice for owners who wish to handle their pets frequently.
- All reptiles will struggle if not well supported during handling and may cause injury to themselves (e.g., loss of tail or damage to vertebrae) or to the handler. Most lizards, will exhibit a serpentine motion when struggling that can be minimized if both the thoracic and pelvic girdles are well supported and firmly but gently restrained.
- Other companion pets, such as cats, dogs, and birds that roam free in the house in which reptiles are kept, may be perceived as predators and create psychologic stress leading to immune suppression and failure to thrive if not addressed.
- Diurnal species fare best if given radiant heat sources from above with an appropriate day-night cycle. Nocturnal species thrive best when under-tank heaters are provided.
- Knowledge of whether a species is arboreal, terrestrial, or aquatic is necessary in order to provide the best environment. For example, many owners and practitioners do not know that green iguanas are arboreal in nature and should be provided with limbs on which to climb. Iguana cages should be elevated to resemble height. Rock iguanas (*Cyclura* species), on the other hand, are ground dwellers and look for places to dig and burrow. These behaviors should be taken into consideration when creating and furnishing enclosures appropriate for reptiles.

BOX 3-1 How Behavior Relates to Captivity—cont'd

- Many lizards will become more active and even aggressive when exposed to natural sunlight, and owners must be warned that they may become dangerously aggressive. It has been the experience of many that once the lizard is back inside out of the sunlight, the aggression is diminished.

Adapted from Bradley TA: Reptile behavior basics for the veterinary clinician. In Proceedings of the ARAV Annual Conference, Reno, Nev., 2002.

green anole lizard *(A. carolinensis)*. The dominant male anoles showed reduced somatic indicators of stress, including a progressive darkening from green to brown coloring and expression of a black postorbital eyespot, than subordinate males. They also recovered more quickly from the stress.[102]

It is important to know which lizard species are naturally social or gregarious and which prefer to be solitary. It is very stressful and often dangerous to intermix species or to house conspecifics together if they are solitary in nature such as the adult green iguana *(I. iguana)*. However, several species can be housed in groups with a single male with multiple females including bearded dragons *(P. vitticeps)* and leopard geckos *(E. macularis)*. Occasionally, lizards that have been housed together for months to years may become aggressive toward one another and should be separated if such behavior is noted. Chameleons should be housed such that males do not have visual contact with each other.

The signs of social stress can be very subtle and may not be clinically evident to an owner or clinician. Often an owner must be convinced that such stress exists and must be eliminated in order to keep the reptiles healthier. Social stress can be minimized when housing nongregarious reptile species together in environments by providing sufficient space and appropriate hiding spaces. It has been theorized that basking placement in reptiles in the wild can indicate hierarchic position in a group, whereby the most dominant is at the highest basking position. For example, in a study of captive juvenile male green iguanas *(I. iguana)*, housed where supplemental heat and perch sites were limited, a divergence in growth and behavior was noted within 1 to 2 months.[101] It was shown that dominant males grew more rapidly and used the supplemental heat sources twice as often as the subordinate males. Because onset of adult behavioral patterns is related to body size, the dominant males also displayed adult behaviors much sooner. Providing multiple basking areas for groups of reptiles may minimize some of this social stress.

Most reptiles are not considered to be social animals, and relatively few reptiles live constantly in social groups and establish a social hierarchy. The social tendencies of reptilian behavior vary with species and age. Although many reptiles show a significant increase in social behavior at breeding time, for the majority of the year even these species prefer a solitary lifestyle. For instance, large social aggregations of garter snakes and other snake species have been documented in preparation for the breeding season, whereas for the rest of the year they prefer a more solitary existence.

Juvenile reptiles, however, often exhibit a more social lifestyle with conspecifics than do adults. As long as the animals are not yet sexually active and sufficient food is available, juveniles will aggregate without agonistic behaviors. This is evident in juvenile green iguanas, which tend to stay on the ground and live under thick shrubbery in groups (exhibiting the safety-in-numbers theory). They often sleep with their heads pointed toward the outside of the brush to allow early detection of predators. It has been documented in different reptile species that food consumption is significantly increased when young animals are housed in groups versus individual enclosures.[127]

Although snakes are commonly considered to be the least social reptiles, recent data suggest that this might not be accurate. Rattlesnakes, for instance, exhibit characteristics consistent with advanced sociality, including group defense, conspecific alarm signals, and maternal defense of young. These findings reinforce the notion that rather than being solitary and asocial, some snake species may form family groups.[21] Another research study revealed that Australian black rock skinks (*Egernia saxatilis*) exhibited long-term monogamy, stable social grouping, and evidence of "nuclear family" systems, attesting to the fact that the social organization of some reptiles may be more complex than previously suspected.[97]

Agonistic Behaviors

Recognition of defensive and aggressive behaviors is probably one of the most important observations in the veterinary clinic. Defensive aggression in reptiles can represent a safety hazard for the staff if employees are not instructed in proper restraint and handling. The ability of reptiles to inflict injury must be emphasized and reinforced. Early recognition of a stressed individual can help to deescalate the situation or to anticipate the next step and to avoid injury to the animal, the handler, and the examiner.

When appropriate, and with the permission of the owner, the reptile patients nails should be trimmed before examination and handling to minimize trauma to staff and the clinician. Also, many lizard species will not let go when they bite and may actually bite more assertively as the "victim" struggles. The different reptile species demonstrate a wide variety of defensive behavioral patterns, and extensive handling experience is needed in order to read the behaviors accurately.

Because of the prevalence of iguanas as pets and their ability to inflict injury to the handler, a more detailed discussion of this species' defensive aggressive behaviors in the animal hospital is included. Unlike parrots, which become more subdued when in a strange territory, normally docile iguanas may become fearful and therefore aggressive. Also, owners are prone to kiss their iguanas on the lips and pet them on the head in an attempt to soothe them. The veterinarian or staff members must forewarn the owners that the iguana, when agitated, may bite them and that the owners must refrain from these dangerous activities.

Despite precautions, it is likely that at some point an iguana bite will occur in the hospital. Attempts to pry the mouth open only increase an iguana's bite force. If after several seconds to minutes (depending on the severity of the bite and the pain tolerance of the victim) the iguana does not release its grip, then the iguana and the attached person should be lowered to the floor. Most iguanas will immediately release whatever they are biting and either assume a defensive posture (as described below) or flee. Applying alcohol to the nose has been reported by some to cause iguanas to release their grip, but in some practitioners' experience, it increases the iguana's fear and therefore its bite force.

Tame, visibly calm iguanas may be handled as described later in this chapter. Many pet iguanas are comfortable resting with their heads over the handler's shoulder and their body supported against the handler's body, while being transported in the hospital. Less-tame iguanas should be held by grasping the shoulder and pelvic girdles and holding the tail close to the handler's body. This helps to decrease the serpentine motion they exhibit when trying to escape. However, the potential for biting, the production of severe lacerations from extremely sharp nails, and tail whipping still exists if the iguana becomes fearful or agitated.

Provoked defensive aggressive behaviors in reptiles include posturing that makes the aggressor appear to be more threatening, such as inflation of the body, standing more erect on all four legs, broadside posturing, dewlap extension, open-mouthed threat, and head bobbing (Figure 3-2). Biting, striking, and tail whipping may also be seen. Male frill-necked lizards *(Chlamydosaurus kingii)* will also kick and bite at one another while displaying extension of the frill around their necks. Some species of reptiles are able to produce a noxious substance to deter aggressors or predators, including the spraying of urine, feces or musk.

Other unusual behaviors reported in reptiles include a reaction that could be mistaken for pathologic central nervous system signs. When

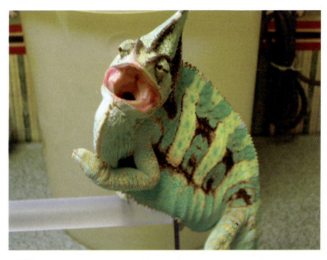

Figure 3-2
A chameleon exhibiting an open-mouth threat display in response to being handled. (Courtesy Teresa Bradley Bays.)

confronted by an ophiophagous (snake-eating) kingsnake, venomous snakes of the subfamily Crotalinae exhibit a suite of defensive responses including head hiding, thrashing, and other unusual responses.[59] Many of these behaviors are discussed in further detail in the sections that follow.

Territorial Defense

Territorial defense is usually an intraspecies behavior, as an individual will only defend its territory from a conspecific. This behavior has not been recorded in the snake but has been observed in certain turtle and lizard species. Turtles appear to be solitary for most of the year and live socially only during the breeding season. Therefore it might be advisable to house sick or injured chelonians individually, as the presence of another animal might be a stressor to these animals.

The strongest territorial defense reaction can be seen in the more social reptile species. Aggressive behaviors in the wild are stimulated in response to predators and to establish territories. Male leopard geckos, although easy to handle as pets, can be quite aggressive to male conspecifics and have been known to kill one another. The same is true of mature male iguanas. Unless an appropriate amount of space is provided in enclosures with multiple lizards in which more than one male is kept, the subordinate male will often grow at a much slower pace and may not thrive.

Defending a territory comes at a price, and the benefits must outweigh the cost. Food abundance appears to be one of the key factors in territorial defense. It has been hypothesized that the lack of home range defense in certain herbivorous and omnivorous lizards and turtles is directly related to the concentration of resources available to these species in their environment.[103] Defending these resources does not outweigh the potential dangers associated with aggression. During a sudden abundance of food, defending a home range appears less important, and individuals that would defend their food source will readily share the food. For example, when feasting on a large carcass, Komodo dragons will readily share the resource peacefully,[103] although they are usually considered solitary animals. Of all the reptile species studied to date, home range defensive behavior appears to be most prevalent in the iguanian and gekkotan lizards.[103]

Reptiles that feed on resources that are distributed in a sparse pattern and therefore have to cover a large territory will not readily claim and defend a home range or territory. The snake, feasting usually on small vertebrates, is a prime example, and, as mentioned previously, defensive territorial behavior has not been documented in snakes.

However, snakes in captivity do quickly establish territorial markers in the cage, and constant rearrangement of cage furniture or cleaning the cage might add additional stress. It has also been shown that snakes use pheromones on the newspaper bedding in order to mark their territory.[63] This finding might suggest that it is best to change the substrate in a serpent tank only on an as-needed basis rather than on a daily basis in order to decrease stress.

Combat for Mating

Sexually motivated behavior is one of the most commonly observed and described behaviors in reptiles. Few species of reptiles have been shown to be monogamous. Combat for mating occurs between two males of the same species (intrasexual combat) and has been reported in snakes, turtles, and lizards. In contrast to popular belief the fighting usually does not lead to fatalities. The winner will earn the right to mate, and the subordinate animal will have to either leave the group or retreat temporarily. Unfortunately, severe injuries and fatalities are much more common in captivity, because the subordinate male does not have an opportunity to flee.

A snake will use its whole body during combat, intertwining itself with its opponent and trying to keep its head in a superior position in order to press the head of the other combatant down. Combat for mating in lizards has also been well documented and is not surprising considering the social structure of most lizard species. The threat displays of the iguana have been described and are easily recognizable.

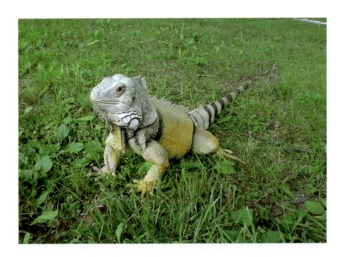

Figure 3-3
Iguanas exposed to natural sunlight can become exceedingly aggressive. Iguanas left outside can escape and may become preyed on by wild or domestic animals. (Courtesy Jörg Mayer.)

Problems with sexual aggression toward humans by reptiles have been reported most commonly with the green iguana *(I. iguana)*[72,88] during the breeding season when hormone levels are fluctuating; such problems are often initiated by the presence of a menstruating human female. Some iguanas will revert back to their normal docile behavior after the breeding season is complete, but others remain aggressive. Certain lizard species may also become more aggressive when exposed to natural unfiltered sunlight, although normal behavior is usually resumed when the reptile is placed back in its enclosure (Figure 3-3). Any reptile that is approached too quickly or handled inappropriately may also show signs of aggression.

It has been suggested that sexually mature male iguanas that are showing signs of aggression may have some of the behaviors curtailed by decreasing daylight hours, eliminating exposure to other male animals in the house as well as to female conspecifics, and decreasing environmental temperatures slightly. The practitioner should stress to the client, however, that aggression is a normal expected behavior for iguanas, and that efforts to control behavior should not be extreme enough to cause harm to the iguana. Depo-Lupron and Depo-Provera have both been used with mixed results in an attempt to decrease human-directed aggression in male iguanas. Castration of male iguanas before sexual maturity may help to decrease the chance of reproductive-related aggression toward people and other pets.[52] Clients should be counseled that castration before puberty would also decrease the development of secondary sexual characteristics including large jowls and crests.

Defensive Antipredator Behaviors

Different reptile species have developed various behaviors in order to avoid or thwart predators. Defensive behaviors can be separated into passive and active categories. Although most prey species will attempt to avoid detection or flee from the immediate danger zone (passive behavior), sometimes direct interaction and confrontation with the predator is necessary (active behavior). Captive reptiles will usually not encounter any natural predators, but some of the discussed behaviors can be triggered by caretakers, especially if the human-reptile bond is not well established. This is why knowledge of these behavioral patterns is extremely significant in the clinical setting, as the misinterpretation of these behaviors has the potential to result in harm to the reptile as well as the handler.

Passive Defensive Behaviors (Avoidance)
Avoiding Detection (Crypsis). Because reptiles have generally low oxidative metabolic capacities and are incapable of outrunning most predators, they rely heavily on hiding as a form of defense.[103] If the reptile senses a threat or danger and is a considerable distance away, it will try to move out of the area unnoticed in order to avoid detection and fighting. A reptile will always try to avoid detection, as this is the least energy-consuming variation of predator avoidance and allows the animal to remain in the same locale. The animal will usually try to physically hide its body in a crevice or a burrow.

However, mimicry or blending in with the environment is also a strategy used by reptiles, and the chameleon is one of the more popular species using this method of crypsis. When housing a species that relies on visual mimicry, it might be best to use cage furniture that has natural colors in order to afford the animal the opportunity to blend in with its environment.

The physical form of crypsis is easily recognizable and commonly seen in the hospital situation. It is very important that the reptile be given a microhabitat in which it feels secure and can retreat. Hide boxes can be made out of disposable materials such as cardboard tubes or boxes purchased commercially (e.g., Exo-Terra Reptile Den).

Escape Behavior (Direct Evasion). If the reptile does not sense impending danger and is surprised by the sudden appearance of a stimulus, it will try to rapidly move away from the source of potential danger. This can involve leaping out of a tree and diving into water or into rock crevices.

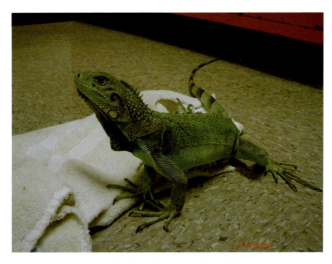

Figure 3-4
This iguana is alert and ready for the fight or flight reaction. Note the elevated stance and the eyes turned toward the object of interest. (Courtesy Jörg Mayer.)

The predator will usually notice the commotion caused by the sudden movement. This sudden and sometimes clumsy flight reaction can be observed in captivity if a lizard is asleep and is startled. This may cause the lizard to fall from a perch or basking area.

The lack of closing eyelids makes the assessment of whether or not a snake is resting more difficult than in other reptiles. However, if the pupils appear to be fixed and do not respond to mild visual clues (e.g., hand movement by the glass), a sudden stimulus can cause a flight reaction in the snake (Figure 3-4).

Lizards that become frightened may roll like a crocodile in attempts to escape restraint or predators. Chuckwallas *(Sauromalus obesus)* will crawl into crevices in rocks to escape predators and then inflate their bodies so that they cannot be pulled out from their hiding place by the predator. Some lizards like the basilisk lizard *(Basiliscus vittatus)* that normally ambulate with all four legs are able to run bipedally on their rear legs to escape predators, even across water. During manual restraint of the snake, the animal will usually exhibit negative taxis to the restrainer and try to work the body out of the grasping hold. The snake achieves this by constant forward movements and/or rotation on its own axis.

Caudal Autotomy (Tail Shed). One of the more commonly known defensive strategies is the partial loss of the tail, known as caudal autotomy.

Many lizards and a very few snakes are able to lose the distal aspect of the tail when grabbed by a chasing predator or by an unsuspecting owner or practitioner. Frequently the piece of tail that falls off will continue to wriggle in order to distract the predator while the reptile is escaping. The tail should therefore never be used to restrain a lizard. Typically little blood loss results from autotomy. The tail breaks at a fracture plane in the center of a vertebra. After several months a shorter cartilaginous rod will replace the bone, and the scales covering it will be irregular and discolored.

Death Display. Another predator defense is to mimic death. One of the best known species to show this behavior is the eastern hog-nosed snake (*Heterodon platirhinos*). The animal turns upside down, opens its mouth, and releases a foul-smelling odor. Other species of snakes also display this behavior, and Eckstein[42] reports that during handling of grass snakes (*Natrix natrix*) approximately one quarter of them pretended to be dead, with this behavior triggered only by touching them. This behavior was not exhibited to the same degree by all snakes. Some of them coiled up with the mouth held slightly open, often with the tongue lolling out of the side of the mouth. Other snakes turned their heads to the side with fixed pupils and mouths opened, sometimes with completely relaxed body muscles. In a more intense reaction the black and creamy colored underside would be presented, showing either the throat area or the entire ventrum. The snakes would pretend to be dead for 2 minutes to half an hour. When the grass snakes did not feel threatened any more, they darted their tongues several times and then they went to a hiding spot (Eckstein, at www.ringelnatter.net).[42] This defense, however, is useful only against predators that are attracted by motion.

Active Defensive Behaviors
Self-Inflation and Vocalization. Several lizard species are able to inhale large volumes of air to expand their circumference, often with the addition of a "hissing" sound and an open-mouth display. It appears that older animals use this display more often than younger (smaller) ones.

A bioacoustic analysis was conducted on the defensive sounds produced by 21 species of snakes. The "typical" snake hiss is described as having a broad-frequency span (from roughly 3000 to 13,000 Hz) with a dominant frequency near 7500 Hz.[132] Whether or not this hissing is also part of a true communication process is still not known.

Symbolic Bite and Biting. If the source of danger is close and a snake is unable to evade using other behaviors, a "fake" strike can sometimes be observed. This symbolic bite usually happens with a closed mouth and is directed in the general direction of the aggressor and often repeated very quickly. This defense is used against larger predators and has significant intimidation potential. It will usually persist until the predator gives up or is confused, and the snake uses this moment to evade the situation by using a flight response. A variation of this defense is the typical "cobralike position." The snake will hold up the cranial third of the body and strike in a forward and downward motion. The snake is able to move while striking and can cover significant distance during this display. Lizards and chelonians will also demonstrate their readiness to bite with an open-mouth display.

Biting is usually the final step in an escalation of behaviors, but it can also happen without warning. Usually snakes will avoid biting for defensive reasons. It has been shown that most of the injuries resulting from snake-human interaction would be avoidable if common sense were used. A study examining snake bites concluded that the majority of snakebite injuries resulted from intentional exposure to snakes in which a variety of factors such as the use of alcohol and lack of protective equipment likely played a role.[94]

Regurgitation. A common observation during inappropriate handling of snakes is regurgitation of food. The frequency of this behavior differs significantly among species. It can be interpreted as a stress response and preparation for flight or as a true defensive behavior to distract the predator. It is extremely important to be able to differentiate this physiologic regurgitation from a pathological presentation. The action of regurgitation in a physiologic situation should always be associated with a direct interaction of the handler and the animal. In captivity, snakes that are overhandled soon after feeding may regurgitate the recent meal. Although regurgitation in snakes as a response to stress is fairly common in certain species (e.g., ball python), it may also indicate diseases that cause mechanical regurgitation such as cryptosporidia, cardiomyopathy, or various metabolic diseases. It is never a normal behavior for chelonians or lizards to regurgitate in response to handling. Occasionally, an owner will report regurgitation in a lizard or chelonian in response to car travel; this is assumed to be the equivalent of motion sickness.

Tail Flicking and Tail Whipping. The rattlesnake is the best known snake that exhibits tail flicking behavior whereby a vibration of the tail of the snake creates sound. Eckstein[42] reported the observation of this tail vibration in the grass snake, *N. natrix*, as well. In the case of the grass snake the end of the tail is hit against grass or other surfaces in order to create sound. Other reptiles, such as the green iguana *(I. iguana)*, show a similar behavior when agitated.

Reptile Behavior 121

Lizards often use the tail to strike out at predators, or if provoked in the examination room. A large green iguana *(I. iguana)* may assume a U-shaped posture with the head and tail presented when defending itself from the suspected predation of the clinician and staff. In this posture the body is protected, the tail can be used as a weapon or sacrificed (see Caudal Autotomy), and the mouth is ready to inflict injury if necessary. Practitioner and staff should be aware of this defensive behavior and be careful in handling such an animal.

Musk Gland Secretion and Elimination. Snakes can empty their musk glands, located in the cloacal area, when angry or frightened. The foul-smelling odor and taste may deter predators. In captivity, the most common species to practice musk defensive behavior is the milk snake. Because of the close proximity of the gland near the hemipenis the structure is often larger in female snakes than in males. Turtles often urinate during handling. This behavior is assumed to be associated with fright, anger, or pain (see Elimination Behaviors).

Miscellaneous Defenses

Reptiles have developed many different defense strategies that are fairly unique to certain species and are too numerous to be discussed adequately. From a veterinary point of view, three additional forms of defense should be mentioned here.

Blood Spurting. The horned lizards, *Phyrnosoma* species, belong to one of several species that are able to restrict blood flow from the head until the blood pressure mounts enough to create rupture of the small blood vessels in and around the eyes. This defense against certain predators results in blood spurting up to 1 meter away.[103]

Coiling Up. The best-known species to use coiling as a defensive behavior is the ball python, but other snakes have also been observed to exhibit this behavior. The snake curls up and may move rapidly in this position or may remain absolutely still (Figure 3-5).

Retraction into Shell. Tortoises and some turtles are able to retract head and legs into their shells to protect themselves from potential predators. This can make administration of medicine and food difficult and may cause harm to the handler if fingers are pinched between plastron and carapace or pulled in up against the projections on the shell, especially in species such as the African spur-thighed tortoise *(G. sulcata)*. Anesthesia is often needed in order to examine and treat these patients.

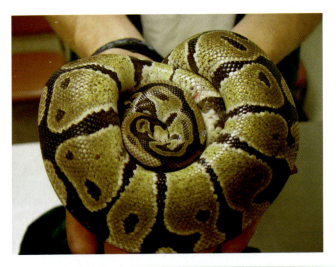

Figure 3-5
The typical defense of the ball python, in which the animal will curl up in a ball, protecting its head. This reaction can be used during the physical examination to assess the mental status and the strength of the animal. (Courtesy Jörg Mayer.)

Taming and Training

Training of reptiles has been successfully done in order to facilitate clinical procedures. The advantages of such training are obvious, as the trainer can condition the animal such that clinical data can be obtained without having to physically interact with the animal. The use of classical and operant conditioning in training for venipuncture and other husbandry issues in Aldabra tortoises *(Geochelone gigantea)* has been described.[129] Similar positive results have been reported in the training of the Nile crocodile[81] and the Komodo dragon.[48] The application of operant conditioning can have significant positive influence on managing a reptile collection and should be considered in species that are dangerous to handle and need to be handled on a regular basis.

As with any species, personality differences can be found among individual reptiles. Some are more easily handled and hand-tamed, whereas others are more nervous and flighty. It has been our experience that some lizards, snakes, and even "pet" crocodilians are able to recognize their owners and act differently around them than they do around other people.

Even a relatively "tame" pet reptile may become fractious when stressed. A nervous lizard tends to flatten itself laterally, widen its eyes, and in some cases extend the dewlap. Lizards may also hold their mouths agape in a threatening gesture if frightened (see Figure 3-2). As described previously, iguanas and other lizards that are placed on an examination table may assume a U-shaped position with the tail pointed toward the practitioner, ready to defend themselves if needed.

For pet reptiles, regular, gentle handling for increasing periods of time may help acclimate them to handling. It is important to realize, however, that some species are more sensitive to handling and may become stressed and immunosuppressed when handled. Chameleons and ball pythons *(Python regius)* are examples of pet reptiles that should not be overhandled, although captive-bred ball pythons seem to be less readily stressed than their wild-caught counterparts when they are routinely and gently handled. It is equally important to remember that as wild creatures reptiles are never domesticated and will act and react instinctively; therefore they cannot be completely tamed.

Sensory Modalities and Behavior

Despite the significant amount of literature available regarding the sensory modalities in reptiles, the application of these findings and how they affect behavior in reptiles is still largely unknown. Some conclusions can be drawn about the relative importance of the various senses from their anatomic descriptions, but much more research on this subject is needed. Many behaviors are dictated by sensory perception, which, depending on the species, can include visual reception using the eyes, chemosensory reception using the tongue, nose, and vomeronasal organ (VO), and infrared detection using the sensory pits.

In order to understand behavioral responses triggered by sensory perception, a minimal understanding of the physiology of the sensory system is needed. It is beyond the scope of this chapter to address the physiologic aspects appropriately, and we recommend *Biology, Husbandry, and Health Care of Reptiles*, edited by Ackerman,[1] for a better overview. As an extremely broad summary, it could be stated that for snakes the chemical pathway is the most important sense for communication with the environment, as snakes make very limited use of the visual system. However, the visual system appears to be the primary sense for communication with the environment for lizards and turtles.

Vomeronasal Organ, Olfaction, and Behavior

It is difficult to separate the VO from the rest of the sensory organs, as it appears to be intricately affiliated with the rest of the olfactory system. We believe that the organ deserves mention since the VO has historically been considered the most important chemosensory organ of reptiles. Research has focused extensively on this organ.[133] Recent scientific evidence indicates that it can act independently and does not depend on the rest of the olfactory system. For example, it has been found that the use of chemical signals by garter snakes in shelter selection and aggregation is mediated by the VO and that neither the olfactory nor the visual system is critical for these behaviors.[63] In a publication investigating the specific stimulation of the VO and the olfactory tract of garter snakes, a significant preference of the VO for nonairborne stimulants like liquids was noted, whereas the olfactory organ was triggered by all volatile test substances.[68]

As previously mentioned, to what degree the different sensory organs influence behavior in different reptiles is still under investigation, but it appears that olfaction plays an extremely important role in reptile biology. Many published reports concerning the importance of olfaction during courtship behaviors and feeding responses are available, and most of these studies investigated the importance of olfaction in snakes and lizards.

Data regarding olfaction and reproductive behavior are available for the garter snake *(T. sirtalis)* indicating that pheromones play a major role in reproductive behavior. Male snakes have been reported to court random objects, if they were laced with female pheromone scents.[85] Also, male turtles of certain species show a variety of courtship behaviors, which are thought to be triggered by pheromone-producing glands of the female turtles.

Squamate reptiles locate conspecifics by scent trailing, and prey is identified and located by tongue flicking; they can apparently locate food using only airborne cues.[24] Chemosensory reception is also important for predator detection and allows the nocturnal, rock-dwelling velvet gecko *(Oedura lesueurii)* to detect the scent of the broad-headed snake *(Hoplocephalus bungaroides)*. As an ambush predator the broad-headed snake benefits by remaining sedentary in rock crevices awaiting the foraging geckos, thereby minimizing the extent of scent distribution on the surrounding rocks.[40]

Another major aspect of how smell affects behavior is related to feeding habits. Predatory reptiles have been shown to use olfaction as a means to find their prey. This was demonstrated in a Y-maze apparatus in which garter snakes were trained to follow an earthworm-extract trail. Correct trailing improved significantly as training progressed using the extract of the prey animal.[75] Foraging behavior of turtles has also been linked to the olfactory system, as a disruption of the olfactory organ impaired the foraging ability in affected turtles.[133]

Odor presentation studies concluded that hatchling iguanas may recognize one another by differences in body odor produced from the femoral glands.[2] Through use of nasal chemosensory systems, lizards have been found to be able to make sophisticated pheromonal discriminations about the reproductive condition of potential mates and sexual rivals as well as the presence of other species.[25]

Vision and Behavior

Most reptilian species do not use vision alone, but rather combine sight with other senses in order to process information. Because so many different reptile species exist, it is not surprising that the structure of the eye differs among them.

For instance, the anatomy of the snake's eye varies significantly from that of other reptiles, and much information has been collected concerning vision in snakes. Grace and Woodward[57] described the cooperation between the visual and heat sensory organs in boid and crotaline snakes. The eye responds to visible light, and the pit organ responds to infrared radiation. Extensive trials in which the animals underwent modification of the different sensory organs showed a cooperation of the two systems in order to improve accuracy. The authors concluded that infrared imaging may allow accurate predatory targeting in the complete absence of visual information; however, both infrared information and visual information are probably normally involved in prey targeting.[57]

Chelonians appear to be very visual and have been shown to react strongly to visual clues during courtship behaviors (e.g., head swaying and coloration displays). Both snakes and turtles have been shown to react with fear responses when the only stimulus was a visual clue.[127] Green iguanas *(I. iguana)* have been shown to have good visual acuity[61] and can distinguish colors.[107] Social status in male anoles *(A. carolinensis)* is influenced by a visual cue whereby dominant males exhibit a darkening of the postorbital skin from green to black. When viewed by other males, this visual cue causes them to be more subordinate.[73]

One of the most diverse and best-developed vision systems can be found in the chameleon. It has been shown that chameleons are able to use their eyes independently from each other, but when the animal tracks prey the eye movements are synchronized.[100] The range of motion in the chameleon eye is 180 degrees horizontally and 90 degrees vertically. In comparison, a rhesus monkey has an ocular range of motion of 60 degrees horizontally and 45 degrees vertically. Given such a high degree of flexibility it is hardly surprising that the chameleon relies extensively on vision, and chameleons appear to have developed a visual communication system.[96]

Hearing, Vocalization, and Behavior

Vibration detection may also play an important role in sensory perception for reptiles. Sleeping iguanas appear to be sensitive to vibration and illumination[109] and will often sleep on the ends of branches over the water so that they can drop into the water if they are disturbed by the vibrations of predators.

For a long time, snakes were considered to be deaf, but scientists have been able to determine that snakes are able to pick up airborne and groundborne vibrations with the whole body and with parts of the inner ear. This specialized form of hearing is referred to as *somatic hearing*. Snakes appear to be most sensitive to airborne vibrations.[134] However, it has also been shown that snakes listen to the ground vibrations created by a prey animal in order to target the prey. For example, studies performed on the Saharan sand vipers, of the genus *Cerastes*, indicated that if vision and olfaction are obstructed, these ambush predators are still able to capture rodents and lizards by using ground-borne vibrations to localize prey.[136] Further evidence suggests that snakes will react strongly to airborne sounds alone in the range of 150 to 450 Hz. Visible reactions to the different frequencies included cessation of body movements, reduction or cessation of tongue flicking, rapid jerks of the head, and rattling.[135]

Research has indicated that lizards respond to lower frequency and stronger stimuli than mammals and will react to audible clues in the 500- to 5000-Hz range.[127] Chelonians appear to be the most sensitive reptiles to frequencies of approximately 50 to 1500 Hz. It has also been documented that aquatic turtles show avoidance responses to low-frequency sound.[127] Geckos have been shown to have a high sensitivity to audible stimuli and respond even to frequencies as high as 10,000 Hz.[133] Experimentally deafened geckos show a decrease in prey capturing, indicating that acoustic location plays an important role in prey location for this species.[133]

Considering the wide range of frequencies detectable by reptiles as well as the capability to "listen" to ground vibrations, it is most likely that the acoustic system is not restricted to the ear alone and receptors are located in other parts of the body. It has been demonstrated that ground squirrels are able to assess the dangerousness (e.g., assess the size) of rattlesnakes solely by the acoustic clues of the rattle.[120] It might therefore be reasonable to conclude that the acoustics of the rattle can also serve a function for interspecies communication and for sizing up conspecific animals during combat or mating. However, few scientific studies exist that examine the communication aspects of acoustic interaction among reptiles.

Communication in reptiles is accomplished mostly using visual cues such as dewlap extension, head bobbing, and open-mouth threat (see Figure 3-2). Audible sighs, however, can be heard from female green iguanas *(I. iguana)* fighting over nesting sites.[109] True vocalization in reptiles includes the barking and growling sounds alligators are able to produce. Young alligator hatchlings also communicate with a high-pitched noise, which might be an interaction with the mother or a signal to other hatchlings. In chelonians sound production has been recorded mainly during mating and courtship rituals. Geckos are one of the most vocal reptiles, and most of the calls are considered alarm or distress sounds. For instance, manual restraint of a tokay gecko will usually be accompanied by a "bark" of the animal. The tokay gecko, in fact, was named for the multipart call that ends in a series of distinct two syllable chirps—"to-kay."

Snakes produce sounds in a variety of ways, and analyses of the proclivity for sound production and the acoustics of the sounds produced within a habitat or phylogeny may provide insights into the behavioral ecology of snakes. The relatively low information content in the sounds produced by snakes could suggest that these sounds are not suitable for intraspecies communication.[134] However, much more research is needed in this field in order to determine if some form of intraspecies or interspecies acoustic communication exists in certain snake species.

Gustation and Behavior

Unfortunately, research on how gustation affects behavioral responses in reptiles may have been neglected because of the significant attention that has been paid to research on the VO alone or because many studies did not separate the two systems from each other. Nevertheless, different taste buds have been documented in all reptiles. Observations about taste predilections have been made in recent years, and different behavioral reactions triggered by taste stimuli have been recorded. Findings in one study suggest that licking may be a response to gustatory stimulation by sugar in the omnivorous lizard *(Gallotia caesaris)* in contrast to previously observed prey chemical discriminations which were shown to require vomerolfaction.[24]

Behavioral responses to plant toxins by omnivorous lizard species *(Podarcis lilfordi)* and the Bonaire whiptail lizard *(Cnemidophorus murinus)* have shown that the animals were able to avoid antinutritive factors in plants (such as saponins) primarily by taste.[25] When presented with cotton swabs soaked in solutions containing components of plant toxins, these lizards exhibited aversion to the swab with decreased tongue flicking responses, avoidance of swabs, short excursion tongue flicks directed away from the swabs, and even rubbing of the snout on the terrarium floor.

Reproductive Behaviors

Courtship and mating behaviors of reptiles are extremely varied, and only a few relevant examples will be mentioned here. Sexual behaviors appear to be influenced and triggered by multiple cues, and usually a variety of sensory organs play key roles in triggering the displays, recognition of the displays, and acceptance or rejection of the displays.

Pheromones play a key role in mediating sexual behavior in the garter snake[85]; however, they are not the only factors responsible for the initiation of the behavior. Pheromones will usually help to locate and identify the correct species, but visual identification of the individual animal is very important in snakes. Krohmer[74] also used the garter snake to demonstrate the presence of sex steroid–concentrating neurons within the pathways regulating courtship and mating. This suggests that sex hormones may be involved in the activation of sexual behavior. Although androgens are elevated on emergence from hibernation, the initiation of courtship behavior and mating appears to be independent of direct androgen control.[74] The conclusion of this paper suggests that hormones may have indirect effects on mating behavior in reptiles.

In order to be able to take an active part in the courtship and mating process, it appears that the physical condition of the animal is very important. Just as with mammals, female snakes must have a certain percentage of body fat in order to remain reproductively active. It was shown that if the body condition in female snakes was below average, these females also had very low estradiol levels and did not show sexual receptivity, whereas males of all body condition indexes had significant testosterone levels and displayed active courtship behaviors.[6] Another example noted in field observations includes a large year-to-year variation in reproductive rates of female red-sided garter snakes *(T. sirtalis parietalis)*, which has led to the suggestion that factors such as nutrition and stored energy reserves significantly modify the effects of mating behavior and ovarian activity.[130]

With respect to energy expenditure, males allocate relatively little to gamete production and are able to reproduce with minor energy investment. In direct contrast, females of many species experience high fecundity-independent costs of reproduction, such as migration to nesting sites and decreased food intake. Females therefore need to amass substantial energy reserves before initiating reproductive activity.[6]

Stress has also been implicated in having detrimental effects on breeding behaviors. Stress has been shown to rapidly suppress mating behaviors in the garter snake.[93] In this study, the authors were able to demonstrate that the exogenous corticosterone had no negative effect on testosterone levels. The data suggest, however, that a mechanism is in place for corticosterone to suppress mating behavior and that these effects do not occur as an indirect effect on plasma levels of testosterone but are attributable more to the direct effect of the hormone itself.[93]

It seems therefore important to recognize when an animal is sexually reproductive and to minimize handling during this time. Close observation of the animal might be needed in order to establish that an animal is sexually reproductive, because sometimes behavior changes are subtle and do not seem directly related to mating or courtship. For example, it has been shown that daily basking periods were lengthened substantially during a breeding period in a natural population of garter snakes.[54]

The successful courtship and mating ritual has been described as an event that can be broken down into three phases.[127]
- Phase one is usually initiated by a chase or direct contact between the male and the female.
- Phase two is initiated if the female is receptive, the two animals accept each other, and physical contact is maximized. The tactile senses play an important part in this phase, and various stimulation tactics exist for the different reptile species.
- Phase three is actual intromission. After a successful mating some male reptiles deposit a plug in the cloacal opening. This plug is most likely formed from secretions from the kidney, and its deposition immediately after insemination probably prevents rival males from copulating with the same female.[36]

Male Reproductive Behaviors

Male courtship behavior can be extremely varied among the different species and appears to involve many different senses. Many lizards use display techniques to draw attention to themselves. Courtship behaviors in lizards may include head bobbing, pushups, and tongue flicking, as well as posturing to make the interested reptile appear larger, including inflation of the body, extension of the dewlap, and broadside posturing.[20,127] The throat of male bearded dragons *(P. vitticeps)* becomes dark black (much darker than in females) during the breeding season.[33]

Although many male lizards will bite the female in the dorsal neck region, male snakes will crawl repeatedly over the females and align their bodies to prepare for copulation. Male boids will press their spurs into the cloacal region of the female to aid alignment. A mix of aggressive and sexual behavior has been documented in observations in which male garter snakes have been seen to forcibly inseminate females.[115]

In some chelonian species the male will also bite the female or, as in the case of the gopher tortoise, will ram his shell into hers (Figure 3-6). Females may become injured during these courtship attempts if they are unable to escape the advances.[65] The male slider turtle will swim backward in front of the female and stroke her face with his long fingernails. During these behaviors the male animal will engage in searching for the tail and localizing the cloaca of the female. Male box turtles, which have a high-domed carapace and a hinged plastron, will mount the female, and once intromission has been accomplished the female will clamp the carapace

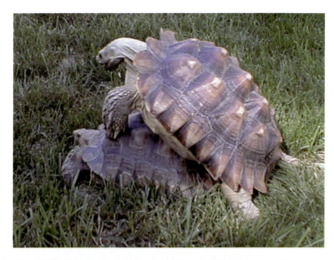

Figure 3-6
Turtles and tortoises that are courting and mating can hurt each other, as the male may aggressively butt the shell of the female. Provide plenty of space and hiding spaces to prevent injury to females. (Courtesy Laurie and Tim Schwab.)

against the male's feet and he will fall backward and remain on his back until mating is complete.

Female Reproductive Behaviors

Female lizards often sustain lacerations from males biting them during copulation. It is important in breeding groups to provide enough space and hiding places to allow the females to escape the attention of the males if necessary. This aggression can also be directed toward the caretaker and can result in severe injuries.[67,77,88]

Initially, gravid female iguanas are often hyperactive. As they become visibly gravid, females of many lizard species tend to become lethargic and anorexic and spend more time basking, and may also become more aggressive. Gravid green iguanas *(I. iguana)*, for example, will protect a nest site by acting aggressively toward cagemates, including biting and hissing. Female chameleons often become darker in color during gravidity. Female bearded dragons *(P. vitticeps)* perform an arm-waving behavior in which they stand on three legs and wave one front leg in a slow circular motion from front to back. It is thought that this is an appeasement display toward aggressive males during the breeding season and during copulation.[33]

In oviparous lizard species that oviposition, the females dig a nest. They often cease feeding approximately 1 to 4 weeks before egg laying and intensely search for a nest site by scratching and digging in various substrates. Female iguanas have been noted to flick their tongues up to three times a minute during early exploration for nest sites and then decrease to one tongue flick per minute in later stages of nesting.[109] The female green iguana *(I. iguana)* will scratch fresh dirt over a larger area than the actual nest in order to distract predators from the nest site. If an appropriate substrate for nesting is not provided, she may become less active and begin feeding again. If this occurs, she may lay the eggs randomly and sporadically or she may develop dystocia and/or retained and mummified eggs.

Parental care is usually defined in other species as behavioral contributions by the parents to offspring survival after oviposition or parturition. In reptiles that exhibit this behavior, the females are primarily involved in parental care behaviors. Different parental behavioral patterns and nonbehavioral patterns in reptiles have been documented. Nonbehavioral patterns of parental care predominate in reptiles but have been shown to be equally as effective as parental behavior.[110]

Parental care documented in reptiles includes nest construction, maintenance, and defense (e.g., crocodilians); true incubation by coiling around the eggs and increasing the incubation temperature by shivering thermogenesis (e.g., rock python); removal of nonviable eggs from the nest; and hydroregulation. Evidence of actual protection of offspring has been limited, but the prehensile-tailed skink *(Corucia zebrata)*, which bears only one live young, has been shown to protect its young for a short period of time after giving birth. An extensive literature overview regarding this issue has been published recently.[117] Crocodilians, both males and females, will guard the hatchlings as they stay close to the water's edge and feed on insects and fish. The hatchlings will dive into the water if they sense that danger is near.

Female reptiles can manipulate the genotypes of their offspring through mate choice and enhanced sperm competition. Offspring phenotypes are influenced through allocation "decisions," behavioral and physiologic thermoregulation, and nest-site selection.[114] The influence of environment on sexual behavioral patterns is often underestimated, and diseases and pathologic conditions associated with reproduction are common presentations to the reptilian veterinarian.[53] The frequency of these medical cases might be significantly decreased once the caretaker truly understands the connection between husbandry and physiology.

Behavior of Hatchlings and Juveniles

Hatchling green iguanas *(I. iguana)* will use the egg tooth to penetrate the shell and will remain in the egg with their heads exposed for up to 24 hours while the yolk is being absorbed. They will shed immediately after hatching and begin eating young leaves in about 6 to 9 days.

Tongue flicking, head bobbing, and dewlap extension as well as rubbing the hind legs and abdomen on substrate can be noted soon after hatching. For the first 6 months they will exhibit head bobbing that is believed to advertise spatial position among conspecifics and may also aid in coordination of group activities. Juvenile bearded dragons *(P. vitticeps)* perform an arm-waving behavior (see Female Reproductive Behaviors) that is believed to serve in intraspecies recognition as well as in an appeasement display toward larger conspecifics.[33]

Juvenile green iguanas *(I. iguana)* have been seen eating the feces of cagemates, as the coprophagy helps to establish bacterial flora for fermentation in the intestinal tract. For the first 6 months iguanas tend to stick together in groups for sleeping, basking, and foraging and appear to exhibit a preference for staying together with siblings most likely through recognition of femoral gland odor.[2] Juveniles in the wild live together mostly in thickets of thorny vegetation and only begin to perch as they get older.

Although occupying the parents' home range may have certain advantages, cannibalism of young animals by their parents has been documented in some lizards; therefore migration into new territory can have significant advantages for the juvenile.[103] Many snake and lizard females will lay their eggs within their home range, and the hatchlings will enter the mother's home range after hatching.[103] Marine turtle hatchlings leave the nest and move immediately toward the sea to fend for themselves.

Eating Behaviors

Historically, two types of feeding behaviors in reptiles have been used: the "sit and wait" approach and the "foraging-hunting" strategy. The alligator snapping turtle *(Macroclemys temmincki)* uses the sit and wait tactic by wriggling a pink fleshy appendage on the tip of its tongue. Once the prey animal comes close enough to investigate, the turtle snaps its large jaws around it. Green iguanas *(I. iguana)* and many other lizards forage actively. However, as more and more data about reptilian feeding habits become available, it seems that these two classifications may be an oversimplification. Changes in feeding habits and diets consumed may also have ontogenetic influences whereby eating strategies change with age. For example, juvenile bearded dragons *(P. vitticeps)* are more insectivorous, whereas adult bearded dragons are more herbivorous.

The act of feeding in reptiles usually involves minimal mastication, although chewing can be observed in carnivorous reptiles. A chewing motion can also be observed in venomous reptiles during envenomation, as the act of chewing delivers significantly more venom than slashing.[119] Insectivorous lizards will chew and crush the exoskeleton of their prey, whereas herbivorous reptiles have small, sharp, perforating teeth that allow them to rip vegetation along the perforations created and swallow with relatively little chewing motion. Iguanian lizards use their tongues to capture prey and rely on wet adhesion and interlocking on the tongue surface. This limits them to smaller food items (Figure 3-7). Chameleons, however, also have a suction component that is created by modified intrinsic tongue muscles that pull the tongue pad inward and allow the chameleon to capture larger prey items, including small vertebrates.[66]

Herbivorous tortoises invariably "taste" their food with a light, incomplete bite before ingestion. This is a good thing in captivity, since they often mistake painted toenails or human clothing for potential food sources. Feeding in snakes is a process involving the whole skeleton. The motion of swallowing can be considered as an "internal" movement or locomotion, as vertebral bends push food from the jaws along a substantial length of the body to the stomach.[92] If disease processes exist that involve the spine, anorexia or regurgitation can be a sequela. This might be most significant in constricting snakes.

A direct correlation between the physiology of digestion and environmental temperatures has been described in the literature. An elevated environmental temperature was associated with a faster and larger meta-

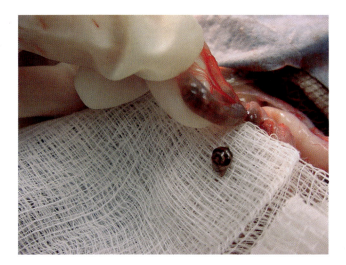

Figure 3-7
It is important to provide appropriately sized prey items to reptiles. This bearded dragon was fed several large grasshoppers, which resulted in an obstruction of the intestines with multiple grasshopper heads that were not digestible. (Courtesy Teresa Bradley Bays.)

bolic increase after ingestion in the Burmese python *(Python molurus)* and the time required to return to fasting metabolic levels was markedly longer at lower environmental temperatures (e.g., 20° versus 35° C; 68° F versus 95° F).[125]

Reptiles are also able to actively increase their body temperature if the physiologic situation requires this. In the South American rattlesnake *(Crotalus durissus)* a feeding-derived thermogenesis caused the surface body temperature of the animals to increase by about 1° C (1.8° F). This temperature change significantly affects the digestive performance. The magnitude of the thermogenesis was greater for snakes fed large meals, as was the corresponding metabolic response.[121]

In many lizards and most snake species, hydration is maintained more from moisture in the diet than from drinking. This is especially true for those on moist and vegetative diets, so appreciable amounts of water may not be consumed. Lizards that do not drink from a water bowl may lap water that has been spray misted on the inside of the enclosures or from a continuous drip system. Water can also be spray misted on food items to help to maintain hydration. Box turtles and many species of tortoises normally drink from water pooled on the ground during and after rain. The water is imbibed by filtering it through overlying vegetation. These tortoises may not recognize or be stimulated to drink from a bowl. A sprinkler system outdoors can be used to simulate rain if lack of water consumption or dehydration is of concern.

Feeding behavior is closely related with the sensory systems, as location of prey and food items has to be accomplished with one or more senses before the actual feeding occurs. Therefore any pathologic conditions affecting the sensory organs can significantly alter feeding behavior. Also, although increasingly more and better data regarding correct nutritional management of reptiles exist[37] and continue to be compiled, diseases directly related to malnutrition are still a common presentation.

Environmental temperatures may also affect feeding behavior. In a study of juvenile green iguanas *(I. iguana)* it was found that as the temperature at the location of a preferred food item decreased, the likelihood of the iguana leaving the warmer temperature to obtain that food also decreased. This was especially true if other, less-preferred food items were available where warmth was provided in the enclosure.[8] Seasonality also affects food preferences. Several species of omnivorous tortoises such as the yellow-footed tortoise *(Geochelone denticulata)* and the red-footed tortoise *(Geochelone carbonaria)* maintained outdoors in subtropical climates are more likely to consume protein in the fall, before temperatures decrease and the animal enters a more torpid state.

The close interaction between basking and nutrition has also been demonstrated in the chameleon. Basking behavior of panther chameleons

(C. pardalis) has been shown to be influenced by nutrition in that lower dietary intake of vitamin D_3 resulted in a positive phototaxis to greater UV-B light[44] (see Environmental Aspects of Behavior).

Social stress from dominant reptiles may keep subordinate reptiles from eating as well or as often and may cause failure to thrive. This is commonly seen in groups of captive lizards and in colonies of aquatic turtles. Multiple feeding stations can reduce competition in enclosures that contain several reptiles. If not enough food or feeding stations are offered, cagemate or tankmate aggression can lead to severe injuries because of competitive feeding behavior. Placing food in open as well as visually protected areas will encourage feeding even in shy species.

Anorexia may occur if species-specific behaviors and tendencies are not known. The most common cause of anorexia in captive reptiles is related to inappropriate environment (e.g., wrong substrate or humidity).[31] Providing inappropriate food items—food of the wrong type or the wrong size—may also lead to anorexia. For example, anecdotal reports claim that wild-caught snakes refused to eat white laboratory rats but would not hesitate to strike at brown rats. Gerbils are often substituted for white mice with smaller snakes, especially ball pythons, for which brown mice are natural prey. Feeding nocturnal species during the day may also lead to anorexia. Knowledge of normal feeding behaviors will also help the owner to pick appropriate prey items and, with some imagination, help with behavioral enrichment of the pet.

If live prey is not readily consumed it should be removed to prevent injury to the captive reptile. Bite wounds inflicted by prey items can create serious medical problems (Figure 3-8). This also applies when insects are fed to reptiles. Excess crickets left in chameleon enclosures commonly perch on the chameleons' periorbital area and "drink" fluid from the eye, causing conjunctival or corneal irritation (Figures 3-9 and 3-10). A case of cricket predation on an anolis lizard *(A. carolinensis)* has been described in the literature.[86]

When preparing invertebrates to be fed to reptiles, a calcium-loaded food source for these insects should always be supplied. We generally recommend feeding only prekilled vertebrate prey to carnivorous reptiles, in order to avoid medical complications and to prevent the suffering of the prey animal (e.g., suffocation by constriction).

Stress and social competition, often caused by the limited space and insufficient visually secure hiding spaces, may lead to anorexia in captivity and is considered part of the "maladaptive syndrome." This has been documented in a colony of lizards that were subclinical carriers of *Salmonella* species at the time of capture; as a result of stress, five developed active overwhelming systemic infections.[70] The initial clinical signs of the problem were decreased activity and anorexia.

136   Exotic Pet Behavior

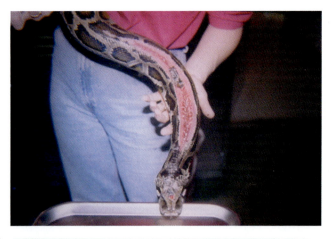

Figure 3-8
Providing live prey items to reptiles can be detrimental if the prey is not consumed in a timely manner. A rat was left in this snake's cage for several days while the owner was on vacation. The rat chewed down on the dorsum of the snake until the vertebrae were exposed. It took approximately 6 weeks for this to heal, and significant scarring occurred. (Courtesy Teresa Bradley Bays.)

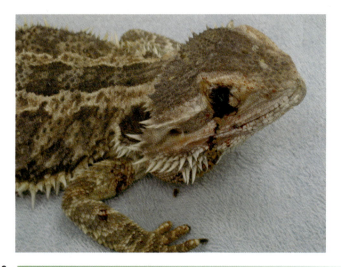

Figure 3-9
The owner of this bearded dragon witnessed crickets apparently "sucking at the fluid of the eye." Cricket predation has been documented, and serious damage can occur if live prey is kept in with captive reptiles for more than 15 to 20 minutes. (Courtesy Teresa Bradley Bays.)

Reptile Behavior 137

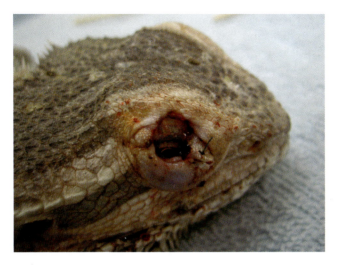

Figure 3-10
The same bearded dragon that suffered from cricket predation. This is postsurgery, after repair of a tear in the lower lid and debridement of what remained of the upper lid. (Courtesy Teresa Bradley Bays.)

As stated earlier, overhandling shy species (e.g., chameleons, ball pythons) can create anorexia as a result of stress, and a common problem in snakes is regurgitation caused by handling shortly after feeding. Therefore it is not advisable to examine or perform diagnostic procedures on a snake shortly after the keeper or owner has fed it, because of increased risk of stress-induced regurgitation.

Undetected disease processes, often evidenced by behavior changes that may go unrecognized by the owner or caregiver, may lead to anorexia. Pathologic conditions of the upper gastrointestinal tract will have a significantly negative impact on the feeding response, and oral, dental, and beak disorders of reptiles are very common presentations in the veterinary clinic.[87] Obesity is a common medical problem encountered in sit and wait predators (especially monitors in captivity), which are offered a high-caloric diet too frequently without the need to exercise in order to obtain food.

Both infectious and noninfectious disease processes often cause anorexia and or regurgitation.* The incubation period of an infectious process in reptiles can be a significantly long period (up to 6 months), making it difficult to associate the anorexia and other clinical signs to the inciting exposure to disease or injury that led to the infection.

---

*References 16,27,64,80,105,122.

Many reptile species become anorexic in cooler temperatures, so it is important to distinguish whether anorexia has a pathologic cause in that species or if it is a seasonal occurrence of the reptile. Advanced gravidity may also lead to anorexia in certain species. Many male reptiles in breeding season have decreased appetites or are anorexic. In natural conditions, it has been shown that most female aspic vipers, *Vipera aspis*, stop feeding during the 2 months of pregnancy.[82]

Healthy lizards kept in proper environments can do well despite weeks of anorexia associated with gravidity. Many captive lizards, however, are already somewhat compromised by poor diet, dehydration, less-than-optimal environment, and parasitism, such that this period of anorexia, even though a result of reproductive necessity, may not be tolerable. Because of the risks associated with reproduction in females, it may be advisable to ovariectomize pet reptiles to avoid compromise created by preovulatory and postovulatory states and gravidity.

In reptile species that flick the tongue or eat prey and food items off of the cage or enclosure floor, it is not uncommon for substrate to be eaten accidentally or intentionally. Even substrates that are designated as safe for reptiles, including bark, corncob, and calcium-containing sands, can cause gastrointestinal problems (including obstruction, perforation, peritonitis, and rectal prolapse from straining) if ingested in large enough amounts. We therefore recommend the use of substrates that are not easily ingested, if at all possible. Although this seems to be particularly common in young bearded dragons, we have also seen it in chameleons, geckos, and uromastyx lizards. Owners must be educated that calcium-containing sand may have nutritional value but can act as a mechanical obstruction.

Elimination Behaviors

The frequency and the amount of elimination varies significantly among the different species of reptiles. In most reptiles urination and defecation happen simultaneously, and normal elimination in reptiles include three parts—clear liquid urine, white chalky urates, and formed greenish to brownish fecal material. The feces of carnivorous and desert-dwelling reptiles are fairly dry and formed, and such reptiles usually have smaller and more infrequent eliminations than equally sized herbivorous reptiles.

The feces of most herbivores are fairly loose and voluminous, and gastrointestinal transit times in herbivorous reptiles (e.g., green iguana) have been shown to be as long as 55 hours.[116] The long transit time in herbivores has been shown to serve as a biologic factor in seed dispersal and as a seed germination agent, as in the case of the Florida box turtle *(Terrapene carolina bauri)*.[78]

In the wild, most reptiles will usually not come into repeated close contact with their eliminations. The situation in captivity is very different, as many reptiles are fed on the bottom of the enclosures where fecal contamination is a common scenario. The constant reinfection with intestinal parasites is a sequela of confined space and suboptimal hygiene conditions. Lizards and tortoises often defecate in their water bowls, so the bowls should be washed and changed daily. Chronic parasitic infestations are difficult to treat with parasitacides, and regular fecal examinations should be part of the routine physical examination. It is imperative that the stool sample be as fresh as possible and that examination of a direct smear be performed, as well as a fecal flotation test.

Diarrhea may be evidenced by fecal material that remains around the cloaca and ventral tail. Constipation is seldom a clinical finding in herbivorous reptiles but is frequently encountered in carnivorous reptiles. In the wild the diet of a carnivorous reptile is varied, but in captivity the reptile is usually being offered the same kind and size of prey animal on a regular basis. This significant lack of variety in diet along with chronic dehydration and lack of exercise might contribute to mechanical obstruction (e.g., too much hair present in gastrointestinal tract at once).

Another form of elimination behavior in reptiles is vomiting. This has been shown to be a protective reflex and a mechanism for removal of indigestible food residues (e.g., fur, claws) from the gut.[5]

Urination in tortoises and turtles can often be observed during clinical examination. When the cloaca is manipulated or during other physical stimuli (e.g., venipuncture), we frequently observe a forceful expulsion of urine. It might be interpreted as a form of defensive behavior to repel a predator or as a part of a flight reaction in order to quickly decrease the body weight. No scientific study regarding this behavior is currently available. It has been proposed that the bladder in tortoises can function as a water reservoir.[69] When the bladder has been forcefully emptied by the animal, it is important to make sure the animal has ready access to water to rehydrate adequately.

The only reptile to date that has been documented to absorb water from the cloaca (cloacal drinking) is the turtle, and reports of observing anal drinking go back as far as 1799.[69] Although soaking reptiles in warm, clean water will encourage drinking and provide a humid environment, they do not absorb water through the skin, and this is not an adequate means of rehydration.

Locomotor Behaviors and Activities

Most lizards ambulate by alternating the feet individually as they move. Some lizards will become bipedal, using only the rear feet, when attempting escape from predators. Juvenile green iguanas *(I. iguana)* and other species such as the basilisk lizards of Central and South America *(Basiliscus species)* are even able to ambulate bipedally for short distances over the surface of water if pushed to do so. Iguanas and other lizards can also swim well using the tail to propel them through the water with the legs pressed against the sides of the body. Aquatic chelonians have webbed feet to aid in underwater propulsion, and sea turtles have flippers.

Crocodilians have a flattened tail that propels them through the water with lateral strokes. The tail is strong enough to propel them straight up out of the water to snatch prey from limbs that hang over the water. On land, crocodilians will belly slide over the muddy areas in a serpentine motion, and in dry areas they walk with their legs beneath them and the abdomen held high off the ground.

Movement in snakes is aided by more than 400 vertebrae, making them very flexible. Most snakes move by lateral undulation on the ground and when swimming, and can reach speeds up to 10 km/hr (6 miles/hr).[22] Rectilinear locomotion, like that of a caterpillar, is used on smooth surfaces or when sneaking up on prey in open areas. Sidewinding and concertina locomotion are used on soft substances such as sand.

Reptiles in general are particularly prone to exhaustion during vigorous activity, especially in comparison with mammals.[11] When not in breeding mode, most reptiles spend a majority of their time immobile, basking and resting. Iguanas, for instance, spend greater than 90% of their day inactive.[123] Any activity can use up precious reserves needed for escape from predators. It has been shown that nocturnal geckos actively forage at low temperatures, and in experiments with the frog-eyed gecko *(Teratoscincus przewalskii)* it was noted that intermittent locomotion could increase the endurance of the lizard's movement.[128]

Even agonistic behaviors such as broadside posturing, dewlap extension, and body inflation that are used to establish territory between reptile conspecifics can negatively affect the endurance capacity of that reptile (Figure 3-11). For example, male side-blotched lizards *(Uta stansburiana)* experience a lateral compression of the thorax when exhibiting the threat display, which causes a concurrent increase in anaerobic metabolism. By restricting aerobic metabolism, the concentration of lactate increases, which then diminishes the locomotor capacity and endurance of the displaying lizard.[15]

Gravidity can also compromise locomotor ability and endurance, which increases the risk of mortality. Studies in side-blotched lizards *(U. stansburiana)* indicated that all females had lower endurance when gravid and that experimental yolkectomy (creating a 30% decrease in fecundity) resulted in an increase in endurance in the gravid females during gravidity and, surprisingly, also in the postovipositional lizard.[89]

Reptile Behavior 141

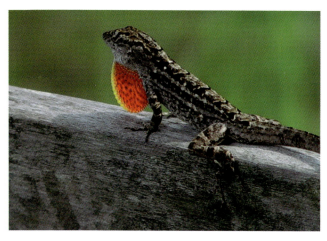

Figure 3-11
An anole displaying its dewlap as a method of communication. This behavior is usually combined with a repeated head bob. (Courtesy Jörg Mayer.)

Veterinary practitioners are often presented with a reptile patient that has been kept for years as a single pet. Often these owners or caretakers do not realize that their lizard, tortoise, or snake is not appearing, behaving, or ambulating normally as they have nothing with which to compare them. Because changes in body condition, locomotion, and behavior can occur very gradually, it is even more difficult for the caretakers to recognize abnormalities in the pet. This is one reason to stress to owners the need for wellness examinations at least twice per year. The practitioner will then have the opportunity to recognize problems early and to make the necessary corrections.

Grooming Behaviors

Few reptiles actually groom themselves; however, geckos will use their tongues to wipe their spectacles (eyecaps) to keep them clean. Reptiles periodically slough their skin, and, depending on the species, the shedding will occur all at once or in pieces. For snakes, shedding should be accomplished in one piece and include the spectacles. The old keratin layer sheds after the new keratin layer beneath has completely formed. Reptiles often rub against hard surfaces such as rocks in order to free themselves from the old skin. A growing reptile usually sheds more frequently. It is advisable not to handle them just before a shed. Often a reptile will refuse to feed at this time.

In snakes that are preparing to shed, the eyecaps often become opaque, and the snake may be more apt to strike, probably because of decreased vision during this time. After a few days, the eyecaps will clear and the skin over the entire body may appear dull. Snakes that have light-colored ventrums may also have a mild pink blush to their undersides during this time. The shed usually occurs shortly thereafter and usually as a single shed skin. In larger boas and pythons, however, the shed may be torn because of the mass of the snake. If this occurs in the animal hospital, it is wise to retain the shed skin to return to the owners if requested, as these may be of either financial or personal value. Crocodilians, turtles, and tortoises will periodically lose horny scutes as they shed.

Unhealthy reptiles or those maintained where temperatures and humidity are not optimal, may experience dysecdysis, in which shed sloughs in an irregular manner. The shed skin may also remain on limbs, tails, or toes. As the shed dries it becomes firm and can cause strictures that compromise the blood supply to the affected extremities. These appendages can become necrotic or infected because of avascularization from constriction.

Sneezing

Many lizard species, including green iguanas, sneeze frequently, expelling a concentrated salt solution, which is secreted by glands in the nasal cavities. Crusts may form around the nostrils, but a healthy iguana will wipe these crusts on rocks and other cage furniture. This crystalline white substance may be seen on glass enclosures and can contain chloride salts of sodium and potassium. As with other species, any sneezing that results in a nasal discharge composed of mucus or discolored yellow or green is not normal, and the animal should be treated by a veterinarian knowledgable in reptile health care.

Coloration and Behavior

The coloration of reptiles and ability to readily change colors in some species may serve as both a form of social interaction including that used for courtship and as camouflage to aid reptiles in the avoidance of predators as well as in the acquisition of food (Figure 3-12). Changes in coloration can also indicate stress and illness. In addition, color changes affect thermoregulation by increasing or decreasing reflectivity.

In many reptiles the males are the more colorful, most likely because they have less parental involvement than the females. Often, vivid colors are located less conspicuously—either ventrally or ventrolaterally—and visible only if specific postures are assumed to show them off during

Reptile Behavior 143

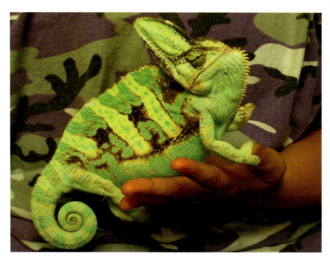

Figure 3-12
This chameleon is changing colors in response to its environment and to its level of stress. (Courtesy Teresa Bradley Bays.)

appropriate times. An example of this is the extension of the dewlap during courtship or fighting. Bearded dragons *(P. vitticeps)* often flash their yellow oral mucous membranes in an attempt to chase away predators. Many bearded dragon males will develop a dark black "beard" when sexually aroused, in pain, stressed, or severely ill.

Thermoregulatory Behaviors

Thermoregulatory behaviors must be considered one of the most important manifestations of behavior in poikilothermic animals. It is evident from many of the other sections in this chapter how critical environmental temperature is for reptiles. Before 1944 it was thought that the body temperature of reptiles reflected the environmental temperature. It then became known that without the ability of the animal to exist in the preferred optimal temperature zone (POTZ), metabolic processes would not function optimally.[26]

Roughly two types of behavioral thermoregulation exist. Reptiles that are heliothermic bask in the sun for heat regulation, and those that are thigmothermic absorb heat by conductance from objects in the environment. The specific behaviors of the reptile species that are kept in captivity must be known in order for an appropriate captive environment to be provided. During a 24-hour period reptiles will alter their behavior in order to achieve the needed body temperature required for various metabolic processes.

Lizards and snakes practice behavioral thermoregulation more than chelonians, which have a shell to retain heat.[98] Thermoregulation is achieved in many ways. Postural changes aid in thermoregulation by changing the surface area exposed to the sun. Extension of the dewlap, for example, helps to maximize the surface area of exposure. To increase exposure, the long axis of the body will be angled perpendicular to the sun, and to cool down the reptile will face the sun.[104] Snakes will coil to conserve heat and cool by uncoiling.[98]

Open-mouthed breathing may be used to regulate body temperature, as can gular fluttering, whereby the throat is vibrated with the mouth open in order to cool the blood in that area through evaporation of water.[9] Burrowing and movement between microclimates are also used to accomplish thermoregulation. Desert lizards will raise themselves up on their toes to reduce heat conduction.[98] Desert tortoises might also hypersalivate or urinate for emergency cooling by evaporation.[10,90]

It has been shown that reflectance, which is affected by coloration, strongly affects the warming rates of animals exposed to solar radiation (heliothermy). This is the principle of the heat lamp as it is applied in captivity. Several lizard species, such as chameleons, are able to change colors in order to thermoregulate by increasing or decreasing reflectance.

Another form of thermoregulation is by convection, whereby the movement of warm air over the exposed body will provide an effective means to increase the body temperature. This method is the core principle of use of a hair dryer or use of a Bair Hugger[1] during anesthesia, which can be applied to warm a cold reptile in the veterinary clinic.

The third way to increase body temperature is by conduction. The reptile will rest on a large stone or rock that has been heated by the sun (thigmothermy). This concept is mimicked in captivity by the under-tank heater.

The temperature range in which reptiles and other ectotherms live is governed by the environmental temperatures in that range. It is easy for animals in the wild to avoid extremely high temperatures by using cryptic behaviors such as burrowing underground. Cold temperatures, however, represent a more critical situation for survival. The critical temperature minimum (CTMin) can be used as a measure of thermal tolerance to the environment. CTMin is defined as the temperature at which an animal has lost the righting reflex.[39] This can be considered as the "ecologically lethal" temperature point, as it is the point at which the animal has lost the ability to escape from lethal threats.

The body temperature in the reptile is not uniform, and it can vary significantly between the head and the rest of the body.[38] This study documented that the temperature of the head appears to be maintained in a narrower spectrum than the rest of the body. If the environmental temperature was below the optimum for the examined species, the head was warmer than the rest of the body. In cases in which the environmental temperature was above the POTZ, the animal was able to keep the temperature of the head lower than the temperature of the rest of the body.

In a study using several species of basking lizards it was determined that the surface temperature of the lizard's body correlated with superficial blood flow and that the core temperature of the lizard correlated more closely with the heart rate.[41] Changes in the heart rate, whereby the rate is faster during heating than during cooling, have been shown to be important for thermoregulation in the monitor lizard *Varanus varius*[112] and in the free-ranging lizard, closely related to our common bearded dragons, *Pogona barbata*.[58]

Certain behaviors require fairly high temperatures—30° to 37° C (86° to 99° F)—including foraging and locomotion. Halliday[60] considers these higher temperatures "activity temperatures." His research indicated that for the Western garter snake *(Thamnophis elegans)*, activities such as swimming, digestion, tongue flicking, crawling, and oxygen consumption were at 100% activity level in temperatures of approximately 28° to 35° C (82° to 95° F). Most of these activities were reduced to a 60% activity level with temperatures of approximately 20° C (68° F).

The ability to achieve the required body temperature in lizards is well developed, as many have been shown to be highly selective of the diameter and degree of shading of their selected rocky retreat sites. These two variables have been found to significantly influence the thermal conditions beneath rocks.[71] Field studies with the Stephen's banded tree snake *(Hoplocephalus stephensii)* showed that a snake's height in the tree was positively correlated with its body temperature because of the increased exposure to solar radiation.[46] It was also noted that a circadian rhythm of temperature selection occurs for the Tokay gecko (*Gekko gecko*) in that during the light phase of a light-dark cycle this nocturnal species would select higher temperatures during a time when locomotor activity was lessened,[106] most likely to store energy for hunting.

Body appendages such as a large dewlap are also thought to help in increasing body temperature. Computer modeling using the pelycosaurus, which has a significantly large dorsal fin, has shown that having a body appendage is an asset because the appendage warms up more quickly in the morning in colder environments.[50]

An increase in body temperature as an immune response has been demonstrated in reptiles. A feverlike response to the injection of dead bacteria into the coelomic cavity has been well documented.[2,99] This fever has been shown to be dose dependent; animals were able to raise the body temperature by over 4° C (7° F), and the elevated temperature was recorded for over 5 days. Reptiles exposed to infection will seek out heat.[45] An increase in body temperature as a stress response has also been documented in the scientific literature. For example, a stress fever during handling has been seen in the wood turtle *(Clemmys insculpta)*.[19]

Thermoregulatory behavior has also been shown to modify the sex of the offspring of female viviparous lizards (*Niveoscincus ocellatus*). Both in the field and experimentally, the extent of basking by the female influenced the sex of the offspring. Reduced basking time produces more male offspring.[126]

Certain metabolites have also been shown to have direct effect on thermoregulation in reptiles. In the bearded dragon *(P. vitticeps)* it has been demonstrated that the injection of prostaglandins will significantly increase the heart rate, which is a key factor in thermoregulatory behavior.[111] The authors also noticed that in cases in which cyclooxygenase (COX) 1 and 2 enzymes were inhibited, heart rates during heating were not significantly different from those during cooling episodes. This information might be of interest, as chronic nonsteroidal antiinflammatory therapy is commonly used in reptiles, inhibiting the COX pathways. Prostaglandins (mainly PGF_{2a}) are frequently used in cases of egg binding and therefore potentially interfere with thermoregulation and the cardiovascular system.

Although a significant amount of research on the physiologic dynamics of thermoregulation in reptiles has been reported in the herpetologic literature, only a fraction of this knowledge has been "discovered" by the veterinary market. It cannot be overemphasized that a complete understanding of the natural history of the species is essential when designing a captive habitat or when dealing with injured reptiles. Fitzgerald and Shine[46] noted a difference in temperature preferences of reptilian species in the laboratory versus what was preferred in the field. Fitzgerald warns about the danger of potential complications when extrapolating information from one environment (e.g., the laboratory) to another (e.g., the natural environment).

Reptiles in captivity should always be provided with a temperature gradient from one end of the enclosure to the other (both a horizontal and vertical gradient are preferred). The authors of this chapter usually recommend a temperature gradient of 10° to 15° F (approximately 5° C) in a housing area or enclosure. Hiding spots or protected areas, where the reptile(s) can avoid direct exposure to both light and heat, should also be provided.

Hibernation and Estivation

Hibernation in reptiles is regulated by temperature, as they lack internal thermogenesis, brown fat, and shivering mechanisms.[98] Reptiles that live in temperate climates and high altitudes have to hibernate when temperatures drop.[98] Captive reptiles maintained in warm environments may not hibernate, although other factors govern hibernation, including the stage in the reproductive cycle, available food supply, body size, and photoperiod, as well as possibly other endogenous rhythms (Box 3-2).[98]

Hibernation helps to synchronize reproductive cycles, and the rising temperatures also stimulate mating. It is important to ensure that a captive reptile is healthy before hibernation, and weight should be monitored carefully during the hibernating months. A healthy reptile will not lose more than 10% of its body weight from water loss and reduction in lipid and glycogen stores during hibernation. Reptiles that appear unthrifty or experience weight loss greater than 10% should slowly be brought out of hibernation and supported appropriately.

Aquatic species hibernate at the bottom of ponds, where the water is less likely to freeze because of its increased density.[98] Anaerobic metabolism is used, and they breathe the oxygen dissolved in the water through their skin.[113] Desert species become inactive or estivate to conserve water, often burying themselves during this time.[98]

Burrowing Behaviors

Burrowing behaviors are noted in certain reptile species and are performed to aid in thermoregulation and egg laying, and to avoid predation. Burrowing reptiles should be provided with substrates that will allow this behavior as well as with hide boxes to simulate this behavior. Those species that have a tendency to burrow should not be provided with under-the-cage heaters, as they may burn themselves when burrowing beneath the substrate provided.

BOX 3-2 Hibernation Stages

1. Decreased temperatures inhibit appetite.
2. A hibernaculum below the frost line that provides moisture to prevent dehydration is sought.
3. Metabolism slows, and lipid reserves from fat stored in the liver, tail, and fat bodies in the coelom are used as an energy source. Most of this is depleted by emergence in the spring.
4. Rising temperatures trigger emergence.

Modified from O'Malley B: General anatomy and physiology of reptiles. In O'Malley B (editor): *Clinical anatomy and physiology of exotic species*, London, 2005, Elsevier.

Behaviors Associated with Pain

Reptiles have neurologic components to perceive pain that are similar to those found in cats and dogs, as well as other domestic species.[118] However, reptiles and other exotic prey species are less likely to exhibit overt pain-associated behaviors, in order to decrease the likelihood of being recognized as ill by predators (Figure 3-13).[79] Also, because immobility is a common survival tactic for prey species presented for examination, it is more challenging to assess if pain is present in reptile patients.[47]

Behaviors that may be associated with pain in reptiles include, but are not limited to, those stated in Box 3-3. These are behaviors that can be noted in lizards, snakes, and chelonians with any disease process (Figure 3-14). However, if pain is a potential component of the disease process or procedure, it should be managed appropriately.[13] A pet owner's assessment of pain and anxiety in their reptile pet should not be discounted, as owners may be the most aware of what normal behavior is for that pet.[13] Preemptive analgesia should be used where appropriate; as with all species, multimodal pain therapy often creates the best response.

Behavioral Enrichment

Unfortunately, many new and uneducated reptile owners may make poor choices for enclosures, environmental temperature, and humidity, as well as food, based on items that are sold at pet stores and advice from outdated

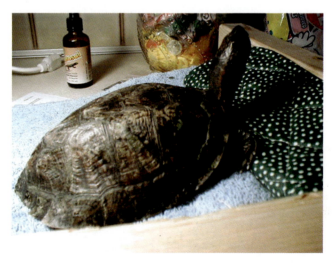

Figure 3-13
This is a classic posture of a turtle or tortoise exhibiting pain and distress. The head is intermittently and repeatedly raised and arched backward. (Courtesy Laurie and Tim Schwab.)

BOX 3-3 Clinical Signs That May Indicate Pain in Reptiles

Lizards
- Immobility or reluctance to move
- Dull and half-closed eyes
- Biting at the affected area
- Anorexia
- Agitation or restlessness
- Hunched posture
- Aggression in a normally passive animal
- Color changes (especially darkening)
- Rapid respiration
- Stinting on palpation
- Avoidance or withdrawal
- Polydipsia
- Lameness
- Continuous swallowing and aerophagia
- Scratching or flicking foot at affected area
- Elevated extended head
- Assumption of abnormal or strained postures
- Absence of normal behaviors

Snakes
- Anorexia
- Holding body less coiled at site of pain
- Stinting on palpation
- Affected area tucked up, with writhing
- Avoidance of handling
- Aggression in normally passive animal
- Withdrawal
- Easily startled, agitated
- Restlessness
- Flight response
- Immobility
- Lethargy
- Absence of normal behaviors

Chelonians
- Anorexia
- Stinting on palpation
- Hunched posture
- Lameness or ataxia

BOX 3-3 Clinical Signs That May Indicate Pain in Reptiles—cont'd

- Avoidance
- Withdrawal
- Closed or squinted eyes
- Flight response
- Immobility
- Biting at affected area
- Lethargy
- Intermittent pulling of head into shell, then extension of the neck out and up
- Absence of normal behaviors

Adapted from Bradley TA: Pain management considerations and pain-associated behaviors in reptiles and amphibians. In Proceedings of the ARAV Annual Conference, Orlando, Fla., 2001.

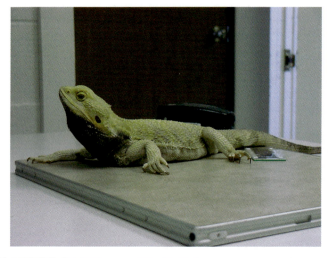

Figure 3-14
This bearded dragon is exhibiting behaviors associated with pain and stress, with its head elevated, ventrum pressed to the table, and a blackened ventral neck area. It was later discovered to be suffering from an intestinal obstruction (see Figure 3-7). (Courtesy Teresa Bradley Bays.)

texts, well-meaning friends, and "breeders." Decisions are also guided by the wish to make the enclosures aesthetically pleasing without knowledge of species-specific needs or behaviors that should be considered when making choices concerning substrate, prey items, and heat, light, and humidity sources.

Encouraging natural behaviors can be accomplished by providing safe enclosures and substrates that mimic natural materials but still allow for

Reptile Behavior 151

efficient management and cleaning. Before deciding which reptile species to obtain, owners should consider the necessary enclosure size, as well as husbandry issues such as light, temperature gradient, humidity (or lack of humidity if appropriate), and adequate hiding places.

Providing a variety of prey species can create a more balanced diet and provide behavioral enrichment. Occasionally adding to or making minor alterations in the cage furniture may also stimulate reptile pets to explore their environment. Providing natural unfiltered sunlight or artificial full spectrum UV lighting may also stimulate activity. In the laboratory setting, environmental enrichment in the form of "play" objects has been shown to reduce self-injurious behavior in the Nile soft-shelled turtle *(Trionyx triunguis)*.[127] Physical comfort decreases stress and the associated immune compromise that can occur in debilitated reptiles. (Figure 3-15).

Medical Implications of Abnormal Behaviors

Abnormal demeanor may be exhibited by half-closed, unfocused eyes, inability or unwillingness to move, extended head and limbs, depression, lack of interest in the surroundings, and the lack of righting and proprioceptive reflexes (Figures 3-16 and 3-17). Many lizards will sit quietly with head extended, eyes closed, and feet planted firmly when being handled or placed on an examination table. Clients often assume that this behavior is indicative of contentment. It is more likely, however, that this behavior is associated with submission, fear, or illness. The lizard may be "zoning

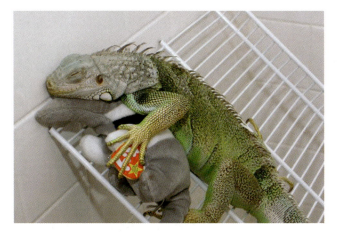

Figure 3-15
This iguana boarded along with its favorite stuffed toy, which it carried up to this basking spot to lie with. (Courtesy Teresa Bradley Bays.)

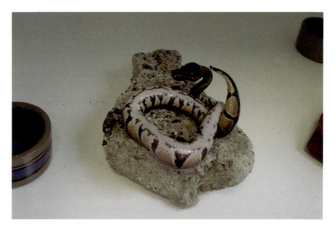

Figure 3-16
The righting reflex in snakes should be evaluated at each examination. This snake is not able to right itself, indicating severe neurologic problems. (Courtesy Jörg Mayer.)

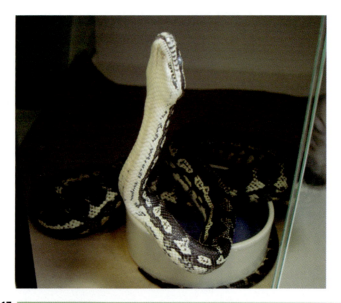

Figure 3-17
Stargazing in snakes is another abnormal behavior indicating neurologic problems. If the animal remains in this position for a prolonged period of time, diagnostic tests should be run to rule out common neurologic diseases such as inclusion body disease, which can be found in the Boidae family. (Courtesy Jörg Mayer.)

out" because of the stress of a strange environment riddled with strange sounds and smells and potential predators. This may be a lizard that is too ill to respond with curiosity to a new environment. This could also be a lizard that will readily strike if provoked—using teeth, claws, and whipping tail to defend itself against predators (as the clinician and staff may be perceived). This lizard may be closer to death than it would appear, and any stressor such as handling, diagnostic procedures, or treatment may prove fatal.

As with any species, when natural behaviors are not understood and addressed, reptiles kept in captivity will experience stress that results in elevated endogenous cortisol. Chronic elevations of cortisol will lead to immune suppression and increased susceptibility to disease. Overhandling of shy species, excessive noise or foot traffic in the area of the enclosure, the presence of other domestic pets that are perceived as predators, and inappropriate diet and environment are all stressors that can affect cortisol levels and thereby create immune suppression.

Reptiles that are not provided radiant heat to bask in will seek out a heat source, especially when they are ill, and they may burn themselves if a hot rock or other in-the-cage heating element is the only heat source that is provided. It is believed that heat receptors are not the same as pain receptors so the lizard does not perceive the pain until it is too late.

Shyer lizard species such as chameleons may remain hidden rather than expose themselves and therefore may not bask or eat. This should be taken into consideration when setting up the enclosure.

Specific knowledge of cage setup may allow the practitioner to understand environmental stressors that may be leading to anorexia, immune suppression, and disease. Because reptile enclosures are often too large to bring into the veterinary clinic, it may be helpful to train your front desk staff to encourage clients to bring in pictures of enclosures so that they can be evaluated.

As discussed earlier (see Eating Behaviors), many conditions lead to anorexia. If anorexia is a presenting complaint, it is important for the clinician to be able to distinguish whether it is pathologic, environmental, or associated with intense breeding condition in males or gravidity in females. In final stages of gravidity, as a place for laying eggs is sought, anorexia, aggression, and increased activity may be noted. It is imperative to assess whether the reptile is in adequate physical condition to undergo what would be a normal period of anorexia associated with gravidity in that species. Also, as stated previously (see Female Reproductive Behaviors), gravid females not provided with a proper place or substrate in which to lay eggs or kept under conditions of inappropriate temperature, humidity, and diet will often suffer from preovulatory stasis, egg binding, or dystocia.

Anorexic reptiles that are hospitalized should be supported with species-appropriate food items. Syringe feeding supplements are now available for herbivores (Critical Care, Oxbow Pet Products), carnivores (Carnivore Care, Oxbow Pet Products), and insectivores (Insectivore Diet, Walkabout Farms). Esophagostomy tubes can be placed for long-term supplemental feeding or in those species that are difficult or dangerous to feed orally. Anesthesia and analgesia appropriate for the patient's level of compromise should be used when these tubes are placed.

Stereotypic behaviors related to escape attempts can cause rostral abrasions and other lesions in captive lizards. Chinese water dragons *(Physignathus concincinus)* are particularly prone to escape attempts that create rostral snout wounds. Placing black tape on a transparent enclosure and minimizing glare and reflection in an enclosure as well as providing adequate space and hiding places may decrease this behavior. Also, many owners do not realize that all reptiles must be provided a day-night cycle in order to thrive; therefore, educating clients in this regard is critical.

When collecting history and information from the owner, it is important to ask where the lizard spends most of its time in relation to heat and light sources. This may give the practitioner clues to environmental conditions that are causing immunosuppression and disease. For instance, if a reptile is spending most of its time in a water bowl, temperatures may be too high or humidity may be too low (Figure 3-18). If a "shy" reptile is

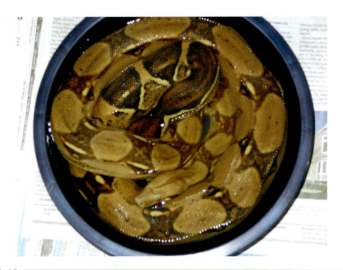

Figure 3-18
Snakes will occasionally spend time in a water bowl. A snake that spends an excessive amount of time in a water bowl, however, may have a problem with parasites, or the environment may be too hot. (Courtesy Jessie Mead and Brad Shrout.)

spending most of its time in a hide box that is placed on the cooler side of the tank, then it may not thermoregulate, as the need for security may outweigh its desire to spend time basking. Behavior modification that will improve health can be achieved by providing an environment that will address these behavioral tendencies.

Although scientific research of chemical alteration of behavior in reptiles exists, it currently has a very limited clinical application, as many drugs used in this field are not commercially available. A large field of behavioral research in reptiles includes the modification of aggressive displays. This might be a result of the relatively easy method of monitoring the impact of the drug and the dramatic displays shown by anoles, which are commonly used in the laboratory setting. Research data obtained using the anole showed that aggression is predominantly controlled in the right hemisphere of the brain and that acute stress or chronic alcohol consumption can significantly reduce territorial aggression.[35] The use of experimental drugs increasing serotonin (e.g. tetralin, quipazine) in the brain also showed a significant decrease of territorial aggression. Using a commercially available drug (fluoxetine [Prozac] at 60 mg/kg) in order to enhance serotonin levels in *A. carolinensis* markedly reduced aggression.[34] In a pilot study, drug dosages of fluoxetine of up to 100 mg/kg have been administered to reptiles without significant side effects; at this dose the only side effect noted was mild respiratory depression.

Euthanasia

Unfortunately reptiles are currently being brought to shelters and to rescue groups on a regular basis, as they become too big for their owners and too difficult to care for. Because most of these are euthanatized, it is best to try to educate clients not to make impulse purchases of reptiles. It is imperative to counsel them on the environmental and medical needs of the species in which they are interested, how big the reptile will get, and how long it will live. Also, adopting reptiles rather than purchasing them should be encouraged.

In the event that a reptile needs to be euthanatized to prevent suffering, injectable euthanasia solutions that are available for dogs and cats can be given intravenously or by intracardiac injection. Intraperitoneal injection is a less preferred method. Ultrasound or doppler can be used to help to locate the heart if necessary. *Euthanasia by cooling or freezing the reptile is not acceptable and is inhumane, as hypothermic conditions decrease the nociceptive threshold causing an increased sensitivity to pain.*[7,23,84]

It is often difficult to tell when a euthanized reptile is deceased, as the heart will often continue to contract for a period of time after the animal has been euthanatized. For this reason, we recommend that the euthanatized patient be kept in a warm environment for 12 to 24 hours before it is given to the owner for home burial, placed in a freezer, or cremated.

Acknowledgment

The authors would like to thank Richard Funk, MS, DVM, for his review of this chapter.

References

1. Ackerman L: *Biology, husbandry, and health care of reptiles: the biology of reptiles*, Neptune, N.J., 1998, TFH Publications.
2. Alberts AC: Chemical and behavioral studies of femoral gland secretions in iguanid lizards, *Brain Behav Evol* 41(3-5):255-260, 1993.
3. Alberts AC, Pratt NC, Phillips JA: Seasonal productivity of lizard femoral glands: relationship to social dominance and androgen levels, *Physiol Behav* 51(4):729-733, 1992.
4. Alberts AC, Pratt-Hawkes NC, Phillips JA: Ontogeny of captive and wild iguanas: from emergence to mating. In Jacobson ER, editor: *Biology, husbandry and medicine of the green iguana*, Malabar, Fla., 2003, Kreiger.
5. Andrews PL, Axelsson M, Franklin C, Holmgren S: The emetic reflex in a reptile *(Crocodylus porosus)*, *J Exp Biol* 203(10):1625-1632, 2000.
6. Aubret F, Bonnet X, Shine R, Lourdais O: Fat is sexy for females but not males: the influence of body reserves on reproduction in snakes *(Vipera aspis)*, *Horm Behav* 42(2):135-147, 2002.
7. American Veterinary Medical Association (AVMA) Panel on Euthanasia: 2000 Report of the AVMA Panel on Euthanasia, *J Am Vet Med Assoc* 218:669-702, 2001.
8. Balasko M, Cabanac M: Behavior of juvenile lizards *(Iguana iguana)* in a conflict between temperature regulation and palatable bait, *Brain Behav Evol* 52(6):257-262, 1998.
9. Bartholomew GA: Physiological control of body temperature. In Gans C, Pough FH, editors: *Biology of the Reptilia, vol 12, Physiology C*, London, 1982, Academic Press.
10. Bellairs A: The internal economy. In Bellairs A: *The life of reptiles*, Vol 1, Weidenfeld and Nicholson London, 1969, Weidenfeld and Nicholson.
11. Bennett AF: Exercise performance of reptiles, *Adv Vet Sci Comp Med* 38B:113-138, 1994.
12. Bernheim HA, Kluger MJ: Fever and antipyresis in the lizard *Dipsosaurus dorsalis*, *Am J Physiol* 231(1):198-203, 237-239, 1976.
13. Bradley T: Pain management considerations and pain-associated behaviors in reptiles and amphibians. In Proceedings of the Association of Reptilian and Amphibian Veterinarians and American Association of Zoo Veterinarians, Orlando, Fla., 2001.
14. Bradley T: Reptile behavior basics for the veterinary clinician. In Proceedings of the Annual meeting of the Association of Reptilian and Amphibian Veterinarians, Reno, Nev., 2002.
15. Brandt Y: Lizard threat display handicaps endurance, *Proc R Soc Lond B Biol Sci* 270(1519):1061-1068, 2003.

16. Brownstein DG, Strandberg JD, Montali RJ, et al: Cryptosporidium in snakes with hypertrophic gastritis, *Vet Pathol* 14(6):606-617, 1977.
17. Burger J: Antipredator behaviour of hatchling snakes: effects of incubation temperature and simulated predators, *Anim Behav* 56(3):547-553, 1998.
18. Burger J, Carruth-Hinchey C, Ondroff J, et al: Effects of lead on behavior, growth, and survival of hatchling slider turtles, *J Toxicol Environ Health* 55(7):495-502, 1998.
19. Cabanac M, Bernieri C: Behavioral rise in body temperature and tachycardia by handling of a turtle *(Clemmys insculpta)*, *Behav Processes* 49(2):61-68, 2000.
20. Carpenter CC, Ferguson GW: Variation and evolution of stereotypical behavior in reptiles. In Gans C, Tinkle DW, editors: *Biology of the Reptilia, vol 7. Ecology and behavior*, London, 1977, Academic Press.
21. Clark RW: Kin recognition in rattlesnakes, *Proc R Soc Lond B Biol Sci* 271 (suppl 4):S243-S245, 2004.
22. Cogger HR, Zweifel RG: *Encyclopedia of reptiles and amphibians*, San Diego, 1998, Academic Press.
23. Cooper JE, Ewbank R, Platt C: *Euthanasia of amphibians and reptiles*, London, 1989, Universities Federation for Animal Welfare and World Society for the Protection of Animals.
24. Cooper WE, Perez-Mellado V: Chemosensory responses to sugar and fat by the omnivorous lizard *Gallotia caesaris*: with behavioral evidence suggesting a role for gustation, *Physiol Behav* 73(4):509-516, 2001.
25. Cooper WE Jr, Perez-Mellado V, Vitt LJ, Budzinsky B: Behavioral responses to plant toxins by two omnivorous lizard species, *Physiol Behav* 76(2):297-303, 2002.
26. Cowles RB, Bogart CM: A preliminary study of the thermal requirements of desert reptiles, *Bull Am Museum Nat Hist* 83:265-296, 1944.
27. Cranfield MR, Graczyk TK: Experimental infection of elapid snakes with *Cryptosporidium serpentis* (Apicomplexa: Cryptosporidiidae), *J Parasitol* 80(5):823-826, 1994.
28. Crews D: Effects of early sex steroid hormone treatment on courtship behavior and sexual attractivity in the red-sided garter snake, *Thamnophis sirtalis parietalis*, *Physiol Behav* 35(4):569-575, 1985.
29. Crews D, Camazine B, Diamond M, et al: Hormonal independence of courtship behavior in the male garter snake, *Horm Behav* 18(1):29-41, 1984.
30. Crews D, Sakata J, Rhen T: Developmental effects on intersexual and intrasexual variation in growth and reproduction in a lizard with temperature-dependent determination, *Comp Biochem Physiol C Pharmacol Toxicol Endocrinol* 119(3):229-241, 1998.
31. de Vosjoli P: Designing environments for captive amphibians and reptiles, *Vet Clin North Am Exot Anim Pract* 2(1):43-68, 1999.
32. de Vosjoli P: Essential concepts of herpetoculture, using the five stages to improve veterinary care, *Exotic DVM Magazine* 3(6):33-36, 2002.
33. de Vosjoli P, Mailloux R: General information—behavior. In *General care and maintenance of bearded dragons*, Santee, Calif., 1997, Advanced Vivarian Systems.
34. Deckel AW: Behavioral changes in *Anolis carolinensis* following injection with fluoxetine, *Behav Brain Res* 78(2):175-182, 1996.
35. Deckel AW, Fuqua L: Effects of serotonergic drugs on lateralized aggression and aggressive displays in *Anolis carolinensis*, *Behav Brain Res* 95(2):227-232, 1998.

36. Devine MC: Copulatory plugs in snakes: enforced chastity, *Science* 187(4179):844-845, 1975.
37. Donoghue S: Veterinary nutritional management of amphibians and reptiles, *J Am Vet Med Assoc* 208(11):1816-20, 1996.
38. Dorcas ME, Peterson CR: Head-body temperature differences in free-ranging rubber boas, *J Herpetol* 31(1): 87-93, 1997.
39. Doughty P: Critical thermal minima of garter snakes *(Thamnophis)* depend on species and body size, *Copeia* 2:537-540, 1994.
40. Downes S, Shine R: Sedentary snakes and gullible geckos: predator-prey coevolution in nocturnal rock-dwelling reptiles, *Anim Behav* 55(5):1373-1385, 1998.
41. Dzialowski EM, O'Connor MO: Physiological control of warming and cooling during simulated shuttling and basking in lizards, *Physiol Biochem Zool* 74(5):679-693, 2001.
42. Eckstein HP: Jb. für Feldherpetologie, Beiheft 4, 145 Seiten (69 Abb. u. 42 Tab.), Verlag für Ökologie u. Faunistik, Duisburg, 1993.
43. Elf PK, Lang JW, Fivizzani A: Dynamics of yolk steroid hormones during development in a reptile with temperature-dependent sex determination, *Gen Comp Endocrinol* 127(1):34-39, 2002.
44. Ferguson GW, Gehrmann WH, Karsten KB, et al: Do panther chameleons bask to regulate endogenous vitamin D_3 production? *Physiol Biochem Zool* 76(1):52-59, 2003.
45. Firth BJ, Turner JS: Sensory, neural and hormonal aspects of thermoregulation. In Gans C, Pough FH, editors: *Biology of the Reptilia, vol 12, Physiology C*, London, 1982, Academic Press.
46. Fitzgerald M, Shine R, Lemckert F, et al: A reluctant heliotherm: thermal ecology of the arboreal snake *Hoplocephalus stephensii* (Elapidae) in dense forest, *J Therm Biol* 28(6-7):515-524, 2003.
47. Flecknell PA: Advances in the assessment and alleviation of pain in laboratory and domestic animals, *J Vet Anesth* 21:98-105, 1994.
48. Fleming G: Husbandry and medical management of Komodo dragons *(Varanus komodensis)* at the White Oak Conservation Center. In Proceedings of the Association of Reptilian and Amphibian Veterinarians, Sacramento, Calif. 1997.
49. Flores D, Tousignant A, Crews D: Incubation temperature affects the behavior of adult leopard geckos *(Eublepharis macularis)*, *Physiol Behav* 55(6):1067-1072, 1994.
50. Florides GA, Wrobel LC, Kalogirou SA, Tassou SA: A thermal model for reptiles and pelycosaurs, *J Therm Biol* 24(1):1-13, 1999.
51. Frye FL: Feeding captive reptiles. In Frye FL: *Reptile care: an atlas of diseases and treatments*, Neptune, N.J., 1991, TFH Publications.
52. Funk RS: Early neutering of male green iguanas—an experiment. In Proceedings of the Association of Reptilian and Amphibian Veterinarians Annual Conference, Reno, Nev., 2000.
53. Funk RS: Lizard reproductive medicine and surgery, *Vet Clin North Am Exot Anim Pract* 5(3):579-613, 2002.
54. Garstka WR, Halpert A, Crews D: Metabolic changes in male snakes, *Thamnophis melanogaster*, during a breeding period, *Comp Biochem Physiol A* 74(4):807-811, 1983.
55. Gehrmann WH: Reptile lighting: a current perspective, *Vivarium* 8(2):44-45, 62, 1997.

56. Goldstein EJ, Agyare EO, Vagvolgyi AE, et al: Aerobic bacterial oral flora of garter snakes: development of normal flora and pathogenic potential for snakes and humans, *J Clin Microbiol* 13(5):954-956, 1981.
57. Grace MS, Woodward OM, Church DR, Calisch G: Prey targeting by the infrared imaging snake *Python molurus:* effects of experimental and congenital visual deprivation, *Behav Brain Res* 119(1):23-31, 2001.
58. Grigg GC, Seebacher F: Field test of a paradigm: hysteresis of heart rate in thermoregulation by a free-ranging lizard *(Pogona barbata), Proc R Soc Lond B Biol Sci* 266(1425):1291-1297, 1999.
59. Gutzke WH, Tucker C, Mason RT: Chemical recognition of kingsnakes by crotalines: effects of size on the ophiophage defensive response, *Brain Behav Evol* 41(3-5):234-238, 1993.
60. Halliday T, Adler K, editors: *Firefly encyclopedia of reptiles and amphibians,* Toronto, 2002, Firefly.
61. Hamasaki DI: The spectral sensitivity of the lateral eye of the green iguana, *Vision Res* 8:1305-1314, 1968.
62. Head ML, Keogh JS, Doughty P: Experimental evidence of an age-specific shift in chemical detection of predators in a lizard, *J Chem Ecol* 28(3):541-554, 2002.
63. Heller SB, Halpern M: Laboratory observations of aggregative behavior of garter snakes, *Thamnophis sirtalis, J Comp Physiol Psychol* 96(6):967-983, 1982.
64. Helmick KE, Bennett RA, Ginn P, et al: Intestinal volvulus and stricture associated with a leiomyoma in a green turtle *(Chelonia mydas), J Zoo Wildl Med* 31(2):221-227, 2000.
65. Hernandez-Divers SJ: Clinical aspects of reptile behavior, *Vet Clin North Am Exot Anim Pract* 4(3):599-612, 2001.
66. Herrel A, Meyers JJ, Aerts P, Nishikawa KC: The mechanisms of prey prehension in chameleons, *J Exp Biol* 203(Pt 21):3255-3263, 2000.
67. Hsieh S, Babl FE: *Serratia marcescens* cellulitis following an iguana bite, *Clin Infect Dis* 28(5):1181-1182, 1999.
68. Inouchi J, Wang D, Jiang XC, et al: Electrophysiological analysis of the nasal chemical senses in garter snakes, *Brain Behav Evol* 41(3-5):171-182, 1993.
69. Jorgensen CB: Role of urinary and cloacal bladders in chelonian water economy: historical and comparative perspectives, *Biol Rev Camb Philos Soc* 73(4):347-366, 1998.
70. Kalvig BA, Maggio-Price L, Tsuji J, Giddens WE: Salmonellosis in laboratory-housed iguanid lizards *(Sceloporus* spp.), *J Wildl Dis* 27(4):551-556, 1991.
71. Kearney M: Hot rocks and much-too-hot rocks: seasonal patterns of retreat-site selection by a nocturnal ectotherm, *J Therm Biol* 27(3):205-218, 2002.
72. Kelsey J, Ehrlich M, Henderson SO: Exotic reptile bites, *Am J Emerg Med* 15(5):536-537, 1997.
73. Korzan WJ, Summers CH: Serotonergic response to social stress and artificial social sign stimulus during paired interactions between male *Anolis carolinensis, Neuroscience* 123(4):835-845, 2004.
74. Krohmer RW: The male red-sided garter snake *(Thamnophis sirtalis parietalis):* reproductive pattern and behavior, *ILAR J* 45(1):54-74, 2004.
75. Kubie J, Halpern M: Laboratory observations of trailing behavior in garter snakes, *J Comp Physiol Psychol* 89(7):667-674, 1975.
76. LeBas NR, Marshall NJ: The role of colour in signalling and male choice in the agamid lizard *Ctenophorus ornatus, Proc R Soc Lond B Biol Sci* 267(1442):445-452, 2000.

77. Levine EG, Manilov A, McAllister SC, Heymann WR: Iguana bite–induced hypersensitivity reaction, *Arch Dermatol* 139(12):1658-1659, 2003.
78. Liu H, Platt SG, Borg CK: Seed dispersal by the Florida box turtle *(Terrapene carolina bauri)* in pine rockland forests of the lower Florida Keys, United States, *Oecologia* 138(4):539-546, 2004.
79. Livingston A: Physiological basis for pain perception in animals, *J Vet Anesth* 21:73-77, 1994.
80. Lock B, Heard D, Detrisac C, Jacobson E: An epizootic of chronic regurgitation associated with chlamydophilosis in recently imported emerald tree boas *(Corallus caninus)*, *J Zoo Wildl Med* 34(4):385-393, 2003.
81. Lock B, McCaskill L: Operant conditioning for the husbandry and medical management of a large group of adult Nile crocodiles at Disney's Animal Kingdom. In Proceedings of the Annual Conference of the Association of Reptilian and Amphibian Veterinarians, Naples, Fla., 2004.
82. Lourdais O, Bonnet X, Doughty P: Costs of anorexia during pregnancy in a viviparous snake *(Vipera aspis)*, *J Exp Zool* 292(5):487-493, 2002.
83. Lovern MB, Holmes MM, Wade J: The green anole *(Anolis carolinensis)*: a reptilian model for laboratory studies of reproductive morphology and behavior, *ILAR J* 45(1):54-64, 2004.
84. Machin KL: Amphibian pain and analgesia, *J Zoo Wild Med* 30:2-10, 1999.
85. Mason RT, Fales HM, Jones TH, et al: Sex pheromones in snakes, *Science* 245(4915):290-293, 1989.
86. Mayer J: An external communication lesion to the coelomic cavity in a green anole *(Anolis carolinensis)*, *Lab Anim* 33(8):17-19, 2004.
87. Mehler SJ, Bennett RA: Oral, dental, and beak disorders of reptiles, *Vet Clin North Am Exot Anim Pract* 6(3):477-503, 2003.
88. Merin DS, Bush SP: Severe hand injury following a green iguana bite, *Wilderness Environ Med* 11(3):225-226, 2000.
89. Miles DB, Sinervo B, Frankino WA: Reproductive burden, locomotor performance, and the cost of reproduction in the free ranging lizards, *Evolution Int J Org Evolution* 54(4):1386-1395, 2000.
90. Minnich JE: The use of water. In Gans C, Pough FH, editors: *Biology of the Reptilia, vol 12, Physiology C*, London, 1982, Academic Press.
91. Moehn LD: The effect of sunlight on disposition in the Desert Collared Lizard, *Crotaphytus insularis*, *J Herpetol* 10:259-261, 1976.
92. Moon BR: The mechanics of swallowing and the muscular control of diverse behaviours in gopher snakes, *J Exp Biol* 203(Pt 17):2589-2601, 2000.
93. Moore IT, Mason RT: Behavioral and hormonal responses to corticosterone in the male red-sided garter snake, *Thamnophis sirtalis parietalis*, *Physiol Behav* 72(5):669-674, 2001.
94. Morandi N, Williams J: Snakebite injuries: contributing factors and intentionality of exposure, *Wilderness Environ Med* 8(3):152-155, 1997.
95. Mori A, Burghardt GM: Does prey matter? Geographic variation in antipredator responses of hatchlings of a Japanese natricine snake *(Rhabdophis tigrinus)*, *J Comp Psychol* 114(4):408-413, 2000.
96. Necas P: Chameleons: nature's hidden jewels, Malabar, Fla., 1999, Krieger.
97. O'Connor D, Shine R: Lizard in "nuclear families": a novel reptilian social system in *Egernia saxatilis* (Scincidae), *Mol Ecol* 12(3):743-752, 2003.
98. O'Malley B: General anatomy and physiology of reptiles. In O'Malley B, editor: *Clinical anatomy and physiology of exotic species*, London, 2005, Elsevier.

99. Ortega CE, Stranc DS, Casal MP, et al: A positive fever response in *Agama agama* and *Sceloporus orcutti* (Reptilia: Agamidae and Iguanidae), *J Comp Physiol [B]* 161(4):377-381, 1991.
100. Ott M: Chameleons have independent eye movements but synchronise both eyes during saccadic prey tracking, *Exp Brain Res* 139(2):173-179, 2001.
101. Phillips JA, Alberts AC, Pratt NC: Differential resource use, growth and the ontogeny of social relationships in the green iguana, *Physiol Behav* 53(1):81-88, 1993.
102. Plavicki J, Yang EJ, Wilczynski W: Dominance status predicts response to nonsocial forced movement stress in green anole lizard *(Anolis carolinensis)*, *Physiol Behav* 80:547-555, 2004.
103. Pough FH: *Herpetology*, ed 3, Upper Saddle River, N.J., 2003, Pearson Prentice Hall.
104. Pough FH, Andrews RM, Cadle JE, et al: Herpetology as a field of study. In Pough FH, editor: *Herpetology*. Englewood Cliffs, N.J., 1998, Prentice Hall.
105. Raymond JT, Garner MM, Nordhausen RW, Jacobson ER: A disease resembling inclusion body disease of boid snakes in captive palm vipers *(Bothriechis marchi)*, *J Vet Diagn Invest* 13(1):82-86, 2001.
106. Refinetti R, Susalka SJ: Circadian rhythm of temperature selection in a nocturnal lizard, *Physiol Behav* 62(2):331-336, 1997.
107. Rensch B, Adrian-Hinsberg C: Die visuelle Lernkazpazitat von Leguanen, *Z Tierpsychol* 20:34-42, 1963.
108. Rhen T, Crews D: Organization and activation of sexual and agonistic behavior in the leopard gecko, *Eublepharis macularis*, *Neuroendocrinology* 71(34):252-261, 2000.
109. Rodda GH: Biology and reproduction in the wild. In Jacobson ER, editor: *Biology, husbandry and medicine of the green iguana*, Malabar, Fla., 2003, Krieger.
110. Rosenblatt JS: Outline of the evolution of behavioral and nonbehavioral patterns of parental care among the vertebrates: critical characteristics of mammalian and avian parental behavior, *Scand J Psychol* 44(3):265-271, 2003.
111. Seebacher F, Franklin CE: Prostaglandins are important in thermoregulation of a reptile *(Pogona vitticeps)*, *Proc R Soc Lond B Biol Sci* 270(suppl 1):S50-S53, 2003.
112. Seebacher F, Grigg GC: Changes in the heart rate are important for thermoregulation in the varanid lizard, *Varanus varius*, *J Comp Physiol [B]* 171(5):395-400, 2001.
113. Seymour RS: Physiological adaptations to aquatic life. In Gans C, Pough FH, editors: *Biology of the Reptilia, Vol 13, Physiology D*. London, 1982, Academic Press.
114. Shine R: Reproductive strategies in snakes, *Proc R Soc Lond B Biol Sci* 270(1519):995-1004, 2003.
115. Shine R, Langkilde T, Mason RT: Cryptic forcible insemination: male snakes exploit female physiology, anatomy, and behavior to obtain coercive matings, *Am Nat* 162(5):653-667, 2003.
116. Smith D, Dobson H, et al: Gastrointestinal studies in the green iguana: technique and reference values, *Vet Radiol Ultrasound* 42(6):515-520, 2001.
117. Somma L: Parental behavior. In *Lepidosaurian and testudinian reptiles: a literature survey*, Melbourne, Fla., 2003, Krieger.
118. Stoskopf MK: Pain and analgesia in birds, reptiles, fish and amphibians, *Invest Ophthalmol Vis Sci* 35:755-780, 1994.

119. Strimple PD, Tomassoni AJ, Otten EJ, Bahner D: Report on envenomation by a Gila monster *(Heloderma suspectum)* with a discussion of venom apparatus, clinical findings, and treatment, *Wilderness Environ Med* 8(2):111-116, 1997.
120. Swaisgood R, Rowe MP, Owings DH: Assessment of rattlesnake dangerousness by California ground squirrels: exploitation of cues from rattling sounds, *Anim Behav* 57:1301-1310, 1999.
121. Tattersall GJ, Milsom WK, et al: The thermogenesis of digestion in rattlesnakes, *J Exp Biol* 207(Pt 4):579-585, 2004.
122. Valentin A, Jakob W, et al: Cryptosporidiosis in adders *(Pituiophis melanoleucus sayi)*. *Tierarztl Prax Ausg K Klientiere Heimtiere* 26(1):55-60, 1998.
123. Van Marken Lichtenbelt WD, Wesselingh RA, Vogel JT, Albers KB: Energy budgets in free-living green iguanas in a seasonal environment, *Ecology* 74:1157-1172, 1993.
124. Verheijen FJ: Photopollution: artificial light optic spatial control systems fail to cope with. Incidence, causation, remedies, *Exp Biol* 44(1):118, 1985.
125. Wang T, Zaar M, et al: Effects of temperature on the metabolic response to feeding in *Python molurus, Comp Biochem Physiol A Mol Integr Physiol* 133(3):519-527, 2002.
126. Wapstra E, Olsson M, Shine R, Edwards A: Maternal basking behavior determines offspring sex in viviparous reptile, *Proc R Soc Lond B Biol Sci* 271(suppl 4):S230-S232, 2004.
127. Warwick CF, Frye F, Murphy J, editors: *Health and welfare of captive reptiles*, London, 1995, Chapman & Hall.
128. Weinstein RB, Full RJ: Intermittent locomotion increases the endurance in a gecko, *Physiol Biochem Zool* 72(60):732-739, 1999.
129. Weiss E, Wilson S: The use of classical and operant conditioning in training Aldabra tortoises *(Geochelone gigantea)*, for venipuncture and other husbandry issues, *J Appl Anim Welf Sci* 6(1):333-338, 2003.
130. Whittier JM, Crews D: Ovarian development in red-sided garter snakes, *Thamnophis sirtalis parietalis:* relationship to mating, *Gen Comp Endocrinol* 61(1):5-12, 1986.
131. Wiesner CS, Iben C: Influence of environmental humidity and dietary protein on pyramidal growth of carapaces in African spurred tortoises *(Geochelone sulcata), J Anim Physiol Anim Nutr (Berl)* 87(1-2):66-74, 2003.
132. Young BA: Morphological basis of "growling" in the king cobra, *Ophiophagus hannah, J Exp Zool* 260(3):275-287, 1991.
133. Young BA: Hearing, taste, tactile reception, and olfaction. In Ackerman LJ, editor: *The biology, husbandry, and health care of reptiles*, Neptune City, N.J., 1997, TFH.
134. Young BA: Snake bioacoustics: toward a richer understanding of the behavioral ecology of snakes, *Q Rev Biol* 78(3):303-325, 2003.
135. Young BA, Aguiar A: Response of western diamondback rattlesnakes *Crotalus atrox* to airborne sounds, *J Exp Biol* 205(Pt 19):3087-3092, 2002.
136. Young BA, Morain M: The use of ground-borne vibrations for prey localization in the Saharan sand vipers (Cerastes), *J Exp Biol* 205(Pt 5):661-665, 2002.

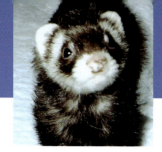

CHAPTER 4

PETER G. FISHER

Ferret Behavior

Natural Behavior and Domestication

The question as to why ferrets were domesticated may be more easily answered than when the domestication process took place and from what molecular phylogeny. This is in part because of the scarcity of written records from 2000 years ago and because of difficulties in identification of which species was actually being domesticated. Vernacular names for the animal we presume to be the ferret frequently varied from geographic district to district, and ancient scientists may have added to the confusion with incorrect translations from one language to another.[43]

Domestication is the process by which human selection and control of breeding results in an animal that provides a service or product that is beneficial to humans. With time, domestication results in physical and physiologic changes from the ancestral species. Animals are domesticated for work, food, or materials for clothing and shelter. Ferrets were in all probability originally used by man to control vermin. The earliest written account of an animal that fits the description of our domesticated ferret dates back to the Greek satiric writer Aristophanes (448-385 BC), who used the term "house ferret" in several of his plays to satirize political opponents. Soon thereafter, in 350 BC, the Greek philosopher and naturalist Aristotle (384-322 BC) also made written reference in a treatise on animals and physiognomy to a polecat that "resembles a weasel; and becomes very mild and tame."[43] It is reasonable to suppose he was referring to the ferret, and the demeanor of the animal described implies a close association with people. These early written accounts coincide with the time (circa 300 BC) when agriculture began to take hold in the civilized regions of the northern Mediterranean region centered around present-day Greece. One theory suggests the Greeks domesticated the indigenous European polecat (*Mustela putorius*) in order to protect grain stores from rodent infestation much in the way the Egyptians domesticated the cat.

Completely carnivorous, the polecat (ferret) will take a wide variety of prey, including hares, rabbits, mice, voles, and rats. The efficiency with which the ferret hunts rabbits brought it into favor with people. Strabo (63 BC–24 AD), a Greek historian, philosopher, and geographer, reported that the Romans used ferrets to control the overpopulation of rabbits on the Balearic Islands: "The ferrets with their claws drag outside all the rabbits they catch, or else force them to flee into the open, where men, stationed at the hole, catch them as they are driven out."[43] By the Middle Ages, man was ferreting rabbits throughout Europe and Asia (Figure 4-1).

Many historians believe that eleventh-century Normans introduced ferrets to Britain, where they were used to chase rabbits out of burrows. The sport of ferreting (hunting for rabbits) resulted in further domestication, as the ferret did not catch its prey but chased or frightened the rabbit out of its hole with its strong musky smell. The fleeing rabbit would then be caught in nets or by dogs or hawks used by the hunters.

This may also explain the ferret's musky body odor. Ferrets with a strong scent would make better ferreters and therefore were bred. The goal was to chase prey, not capture it. Ferrets that caught and ate the rabbits not only would destroy the food source and pelt but also would be more difficult to retrieve from the rabbit burrow. To discourage prey capture, working ferrets sometimes were harnessed with string, had bells attached to their collars, or were muzzled. With time the instinct to hunt *and* kill was bred out of the ferret. The sport of ferreting is still practiced by many people in Europe and Australia but is outlawed in the United States and Canada.

It is believed ferrets were brought to the United States in the late eighteenth century and used to control shipboard vermin on long, transatlantic crossings.[37] In the mid nineteenth century ferrets were bred for their fur, a practice that continued late into the twentieth century. Only recently has fur production fallen out of favor in much of the world.

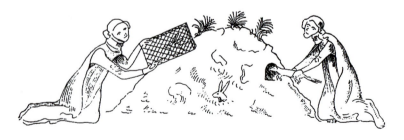

Figure 4-1

Ferreting in the Middle Ages—approximately 1300 AD. (From Thompson AD: A History of the ferret, J Hist Med 6(4):471-480, 1951.)

Ferrets have been kept as companions by historical figures such as Genghis Khan and Queen Elizabeth I; however, their popularity as pets did not increase until the late 1960s. This resulted in additional physical and behavioral changes as ferrets were bred for greater docility, decreased odor, preferred body confirmation, coat color, and failure to thrive in the wild. The last half of the twentieth century also saw the domestic ferret grow in popularity as a laboratory and research animal.

This ferret domestication timeline brings us to the present day, but the precise parent species of the domestic ferret remains uncertain. Ferrets may have been domesticated from the European polecat or from its eastern congener, the steppe polecat *(Mustela eversmannii)*, which has more similar morphology of the cranium. Because *M. putorius* and *M. eversmannii* are occasionally reported to hybridize where they overlap in their distribution, the reality of a true species split has been debated, and several authors have at least considered whether *M. putorius*, *M. eversmannii*, and the endangered *Mustela nigripes* from North America (black-footed ferret) could be viewed as one Holarctic species.[13]

Regardless, in 1758 the domestic ferret was classified by Linnaeus as a separate genus and called *Mustela furo*. At that time it was believed that the steppe polecat was the most closely related to the domestic ferret. In 1970, through the examination of external chromosome shape, it was determined that the European polecat was closer to the domestic ferret than the steppe polecat. When this evidence came to light it was decided *M. putorius* and the domestic ferret were one and the same species, and the domestic ferret was then renamed *M. putorius furo* to distinguish it from the polecat.[5]

In 1998 Davison and co-workers[13] used mitochondrial DNA sequencing to investigate polecat genetic diversity in Britain. Molecular genetics, however, did not resolve whether ferrets were originally domesticated from *M. putorius* or *M. eversmannii*. The degree of nuclear introgression* of domestic ferrets and polecats may be so extensive as to rule out ever tracing their wild ancestors.

It must be emphasized that the behavior of domesticated animals in captivity differs from that of tamed wild animals and that these behavioral differences have arisen as a result of selection by humans.[5] The exact form taken by such selection will, however, depend on the role of the particular domesticated animal in relation to people. Behaviorally there are major differences between domestic ferrets and the ancestral polecat.

---

*Introgression: The introduction of a new gene or genes into a population by crossing between two populations and following with repeated back-crossings to that population while retaining the new gene(s).

Polecats tend to be solitary and very territorial with fighting between males having been observed, presumably over territory and sexual domain. The domestic ferret on the other hand is very social and gregarious, enjoying play activities with conspecifics and preferring to sleep with other ferrets of the same or opposite sex.

The polecat is quick, nervous, and easily frightened and will show fear of people if left with the mother during the critical period of $7\frac{1}{2}$ to $8\frac{1}{2}$ weeks of age.[34] The domestic ferret, however, was initially kept as a pest destroyer, normally raised in confinement and liberated to the field in order to hunt the intended prey. Therefore these ferrets were raised to be easily handled and could not be nervous or fearful of humans. Further resemblance and disparities between the domestic ferret and the wild polecat will be made in other sections of this chapter as we investigate the behavior of today's pet ferret.

Sensory Behaviors

Vision and Behavior

Being domesticated from a crepuscular species, ferrets possess a tapetum lucidum, which allows for more effective vision at low levels of light. They do not see well in pitch dark and have difficulty adjusting to bright light. This means that a ferret must be allowed to adjust to the light and become fully awake before it is removed from under a blanket or from a cozy spot where it is sleeping, or the handler risks being bitten.

Ferrets have binocular vision, and although they can swivel their eyes to look at different objects, most ferrets look forward and turn their heads to see things to the side. The pupil is horizontally slit, which is common in species that chase prey with gaits characterized by a hopping motion[39] and explains the ferret's fascination with a bouncing ball. Ferrets have very good visual acuity at close range, which is important because the ferret uses varying body language and visual displays to communicate.[28] They see less detail at greater distances and as a result pay more attention to complex visual stimuli such as moving objects.

Hearing and Behavior

The ear canals of a ferret do not open until approximately 32 days postnatally (as compared with 6 days in a cat), which coincides with the appearance of a startle response to loud hand claps and the recording of acoustically activated neurons in the midbrain (Figure 4-2).[31] This late onset of hearing may explain why kits produce exceptionally loud, piercing sounds during the first 4 weeks of life. Lactating jills are tuned in to

Ferret Behavior

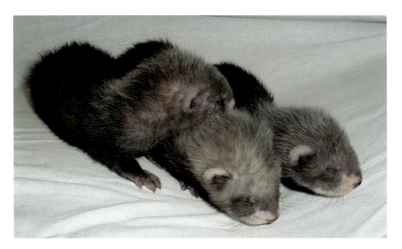

Figure 4-2
The ear canals of ferrets do not open until approximately 32 days postnatally, as compared with 6 days in cats. This late onset of hearing may explain why kits produce exceptionally loud, piercing sounds during their first 4 weeks of life. (Courtesy Peter Fisher.)

kit vocalizations and will respond to high-frequency (greater than 16 kHz) sounds in a maze test, whereas males and nonlactating females will ignore these sounds.[39] Adult ferrets hear best when sounds are within a range of 8 to 12 kHz.[39] This may explain why ferrets love squeaky toys, which produce sounds in this range.

Olfactory Behaviors

Kits of wild polecats have a critical period of learning the scent of prey (olfactory imprinting), which according to Apfelbach (1986) is between 60 and 90 days of age.[1] Except under duress, polecats will refuse to eat any prey whose smell they have not learned by that time.[39] As adults, they will actively search for prey with which they were familiarized during this critical time period and will ignore other prey or food smells. This may explain why certain ferrets will eat only one type of diet and why kits exposed to only one brand of food at 60 to 90 days of age may be opposed to dietary changes later in life. It is therefore recommended that young kits be offered a variety of foods during their first 6 months of life in order to prevent dietary selectivity or olfactory imprinting.

The sense of smell in ferrets is particularly keen. Wild mustelidae hunt down their prey using their sense of smell to home in on the quarry. During exploratory behavior the ferret spends a great deal of time with its nose to the ground investigating its environment. Objects placed directly in front of a ferret will be examined first by smelling, followed by visual or tactile inspection.

Communication Behaviors

Olfactory Communication

Polecats are a solitary species and leave marks throughout their home range by performing a repertoire of scent-marking actions that include wiping, body rubbing, and the anal drag (Figures 4-3 and 4-4).[10] Observations of ferrets in an outside enclosure revealed that anal drags were performed at latrines near den sites and at an equal frequency by males and females throughout the year.[10] Mustelidae also use urine for scent-marking and produce skin oils that are profoundly affected by circulating hormone levels. Hobs (male ferrets) in particular will produce intense seasonal skin oils that correspond to the increased testosterone levels associated with longer day lengths.

Ferret anal scent gland odors are sexually dimorphic, and studies have demonstrated that ferrets can use these variations as a communication tool.[11] Ferrets can distinguish between male and female anal sac odors, among strange, familiar, and their own odors, and between fresh and 1-day-old odors.[11] These results are consistent with both a sex attraction role and a territorial defense role for anal sac odors.

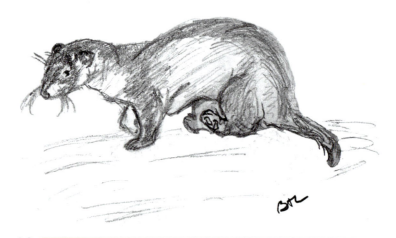

Figure 4-3

The anal drag. The domestic ferret defines its territory by marking behavior such as backing into corners to defecate and following with the anal drag, as illustrated here. (Illustration courtesy Barb Lynch.)

Ferret Behavior 169

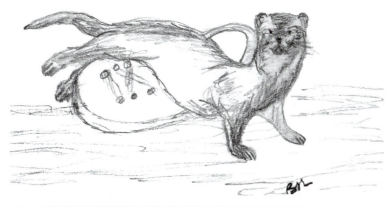

Figure 4-4

Wiping behavior. Domestic hobs possess preputial sebaceous glands that produce oils that they will wipe or mark on household items to communicate sexuality and territoriality. This behavior corresponds to the increased testosterone levels associated with longer day lengths. (Illustration courtesy Barb Lynch.)

Different messages are conveyed by the various marks. Kelliher and Baum[22] showed that in the ferret, olfactory detection and processing of volatile odors from conspecifics is required for heterosexual mate choice.[22] Males perform more body rubbing than females (jills), especially during the breeding season. Anal drags leave an olfactory signature of anal sac secretion for intersexual and intrasexual communication. Olfactory marking behavior also communicates territoriality and gives other ferrets knowledge of the marking ferret's sex and hormonal activity. Wiping and rubbing actions release the ferret's general body odor and may act as a threat signal in agonistic encounters.[10]

The response to olfactory stimuli and the scent-marking behavior of domestic ferrets is much less pronounced than that of their undomesticated counterparts. Domestic ferrets retain the actions of marking that are so important to their wild relatives.[39] The ferret thrives in the company of other ferrets; readily sharing living quarters, hammocks in which they sleep, food bowls, and water bottles. Despite this harmony, ferrets are still instinctively territorial and lay claim to smaller, albeit significant territories within their home environment. Like the wild polecat, domestic ferrets back up and defecate on objects or certain areas (and some even anal drag after defecation) in order to mark their territory. The domestic ferret tends to choose corners in which to defecate that may represent territory perimeters.

When it comes to the postdefecation anal drag, operators of ferret shelters will note that this behavior will increase in some ferrets when a new ferret is introduced to the household or when ferrets become more seasonally hormonal.[25] This innate behavior occurs even in ferrets that are surgically descented (anal sacculectomy), as the ferret is unaware of its missing anatomy. Ferrets also possess perianal sebaceous glands that secrete oils used in scent-marking. The strength of the scent from these glands is reduced in neutered males.

Worth mentioning is the way in which ferrets use their sense of smell in meet-and-greet behavior. When ferrets are introduced they will often sniff each other's anal area and neck and shoulder region (Figure 4-5). This behavior may give a domestic ferret information about the other ferret's sex and hormonal status. This activity may be the domestic ferret's equivalent of the behavior in the wild counterpart by which sexual receptivity is assessed.

Vocalizations

Although quiet most of the time, domestic ferrets do make a variety of vocalizations with which they communicate. In order to determine the meaning of ferret sounds, Shimbo[39] recorded waveforms and sound spectrographs of various domestic ferret vocalizations. Interpretation of these

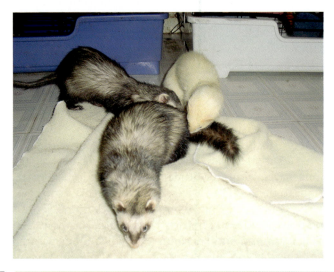

Figure 4-5

Meet-and-greet behavior. When ferrets are introduced, they will often sniff each other's anal area and the neck or shoulder region. This behavior may give the domestic ferret information about the other ferret's sex and hormonal status. (Courtesy Laura Powers.)

auditory studies led to several generalizations such as an increase in tonality on a basic signal indicates heightened excitement, a rising inflection indicates urgency, and a rising pitch of a string of sounds indicates displeasure.[39] Any one or more of these alterations in inflection can be superimposed on any vocalization to alter its meaning. The following are descriptions and the interpretive significance of the most common ferret vocalizations as recognized by many ferret owners.

Dook

Also know as chuckling or "the buck," the dook is the most commonly used ferret vocalization. This vocal signal can be low- or high-pitched and is usually strung together in a series of chortles or chucks in undulating pitches. The dook usually signifies happiness or excitement and is commonly expressed during play and exploratory behavior. The greater the excitement level is, the louder are the intensity and volume.

Hiss

The ferret and most other mustelidae use a hissing sound to convey anger and frustration, but it can also denote fear or be used as a warning signal. It can be a short burst that warns a playing partner, "Hey, that hurt, back off a little," or serves as a fear response, forewarning that "my guard is up, be careful." Prolonged hissing usually indicates frustration.

Scream

A high-pitched screech is used when a ferret is startled, frightened, or in pain. When cornered by another animal, ferrets may scream to startle their opponent and thereby gain escape. Prolonged screaming is an indication that something is seriously wrong and may occur when a ferret is in intense pain; such screaming has also been reported to occur during seizures.[6] All cases of continual or recurrent screaming warrant a medical workup.

Bark

An unusual loud chirp may occur as a defensive vocalization when a ferret is frightened or very excited. Some ferrets bark when they are angry. It is usually easy to discern a happy, curious ferret vocalization from one indicating anger, fear, or extreme pain. Be aware that an apprehensive or distressed ferret may bite, and use appropriate caution with ferrets that are using these verbal signals.

Visual

Ferrets also use body language and a variety of visual displays to communicate moods and feelings. They prefer to follow and attack prey moving

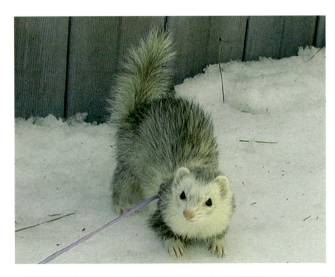

Figure 4-6
Bottle brush tail. Piloerection in the form of a frizzed-out tail may be a sign of anger or excitement, either fearful or joyous. During a display of anger the puffed tail is usually accompanied by an arched back and a vocal hiss or screech. If the display represents excitement and joy, the tail may fuzz out and flick back and forth. (Courtesy Lisa Leidig.)

at a velocity close to the escape speed of a mouse.[45] This may help to explain their fascination with bouncing balls, toys pulled along the ground in front of them, and in general anything that moves. During exploration the inquisitive ferret will periodically demonstrate scouting behavior in the form of erect or alert posturing. This attention response is similar to (and probably stems from) actions shown by the European polecat while investigating unfamiliar surroundings. During this response the neck is raised, the head is held at 90 degrees to the body, the ears are pricked, and the vibrissae are extended.[39]

Piloerection in the form of a frizzed-out tail may be a sign of anger or excitement, either fearful or joyous (Figure 4-6). During a display of anger, the puffed tail is usually accompanied by an arched back and a vocal hiss or screech. If the display represents excitement and joy, the tail may fuzz out and flick back and forth. Piloerection of the tail may also be noted during an anaphylactic reaction such as that seen with a vaccine reaction.

Locomotor Behaviors and Activity

Normal locomotion in a ferret consists of alternating movements of all four feet, although a ferret can be seen to hop or gallop with the rear legs when running or at play. Many repeatable locomotor patterns can be noted that tell us the ferret is a happy, playful pet; these activities have been described and nicknamed by ferret owners.[37] For example, the "dance of joy" or the "weasel war dance" is exhibited by the ferret that is happy and excited. The animated ferret tries to go in several directions at once; dancing from side-to-side, hopping forward, twisting back, flipping and rolling on the floor—all at an energetic pace. There seems to be no apparent reason for this dance other than pure joy and happiness.

The "alligator roll" is a form of intense play or wrestling between two ferrets where one ferret grabs the other by the back of the neck and flips him upside down. Some feel this is a way for one ferret to show dominance.[6] Because wild ferrets are solitary, any form of social hierarchy would be a reflection of domestication and the housing of multiple unrelated ferrets in close captivity. It is obvious that ferrets are energetic, fun-loving animals. As a result of this high energy, ferrets need ample play time (preferably up to 2 hours per day) and benefit greatly from environmental enrichment.

In addition to the "dance of joy" and the "alligator roll" already discussed, play behavior may include other visual displays. During periods of intense play ferrets may suddenly stop, fall to the ground, and slump, with body flattened, eyes open, and back legs splayed. This usually indicates the ferret is worn out and is taking a short break. In a few minutes the ferret will usually engage the rear legs and inch forward by pushing with the hind feet only. Once rested or if teased by a playmate into resuming the fun, the ferret will jump up and again engage in full-blown play behavior. This slumping may stem from the silent stalking of polecat predatory-attack behavior in which the body is held close to the ground. The actual predatory attack in which the ferret springs forward may be elicited by any rapid movement, which initiates a preprogrammed electrical brain stimulation. Therefore further romping on the part of the domestic ferret play partner initiates a return-to-play assault by the "slumping" ferret.

Elimination Behaviors

Because of their high metabolic rate, short gastrointestinal tract, and gastrointestinal transit time of about 3 hours, ferrets defecate frequently and can mark the corners of their cages, much to the aggravation of the conscientious owner who keeps a clean litter box available at all times. It should be stressed that clean to the ferret often means unused, as many ferrets will avoid a litter box that has been soiled only once. Before defecating and urinating, ferrets will usually briefly explore their cage environment in order to find a suitable location in which to void. Most ferrets choose one or two corners within the cage as the favorite location.

Once satisfied with the spot, the ferret will turn around, back into the corner, and, with back slightly arched and tail raised directly over the back, defecate using slight pulsing contractions of the abdomen. Ferrets do not bury their stool but will at times perform a postdefecation anal drag in which they scoot their anus along the floor for a few seconds. When urinating the ferret behaves similarly to find the appropriate site, it then squats with the rear legs spread slightly apart. The urination posture of both males and females is similar, with the only difference being that females squat slightly lower. Ferrets have an innate love for digging, and a clean litter box is a perfect setting for digging and play behavior, often resulting in an unused, tipped-over litter box. See Box 4-1 for litter box tips.

Urine Licking Behaviors

It is not uncommon for ferret owners to report that their ferret licks or drinks its own or a cagemate's urine. Physical examinations and health workups including complete blood count, chemistry panel, and urinalysis are usually unremarkable. It is possible that this behavior stems from the behavior of polecat hobs, which sometimes groom themselves with their own urine to make themselves more desirable to jills.

Reproductive Behaviors

Ferrets usually reach sexual maturity at 8 to 12 months of age. Most reproductive behavior in the pet ferret is suppressed because of surgical sterilization and exposure to artificial, indoor lighting for consistent periods of time averaging 15 hours per day. Knowledge of normal reproductive behavior is important when interpreting certain ferret play and aggressive behaviors as well as understanding the behavioral and physiologic changes associated with adrenal disease.

Researchers have shown that both estrogen and testosterone contribute to masculine sexual behavior in male ferrets[8] and female ferrets.[41] Ferret hormonal activity is strongly influenced by endogenous circadian rhythms, which persist under conditions of constant light and constant darkness. However, these circadian rhythms are usually influenced by external factors such as light, temperature, barometric pressure, and hormones.[20] Of these factors the most important is light, and ferret sexual behavior becomes more evident as natural day lengths increase. As day lengths increase, circulating melatonin levels diminish and hypothalamic gonadotropin-releasing hormone (GnRH) is released in a pulsatile fashion, in turn resulting in the release of pituitary luteinizing hormone (LH) and follicle-stimulating hormone (FSH), which stimulate the release of

BOX 4-1 Litter Box Tips

- Spend some time observing your ferret's habits in the cage. When it backs into a cage corner to relieve itself, pick it up and place it in the corner of the litter box.
- Provide a large litter box that takes up most of the bottom of the cage. This is more likely to encourage use of the box. Punch holes in the litter box and wire it to the cage walls so that it can't be tipped over.
- Offer praise and food treats when your ferret uses the box.
- To discourage digging use newspaper strips in the litter box, and slowly add a little bit of litter. Over a week or more gradually add more litter and less newspaper. Most ferrets learn not to play in the litter fairly quickly. Newspaper doesn't deter odors, so it needs to be changed often.
- Buy a ferret-friendly litter box with one low side and a guard on the higher sides to prevent the ferret from backing up far enough to miss the box.
- Clean soiled corners, inside or outside the cage, with an appropriate pet odor neutralizer such as Urine-Off or Eliminodor.
- Provide litter boxes in corners of rooms ferrets are allowed to explore. More than one litter box is ideal. If your ferret seems to prefer a certain corner, place the litter box there.
- Ferrets do not bury their stool as cats do; therefore only a shallow layer of litter to cover the bottom of the litter box is needed. Avoid fine clumping litters as they are messy and dusty, potentially resulting in respiratory problems.
- Recycled newspaper litter or plain clay litter are good choices. Avoid scented litters, as ferrets may avoid them.
- Change the litter box(es) often to encourage use.
- Most ferrets won't soil their beds or food bowls. Place bedding or food dishes in all non–litter box corners of the cage. Bedding that has been slept in and retains the ferret's body scent works best.
- Before out-of-the-cage play, place your ferret in the cage's *clean* litter box. Continue to place it in the box until it urinates or defecates, then reward it with play.

estrogen and testosterone from the gonads.[38] This results in an increase in sexual activity and interest.

Male Reproductive Behaviors

The onset of puberty in hobs is denoted by development of male sexual behaviors such as showing more interest in jills and the introduction of neck gripping and pelvic thrusting into their play behavior. If exposed only to natural lighting, the hob will become reproductively active a full

1 to 2 months before the jill.[18] A testosterone surge will result in reproductive behaviors associated with attracting the opposite sex and protecting territory.

Hobs in rut will be more aggressive and will scent-mark in order to get the message across to potential breeding partners that they are ready to mate. Male ferrets have preputial gland secretions that they will wipe on objects by dragging their bellies across the ground. Perianal scent glands are also used for scent-marking by dragging the anus or scooting across the ground (anal drag). Numerous dermal sebaceous glands, most prominent at the nape of the neck, are used by rubbing and rolling onto inanimate objects hobs wish to mark. Males have more sebaceous glands than females, and glandular production appears to be under androgenic control.[32] In a natural setting all these reproductive behaviors would allow multiple polecat hobs to stake their territory and fight off any potential competitive male suitors so that by the time the jill becomes sexually receptive they can get down to the business of breeding.

During the mount, the male grabs the nape of the jill's neck with his teeth and will grip her body by wrapping his forelegs around her ribcage. Pelvic thrusts last variable lengths of time up to 3 minutes. Between pelvic thrust bursts are periods of rest during which the male simply lies over the female and holds on with the neck grip. At the point of penetration the male will increase the arch of his back anteriorly, causing his foreleg grip to slip behind the female's rib cage.[30] Holding this position for a variable but usually prolonged period of time is the best interpretation of penetration, at which time pelvic thrusting ceases. Occasionally the male will tense his pelvis, causing the tail to raise for short periods of time. At this time the female will occasionally flinch or remain flaccid.[30]

Variable mating times from 120 minutes to 3 hours have been reported, but in one study mating times recorded in 10 pairs of ferrets lasted from 34 to 172 minutes.[30] These prolonged intromissions appear necessary in order to ensure fertilization. Whether this is to allow for increased sperm deposition as a result of the multiple ejaculations of the male or if it is necessary to stimulate the LH surge and subsequent ovulation in the female is open to debate. Neutered males with adrenal gland disease may display sexual behavior because of production of testosterone by the abnormal glands (see the discussion of adrenal disease).

Female Reproductive Behaviors

Behavioral changes associated with rising estrogen levels and puberty in the female ferret are less pronounced. Some jills may show evidence of being more excitable and nervous, whereas most show no behavioral changes at all. Wheel-running activity was shown to increase during estrus, with the number of wheel revolutions being doubled or tripled as compared with totals in ovariohysterectomized or anestrus ferrets.[14] With the onset of full estrus, food intake may decrease and jills may sleep less and become irritable.[18] Before onset of full estrus, jills will be unresponsive to the advances of a hob in rut. There will be a good bit of anal, genital, and neck sniffing, nose poking, and attempts by the male to grab the female by the neck, but the jill will ignore this behavioral foreplay or when tired of it hiss and nip or attack the male.

Dramatic edematous vulvar swelling in response to estrogen secretion by the ovaries is a clear signal that full estrus has occurred. At this time the jill will demonstrate the above behaviors but with more noise and intensity. These reproductive behaviors are very similar to those in other mammalian species, with much sniffing, genitalia display, and play fighting. When ready to breed, the female becomes flaccid and submissive, and mounting by the hob is allowed.

Being an induced ovulator, the jill will remain in estrus for extended periods if not bred. If breeding does not occur, the vulvar tissue will remain swollen, and hyperestrinism can cause severe anemia that will not abate until ovariohysterectomy or hormonal treatment is instituted. Adrenal disease may also cause a swollen vulva as a result of androgens being oversecreted by the adrenals. Remnants of ovarian tissue may also cause hyperestrinism.

Social and Antisocial Behaviors

As a general rule, patterns of behavior and social relationships are developed through learning as well as heredity, and social animal groups are organized by social status, territoriality, and reproductive activities. The interplay of experience and innate* factors in the development of behavior is very subtle and can be difficult to separate.[16]

European polecat kits are dependent on their mothers to bring them meat meals from the time they are weaned at 6 to 8 weeks to the time they begin to hunt on their own at 10 weeks of age. During this preweaning time kits have been observed to interact socially and play.[24] However, by the time they are 13 weeks old, a time when kits may leave their nests permanently and go out on their own, kits show various degrees of independence from one another.[24] Adult polecats are essentially solitary, with one study finding ferrets to share dens simultaneously with other ferrets on only 7.4% of 706 radio-tracking events.[36] Also, adult ferrets

---

*Innate behaviors are those that do not seem to require specific experiences (learning) for their expression.

demonstrate intrasexual territoriality, with dominant males showing more spatial overlap with females than with subordinate males.[29]

The domesticated ferret, on the other hand, shows much more diurnal activity, and many can be kept in pairs or groups without conflict. The best explanation for the difference in socialization patterns is that familiarization and habituation* play a significant role in the ferret's social response to both man and conspecifics. Familiarization in the form of imprinting may be involved as young polecats removed from their mothers during this critical phase in their development (4 to 10 weeks) become imprinted on their human caretakers. Evidence to support this belief is the fact that young polecats follow their mother on foraging expeditions and that hand-reared ferrets readily follow a human being. It has also been shown that the presence of the mother appears to facilitate the development of fear of humans in the young.[34] In captivity, however, fear of humans does not develop in wild polecats if they are removed from their mother at any time before the second day after their eyes have opened (typically 28 to 34 days).[34] Socialized ferrets are also more likely to show habituation than isolated ferrets,[9] demonstrating that socialization and domestication go hand in hand. Pet ferrets acclimate to their environment and will rise to the occasion when given an opportunity to play, explore, or interact with others. In other words, they become diurnal as their periods of activity coincide with that of their human household.

Most ferrets enter the pet trade at any time from 6 to 10 weeks of age. In the United States most pet ferrets come from a few large commercial breeding farms and therefore are exposed to other ferrets and humans from the time their eyes open. From the above data, and from observing domestic ferrets and their obvious agreeable nature with both humans and cagemates, it seems safe to assume that ferrets, like dogs, do have a critical period of socialization. This period occurs between the time their eyes open at 4 weeks of age to 10 weeks.

Through their observations, most ferret researchers and multiple ferret owners believe that ferrets do not form any kind of social hierarchy and that positioning for dominance does not occur. Nevertheless, ferrets will fight occasionally, especially when exposed to an unfamiliar ferret. Some ferret rescue workers have recommended placing Ferretone on the necks and scruffs of all ferrets being introduced to an unfamiliar ferret. Ferrets consistently like this oily supplement and will likely lick each other in an appropriate manner while being less likely to demonstrate aggression.

---

*Habituation is a decreased response to new objects and environments resulting from prolonged or repeated exposure.

Pet ferrets readily show affection for their human owners through gleeful greeting behavior and willingness to shower owners with ferret kisses. Young ferrets, on the other hand, are not likely to enjoy quiet cuddle time. Their exploratory behavior creates too strong an urge to get off an owner's lap and move on to investigate the environment around them. As ferrets mature, a combination of age, improved socialization, and a decrease in exploratory behavior results in a more staid ferret that enjoys periods of quiet snuggling and petting.

Ferrets have been domesticated for over 2000 years; therefore it seems likely that given the right environment, poorly socialized ferrets can become more affable and gregarious. This suggestion is supported by the fact that intact hobs kept together in a colony situation with minimal human handling can live in harmony outside the breeding season.

Grooming Behaviors

Ferrets will groom their fur through licking and gentle nibbling motions. They normally maintain a smooth and shiny hair coat as long as they are kept on a balanced diet made up primarily of high-quality animal protein and fat. Ferrets have also been known to groom other ferrets to which they are bonded. This grooming is usually around a cagemate's ears and head as the ferrets lie side by side.

Normal ferret skin is smooth and pale without evidence of flaking, scabs, or inflammation. A dry, dull fur coat and evidence of flaking may be a reflection of poor diet or low environmental humidity. In the wild ferrets spend a good part of the day in underground burrows in which the humidity is high and the temperature a consistent 55°F (13°C). The dry warmth of many homes during the winter months may cause the skin to dehydrate, with subsequent flaking and itching. Pruritus may also be a sign of external parasites or adrenal disease.

A ferret's hair coat has a thick cream-colored undercoat covered by longer, coarse guard hairs. It is the color of these guard hairs that defines the various ferret coat colorations—from dark and light sable to cinnamon, silver, or white. Both intact and neutered ferrets undergo a hormonally influenced molt, usually twice a year, in which the hair coat thins in response to photoperiod. As daylight hours and environmental temperatures increase, corresponding with late spring in the Northern Hemisphere as well as ferret breeding season, ferrets may lose most of their guard hairs over a period of several weeks. Ferrets can get trichobezoars from grooming, which can get large enough to cause gastric obstruction or irritation (Figure 4-7). Therefore the use of a hairball remedy in the form of a feline petroleum-based laxative is especially important during this seasonal molt.

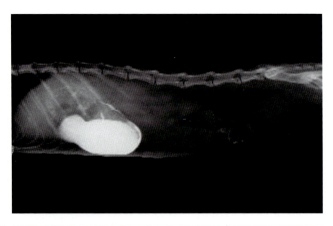

Figure 4-7
This lateral abdominal radiograph was taken 90 minutes after the ferret was given barium. The ferret had a trichobezoar causing a gastric blockage secondary to grooming during molt. As daylight hours and environmental temperatures increase, corresponding with late spring in the Northern Hemisphere and the ferret breeding season, ferrets may lose most of their guard hairs over a period of several weeks. The use of a hairball remedy in the form of a feline petroleum-based laxative is especially important during this seasonal molt. (Courtesy Peter Fisher.)

The skin of the ferret contains numerous sebaceous glands, the secretions of which give the ferret its characteristic musky odor.[32] These secretions also are strongly influenced by seasonal hormonal influences, especially in the male, and may give the coat a greasy feel and an obvious yellow to orange appearance most noticeable over the dorsal shoulder area. In the Northern Hemisphere these secretions are observable in the late spring to early summer, corresponding with the ferret's natural breeding season. If this coat discoloration and increased odor are particularly evident and do not diminish with time, they may be signs of adrenal disease, especially in the male ferret. If associated with adrenal disease, loss of guard hairs may occur concurrently, and areas of obvious alopecia may develop, as well as other systemic signs discussed elsewhere. During this time ferrets may also show increased scent-marking behavior and will rub their backs and shoulders along carpet and furniture to the dismay of odor-conscious owners. Cage walls and bedding readily take on the yellow color and musky odor of these sebaceous secretions.

Feeding Behaviors

The ferret is an obligate carnivore with a short intestinal tract that lacks a cecum and ileocolic valve. The small intestine is approximately five times longer than the ferret's body, and the mean gastrointestinal transit time of food passage from stomach to rectum is 182 minutes.[3] This rapid transit time, along with the ferret's lack of intestinal brush border enzymes, especially lactase, contributes to inefficiency in absorption. As a result, they are less able than cats to absorb sufficient calories from carbohydrates. To compensate for the inefficiency of its digestive tract, the ferret requires a concentrated diet, high in protein and fat and low in fiber.

Ferrets snack and eat multiple small meals throughout the day, and unless regularly fed very high–fat content foods they generally eat as much as they want without becoming obese. Ferrets normally increase food intake approximately 30% in the winter and gain weight by depositing subcutaneous fat. This will reverse as daylight lengthens in the spring. For maintenance, ferrets may consume 200 to 300 kcal/kg body weight daily. Daily food consumption averages 42 g (1.5 oz) and 49 g (1.7 oz) dry matter per kg body weight for male and female ferrets, respectively.[4]

Ferrets are solitary feeders that when allowed free access to food will eat 9 or 10 meals per day, which is true of most species when food is available ad libitum. In laboratory studies in which ferrets had to perform a task (bar press) to gain access to food, it was shown that meal frequency declined.[21] There was a corresponding increase in meal size, allowing the ferrets to maintain a relatively constant total daily food intake sufficient to maintain normal growth and body weight.

These shifts in feeding patterns in response to increased work needed to procure a meal are similar to those in other species and are consistent with an ecologic analysis of foraging behavior.[21] Generally, socially feeding animals increase procurement and consumption rates as food availability decreases, whereas solitary feeders, such as cats and ferrets, do not.[27] This study demonstrates that ferrets could be maintained on meals fed once or twice daily versus a free-feeding situation. Many ferret owners like to offer raisins or other simple carbohydrates as treats, but these high-sugar treats are difficult for the ferret's gastrointestinal tract to digest and may be contraindicated because of the prevalence of insulinoma in ferrets. Instead, small pieces of cooked chicken, Totally Ferret, or N-Bones treats may be offered.

Prey-Catching Behaviors

The predatory behavior of ferrets consists mainly of instinctive behavior patterns that are elicited by external stimuli. In all higher animals a sudden change or stimulation will usually elicit a movement toward the source—a response described as the *orientation response*. The learning of an orientational component plays an important role in the development of functional sequences of behavior. Eibl-Eibesfeldt observed the prey-catching techniques of polecats and found that the normal movements of pursuit, grasping the neck of the prey, shaking it, and turning it over on its back occur the first time an appropriate object is presented.[19] After several experiences the neck bite becomes properly oriented for quick killing of prey. More recently, similar behavior was demonstrated in the black-footed ferret in which maturation, experience, and greater environmental complexity (enriched cage, including encouragement of food-searching behaviors) all increased the likelihood of the ferret's making a successful kill.[44]

This behavior becomes important when the domestic ferret is kept in a household with other exotic pets that it may perceive as prey. It is at this time that the ferret may cross the line from play behavior to prey-catching behavior. Both behaviors can look similar initially, as ferrets at play also demonstrate neck biting, but if stimulated by a perceived prey species (pet bird, lizard, or rodent) the ferret may instinctively go beyond play and inflict harmful or fatal bite wounds on the other pet. Therefore, ferrets should not be left unsupervised with other small exotic pets.

Apfelbach showed that for the ferret the time needed to catch and kill rats depended on the size of the rats in relation to the ferret. Killing success decreases with a relative increase in prey size.[2] This may explain why the domestic ferret tends to live harmoniously in a home with dogs and cats. These larger species do not stimulate instinctive prey catching and killing behavior, but instead the response to the larger animal takes the form of the less-intense, albeit similar, play behavior.

Exploratory Behaviors

A number of investigations have demonstrated the existence in mammals of behavior not motivated by fear, thirst, or hunger and unrelated to general activity level. These have led to postulation of another drive, the exploratory drive.[15] Characteristically, such behavior is aroused by novel external stimulation. It involves either locomotor activity or manipulation of objects, and it declines as a function of time.[15] In general, higher animals will approach and examine strange objects with whatever sensory equipment is available to them, and in a strange environment they usually move around and examine all of their surroundings.

When an animal is exposed to a novel object or environment it will first familiarize itself with the new stimulus or situation. With a strange object, exploration must precede play. As familiarity increases the exploratory behavior decreases and the animal's curiosity of the novelty may with time lead to play behavior. With other new situations fear may lead to rejection instead of exploration. Whether fear or curiosity and subsequent play behavior are elicited depends on various factors, including the physiologic state of the individual animal and the magnitude, intensity, or strangeness of the eliciting stimulus. In general, a small change in the environment elicits investigation, whereas a major change may elicit fear.

Degree of domestication can also affect exploration behavior. In his work on identifying behavioral differences between the domesticated ferret and its wild counterpart, the European polecat, Poole (1972) showed that wild ferrets are less likely to examine and more likely to avoid strange objects than tame ferrets.[34] In this study attention responsiveness to new auditory stimuli was measured, and exploration of new surroundings was observed. The attention response is essentially a method of scanning for stimuli. The European polecat shows extreme caution in exploring an unfamiliar environment; it takes frequent cover, uses definite pathways in the immediate vicinity of its den, and regularly returns to its home area after making forays into unfamiliar territory. The polecat also shows a more rapidly diminished attention response to auditory stimuli.

The domestic ferret, on the other hand, can be moved to a strange cage or placed in an unfamiliar area without showing signs of fear or disorientation. The ferret also shows persistent response to repeated auditory stimuli, a feature that might also be related to the reactivity typical of a juvenile animal. These results again appear to support Lorenz's view that domesticated animals show more juvenile behavior as compared with their wild counterparts.[19] Ehrlich's work with the black-footed ferret[15] demonstrated similar findings: increased handling (equivalent to greater degree of domestication) leads to increased exploration behavior. Those findings may explain why today's domestic ferret shows an intense curiosity and little fear of its surroundings. When allowed to roam, the domestic ferret shows fearless exploratory behavior: Box on the floor? Got to see what's in it. Hole in the floorboard by dishwasher? Got to go inside and explore. Cabinet door ajar? Got to open it and explore what's inside. Any open door or unexplored space is an invitation for scrutiny.

The domestication process has been thorough at removing the ferret's fear response when it comes to exploratory behavior, and the ferret's inquisitive nature and love of exploration are boundless, sometimes to its detriment. As a result of being continuously handled and carried securely without being dropped, or perhaps because of its reportedly poor eyesight, domestic ferrets show little fear of height. This is opposite to what Shimbo[39] found in her personal experience with undomesticated polecats, which appeared very frightened and uneasy when exposed to heights.[39] This apparent lack of fear of heights in the domestic ferret can result in injuries or death if they climb out of an upstairs or apartment window. An open door may also be addressed with fearless curiosity, and the urge to explore can lead the ferret to the outdoors where it is limited in its ability to find food and to protect itself from predators or from extremes of weather.

Play Behaviors

Reflecting on the 1953 Lorenz hypothesis that the behavior of domestic animals resembles that of juvenile individuals of their wild counterparts,[19] it can certainly be said that this holds true when it comes to play behavior. In general, motor patterns used in intraspecies play behavior are characterized by actions that occur frequently in other functional contexts (e.g., aggression, sexual, and predatory behaviors).

In 1966 Poole observed polecats *(Putorius putorius)* at play and demonstrated the incomplete sequence of conflict behavior. Four of the agonistic patterns were absent from intense play behavior—two extreme forms of attack ("sustained neck biting" and "sideways attack") and two extreme fear patterns ("defensive threat" and "screaming").[19] The play behavior imitated patterns of aggression, but in a less-serious and less-threatening manner. Adolescent ferrets' play behavior also imitates sexual behavior, with juvenile male ferrets exhibiting higher levels of neck biting and "stand-over" behavior than females (Figure 4-8). Sex differences in the expression of prepubertal play behavior of ferrets apparently result from the differential exposure of males and females to androgen during the postnatal period.[42]

The same holds true for the domestic ferret. The ferret demonstrates an obvious love of play in a variety of forms, and we can imagine their mer-

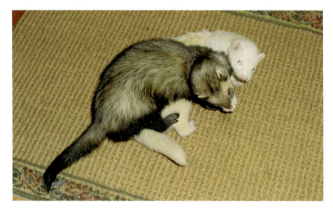

Figure 4-8
Mounting play behavior. Adolescent ferrets' play behavior also imitates sexual behavior, with juvenile male ferrets exhibiting higher levels of neck biting and "stand-over" behavior than females. Sex differences in the expression of prepubertal play behavior of ferrets apparently result from the differential exposure of males and females to androgen during the postnatal period. (Courtesy Peter Fisher.)

riment stemming from predatory, sexual, exploratory, and digging behaviors. The typical sequence for two ferrets at play would begin with the chase, followed by an exaggerated approach or ambush, veering off, and reciprocal chasing, followed by mounting, rolling, and wrestling with inhibited neck biting (Figure 4-9). These mock sexual and predatory behaviors are accompanied by vocalizations that signal both excitement (dooking) and anger (hissing).

The solitary ferret at play also demonstrates various behaviors that stem from normal behaviors seen in its wild counterpart. Predators stalk and chase quarry. Observe the ferret playing with a hard rubber ball or squeaky toy, and you will see the same type of behaviors. Hard rubber balls, such as Super Balls, really stimulate hunt and capture behavior. A rolling or bouncing ball captivates the ferret, which immediately begins the hunt. The ball is aggressively pursued until the ferret "captures" it by grabbing it, then bites hard and shakes it as if it were prey. Keep in mind that ferrets love soft-rubber items and will readily ingest the torn pieces of soft rubber, creating potential for gastrointestinal foreign bodies (Figure 4-10). Therefore any ferret play ball needs to be hard enough and large enough

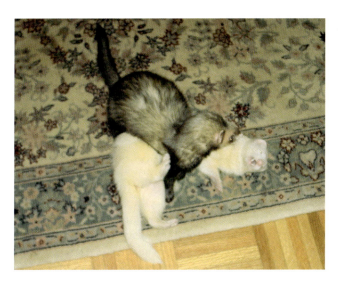

Figure 4-9
Neck-biting play behavior. The typical sequence for two ferrets at play would begin with the chase, followed by an exaggerated approach or ambush, veering off, and reciprocal chasing, followed by mounting, rolling, and wrestling with inhibited neck biting. These mock sexual and predatory behaviors may be accompanied by vocalizations that signal both excitement (dooking) and anger (hissing). (Courtesy Peter Fisher.)

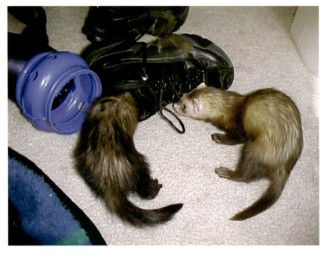

Figure 4-10
Ferrets, especially young ones, love to chew and will eat things that are inappropriate for them and may cause gastrointestinal obstruction. They are especially fond of plastic, rubber, and foam rubber (Courtesy Teresa Bradley Bays.)

that the ferret cannot readily tear off chunks that it might ingest (Figure 4-11).

Playing ferrets also love to dig. This digging behavior comes naturally, as the sharp claws and streamlined body of the polecat were designed for digging and tunneling deep underground in pursuit of game or for making their below-ground burrows. This ancestral behavior may explain why ferrets love to dig at the carpet, the floor, and their litter box and enjoy digging in the soil of potted plants. Some ferret owners satisfy this desire to dig by allowing the ferrets to dig away in a large plastic play box (such as a large cat litter box) filled two-thirds full with rice or potting soil. A neater option is to provide the ferret with tubing to explore. Both flexible (ribbed plastic similar to clothes dryer vent tubing) and rigid (PVC pipe) tubing make for great exploratory amusements.

Because of its keen olfactory sense the ferret explores with its nose. The ferret can be observed searching back and forth across a room with its nose to the ground. When it finds an object of interest, often the ferret will drag it off to its "lair," also known as "ferreting it away" (Figure 4-12). This ferret burrow is usually the most inaccessible location the ferret can find—a small cubby or a hole discovered under the kitchen cabinets or in the back of a closet. The ferret is instinctively seeking out a tight, dark, enclosed space, which mimics its native ancestor's underground burrow.

Ferret Behavior 187

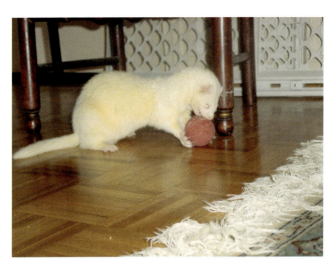

Figure 4-11
Rubber ball play. A rolling or bouncing ball captivates the ferret, which immediately begins the hunt. The ball is aggressively pursued until the ferret "captures" it by grabbing it, then bites hard and shakes it as if it were prey. (Courtesy Peter Fisher.)

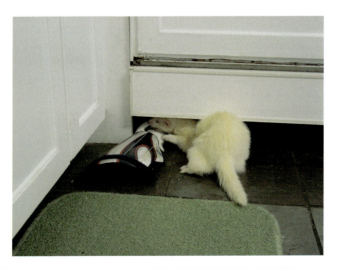

Figure 4-12
Hiding objects. When it finds an object of interest, often the ferret will drag it off to its "lair," also known as "ferreting it away." This ferret burrow is usually the most inaccessible location the ferret can find—a small cubby or a hole discovered under the kitchen cabinets or in the back of a closet. (Courtesy Peter Fisher.)

It is amazing to see the variety of objects the ferret has "stolen and stashed." This hoarding behavior probably stems, once again, from behaviors seen in polecats, which have a very high metabolic rate and energy need; therefore having a readily available food supply is a must. Instead of toys and objects of interest, polecats would build a cache of leftover food items and prey on which to feed while resting in their burrows.

Environmental Enrichment

Studies suggest that environmental impoverishment, whether in the form of physical or social restriction or limitation of play objects, has wide-ranging effects on the overall well-being of ferrets. Chivers and Einon[9] found that some of the isolation-induced effects on behavior seen in rats also occurred in ferrets, with deprivation of rough and tumble social play causing hyperactivity that persisted into adulthood.[23] Work done by Korhonen (1992) showed that overall health, reflected by optimum weight and fur coat quality, occurred when ferrets were provided with increased housing floor space and compatible cagemates and when offered balls and bite cups with which to play.[23]

Although adult ferrets may appear perfectly content sleeping in their hammocks 20 hours a day, this certainly is not mentally and physically stimulating. Unsupervised free time in a "ferret proof" room is always recommended. Keep in mind that ferrets love human interaction, like to explore new places and objects, have a keen olfactory sense, and enjoy digging. A ferret that jumps back and forth in front of you and nips at your feet is telling you it wants to play. Simply getting down on your hands and knees and chasing a ferret will stimulate more ferret dancing and happy vocalizations, chuckling, or dooking.

If the ferret is *not* prone to biting, try playing tug-of-war games with an old washcloth or favorite plush toy (Figure 4-13). If the ferret is other-ferret friendly, try taking it to a fellow ferret fancier's ferret-proofed home for some exposure to a whole new environment complete with sights, smells, and ferret friends. Transmissible diseases, especially the gastrointestinal infection likely caused by a coronavirus and commonly referred to as epizootic catarrhal enteritis (ECE), should be considered when allowing initial contact between ferrets.

Digging can be encouraged by hiding toys in a children's sandbox or in a litter box (Figure 4-14). Remember, however, to never leave ferrets unsupervised outdoors, as they tend to wander and may get lost. They are also relatively intolerant of extreme heat or cold.

Inactive ferrets are prone to weight gain and its subsequent effects on overall health. Constant captivity in an enclosed space may also lead to behavioral problems such as biting and conspecific aggression. It is the

Ferret Behavior 189

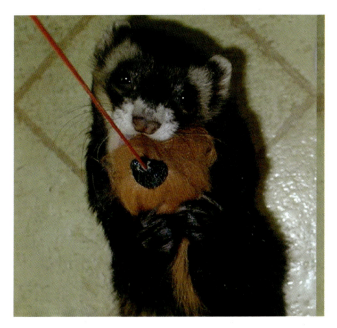

Figure 4-13
Environmental enrichment. Fuzzy plush toys on an elastic string make a great play toy that keeps the playful ferret entertained. Play with these types of toys should be supervised. (Courtesy Lisa Leidig.)

ferret owner's responsibility to ensure that this active, energetic pet's mental, physical, and sensory well-being is routinely stimulated so that it may lead a full and robust life. Not all activities require human interaction, nor do they require a big monetary investment. Many just require a little time, creativity, and imagination. Box 4-2 describes some activities created by ferret owners—suggestions for inexpensively creating a fun and stimulating ferret household environment.

Aggressive Behaviors

Conspecific Aggression

The primary function of aggressive behavior between conspecifics is to determine and maintain rank or territory. Aggressive actions are among the most prominent social activities of animals, with patterns of aggressive behavior differing from species to species. Although such actions often appear antisocial, the fighting, bluffing, and threatening serves to promote survival of the species. It appears that a species disposition to

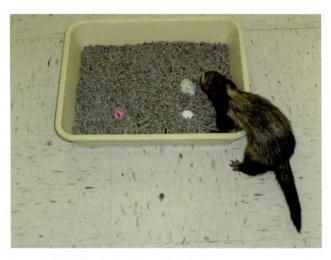

Figure 4-14
Environmental enrichment. Filling a large plastic litter box with recycled newspaper pellets or rice and hiding objects for the ferret to find helps satisfy their innate digging behavior. Ferrets that enjoy playing in their water bowls will also enjoy recreation in a small wading pool with added Ping-Pong balls coated with Ferretone. (Courtesy Peter Fisher.)

aggression is innate, but many details of the aggressive behavior are learned or perfected through experience.[12]

In most animals early social experience greatly affects subsequent aggressive behavior. True fighting behavior between domestic ferrets is similar to that described by Poole in his study of European polecats[33]—as an incident during which each animal attempted to bite the back of its opponent's neck with a sustained, immobilizing hold. Successful bites (i.e., those during which the opponent was unable to break free) were sometimes accompanied by shaking or dragging of the immobilized animal. When the attacked animal was able to break free, it sometimes displayed evidence of intimidation, including screaming, defensive biting, hissing, fleeing, urinating, or defecating. However, serious injury did not usually occur.[40]

Staton and Crowell-Davis[40] reported on the results of an experimental protocol to evaluate the effects of four factors on the fighting behavior between pairs of domestic ferrets: familiarity (pairings of cagemates versus strangers); time of year (pairings during winter versus spring); sex (male-male, male-female, and female-female pairings); and neutering status (intact-intact, neutered-intact, and neutered-neutered pairings).[40] Awareness of factors that might affect the potential for aggression between

BOX 4-2 Environmental Enrichment Ideas

- Use food as treats, with the following caveats. Keep in mind that ferrets are strict carnivores with high protein requirements. They use fats more so than carbohydrates for energy needs. However, excessive high-fat treats will result in the ferret's caloric needs being met with minimal food intake and as a result protein requirements may not be met. So if treating with high-fat oils such as Ferretone, remember to use them in small quantities.
  - Try rubbing a little Ferretone on Ping-Pong balls and floating them in a shallow pan of water.
  - Place a few pieces of food or desirable treat in an egg carton, tape the lid shut and cut a small hole in the top. Make the ferret work for the treat. The same idea can be used with a milk carton.
  - Place a few pieces of good-quality ferret food (try a different variety from its normal everyday food) in an 8-ounce (237 mL) plastic soft-drink bottle, leave the top off, and let the ferret roll and play with it trying to make the treats come out.
- Create handmade toys and amusement centers.
  - Make tunnels from PCV pipe or empty oatmeal containers with the bottoms cut out and taped end to end.
  - Tape cardboard boxes together, and cut holes in various locations for exploration.
  - Glue a small bell inside a plastic Easter egg.
  - Make a ferret maze out of a large appliance box. Fill the box with scrap cardboard rolled and taped into round or triangular tubes. Hide food items at various spots within the box.
- Fill a box with potting soil, rice, hay, plastic balls, or crumpled paper balls, and let the ferret fulfill its instinctive digging needs.
- Use old towels to give a ferret a "magic carpet ride," or just twirl the towel around and over the ferret.
- Use dryer hose to satisfy instinctive tunneling behavior. Some owners like to stretch the hose out, using a beanbag chair to hold one end in place.
- Obtain a bottle of deer or boar scent from the hunting section of a sporting goods store, and rub a drop or two on a favorite toy.
- Tie plastic or a Ping-Pong ball to a piece of sturdy string and hang it from the ceiling to 2 in (5 cm) above the ground.
- Put empty paper grocery bags on the floor. Some of the bags can be filled with crumpled paper, Ping-Pong balls, or food treats.

unfamiliar ferrets may predict likelihood of a fight. Results of the Staton and Crowell-Davis study suggest that familiarity, sex, and neutering status are all important determinantes of aggression between ferrets. Sixty percent of the attempts of pairing strangers resulted in combative behavior, whereas none of the familiar cagemates fought.

Based on previous information on aggressive behavior in intact male ferrets[33] and that shown in studies of other species, it was thought that intact male ferrets would, in general, be more aggressive than neutered animals. However, the study showed that intact male ferrets were not indiscriminantly aggressive and that pairs of neutered males were just as likely as pairs of intact males to fight. In addition, the study showed that females were in general not less aggressive than males, with pairings of unfamiliar neutered female ferrets likely to result in aggression. The study also showed that if unfamiliar neutered ferrets are introduced, the pairing of two males or a male and female would result in the lowest levels of aggression.

It is also interesting to note that time of year (winter versus spring) did not affect the incidence of fighting behavior, even for intact animals in which circulating hormone concentrations are likely to change with seasons. This may have been a result of the fact that animals in this study were housed under artificial lighting and that this amount of light was not altered to mimic the increase in daylight that stimulates the breeding season in ferrets. The fact that 60% of unfamiliar pairings did fight illustrates the difficulties faced by pet owners attempting to introduce a new ferret into the household or in ferret shelters in which new additions and limited space result in frequent pairings of strange ferrets.

Studies with kangaroo rats, pigs, and mice have shown that olfactory exposure, visual exposure, and sharing a common substrate may all play a key role in establishing familiarity between strangers and thus reduce fighting behavior.[40] A second part of the Staton and Crowell-Davis study showed that this was not the case with ferrets. Housing strange ferrets next to each other for 2 weeks where they shared visual and olfactory stimuli did not reduce fighting when the ferrets were later introduced. However, ferret owners claim that housing a new ferret next to an existing ferret or ferrets for a period of time before introduction does help. If introducing a female to a bonded male-female pair, experienced ferret owners advocate housing the new female with the male for a few days, as they are more likely to get along. If they get along, then putting all three together inside the original cage with additional sleeping arrangements can be tried. Make sure close supervision is provided during these introductory periods.

In addition, ferret shelter managers have found that a 4- to 5-day introductory period works best when familiarizing a new ferret to a multiple-ferret household. A small open room with a minimum of hiding areas and one that does not house other ferrets works best as a neutral meeting site. The new ferret member is introduced to the most congenial ferret in the household, usually an older, easygoing male, for 30 minutes of chaperoned meet-and-greet time. If the ferrets seem to get along, then the time together is extended. Once the new ferret has accepted the introductory ferret, other ferrets are slowly introduced to see if the new ferret is capable of cohabiting with the group. Ferrets are individuals, and this bonding procedure does not always work; some ferrets just prefer living alone.

Aggression and Biting Behaviors

Ferrets use their mouths in many behaviors, including play, attention seeking, defense, "hunting," fear, and response to pain. Watch young kits wrestle and play and you will see them bite each other's necks and drag each other around while grasping any loose skin with their mouths. Mother ferrets use their mouths to pick up and move their kits if they have wandered too far and to discipline them with gentle nips. Ferrets playing with a toy will usually pick it up, grab it, and drag it around with their mouths.

Inappropriate nipping or biting may occur when ferrets perceive people as playmates, as an attention-getting device, or when ferrets are in pain or hungry. Depending on the message they are trying to convey, ferrets may give a friendly nip or grab a human's hand or foot, bite down, hold on, and shake their heads. This is how they would respond to another ferret, whose naturally thick skin and fur would lessen the intensity of the bite. To humans, however, the bite can be both painful and alarming.

In ferrets with a history of consistent biting behavior, it is ideal to try to determine the cause. This begins with collecting a behavioral history and in problem cases having the owners fill out a behavioral questionnaire (Box 4-3). Once the type(s) of aggression and most probable causes for the aggression have been identified, the goal is to avoid situations that elicit the biting behavior and to diminish biting behavior if it occurs.

Box 4-4 summarizes the various causes of ferret aggression and potential situations in which biting behavior may occur. Recently purchased or adopted ferrets may be especially problematic, as they come with limited socialization, training, or handling. These (often young) ferrets may bite as a fear response to sudden movements and noise. This is probably a reflex response that stems from the ferret's wild counterparts who were preyed on by larger mammals or birds of prey. If frightened or startled the ferret may show a defense reaction much like the frightened submissive dog—it will arch the back and fluff out the tail and body fur (piloerection) to look larger and stronger, open the mouth in a threatening way, and hiss or

> **BOX 4-3 Behavioral Questionnaire for the Biting Ferret**
>
> - How long have you owned your ferret?
> - Are there certain situations that initiate the biting behavior?
> - Is this your first pet ferret?
> - Describe your ferret's environment?
> - Is there a new pet in the household?
> - Has the amount of "free time" and exercise your ferret gets recently changed?
> - Have there been any lifestyle changes that may be reflected in the ferret's behavior?
> - Have you experienced a recent move or change in living arrangements?
> - Have any new ferrets been brought into the household?
> - Do young children routinely handle your ferret?
> - What do you do when your ferret bites?
> - What forms of behavior modification have you tried? What is the response?
> - Are there situations or objects that stimulate biting behavior?
> - Do you smoke?
> - Do you apply hand cream to which the ferret may be attracted?

screech in order to frighten the perceived attacker or alarm other ferrets in the area. If not descented the ferret may empty or express its anal sacs, again much as a frightened dog would do. Depending on the level of socialization of the ferret, this fear response may also lead to biting.

It is best to try and prevent this defense response by letting the fearful ferret know your whereabouts and intentions when handling. To ensure that the ferret will not be startled, make noise outside the cage or rattle the cage door so they are aware of your presence, and when approaching talk in a soothing manner. If the ferret continues to appear fearful, give it time to adjust to your presence before handling, then use a towel to pick it up while talking to it quietly.

If a ferret is possessive of a particular toy, take away the guarded object, and discourage the ferret from obtaining objects that are off limits. If the problem persists, try redirecting the ferret's attention with an alternative activity such as ball chasing, or try desensitizing the possessive ferret with repeated relaxed exposures to the object or toy and reward with gentle praise or a treat when the ferret is not possessive. Be careful not to reinforce this behavior by offering another, possibly more acceptable toy while the ferret is nipping.

With fear-related or maternal aggression, avoid circumstances that might elicit aggression. It is important not to startle or grab fearful ferrets,

BOX 4-4   Causes of Ferret Aggression or Biting Behavior

- Play aggression—The most common underlying cause for biting in ferrets, this is a normal behavior, especially in young ferrets, that needs to be mitigated.
- Possessive aggression—Aggressive behavior directed at humans or other pets that approach the ferret when it is in possession of something it values, usually a favorite toy. May be exacerbated by restricting the ferret's free time and space.
- Fear-related aggression—Occurs when ferret is startled or poorly socialized and not used to handling. This type of aggression can occur as a result of punishment, traumatic experiences, or genetic factors.
- Predatory aggression—A normal innate behavior of the polecat from which the ferret was domesticated. When directed toward people or other pets it results in a behavioral problem that may involve stalking, chasing, grasping, and biting.
- Redirected aggression—Occurs when the harmful behavior is directed toward a person or pet that is not the original stimulus for the aggressive behavior. Occurs when a person or pet interferes with two ferrets that are playing hard.
- Maternal aggression—Refers to aggressive behavior directed toward humans or other pets that approach a jill with her kits.
- Pain-induced or irritable aggression—Caused by an underlying medical condition:
  - Gastrointestinal foreign body, hairball, gastric ulcers
  - Inflammatory bowel disease
  - Hormonal changes associated with adrenal disease
  - Any painful disease process
- Sexual aggression—May explain conspecific ferret aggression in which mating behavior may be accompanied by intense biting.

especially when they are sleeping, and to respect a nursing jill's privacy and innate protective behavior. Ferrets are rarely fearful once they are awake and aware of your presence; however, if they continue to be cautious and nippy, try to replace the fear response with a counteraction such as anticipation of play or food. Extra care should be taken with deaf ferrets that may startle more readily. Congenital deafness occurs in ferrets, and anecdotal reports indicate that an increased incidence of deafness exists in albino and/or black-eyed ferrets.

If a ferret stalks and nips at young children, it may be best to change your ferret's free time to a time when the child is napping or away from home. Owners should be made aware that other household pets (e.g., birds, rabbits, or rodents) may be perceived as prey, and unsupervised contact time with that pet should be discouraged. It is also a good idea to put the pet dog or cat in another room during the ferret's free time until the behavioral interaction of these pets is known.

Overly exuberant play behavior or play aggression is the most common situation in which ferret frolicking can lead to biting. Gentle nips are normal and natural to ferrets, which often bite at other ferrets to encourage play. Therefore it is not uncommon for ferrets to nip their owners gently in order to gain their attention. Play biting in ferrets is similar to the same misbehavior in puppies. Box 4-5 outlines ideas for controlling this behavior problem.

Ferret play can escalate to the point where its frenzied commotion borders on aggressive behavior. One ferret may arch its neck and back and shove itself sidelong into the other in a very characteristic way. This fake challenge is an example of subdued or "domesticated" aggressive behavior turned to play. Nose poking, ramming another ferret with mouth open, and defensive threats in which the ferret stands very erect with back arched and tail possibly brushed up are other examples of playful behaviors that originate in polecat aggressive behavior. The magnitude of the actions and vocalizations differentiates play from aggressive behavior.

Young kits at play are particularly mouthy, as seen with continual biting, mouthing, tugging, and dragging each other. These behaviors are

---

BOX 4-5   Preventing and Managing Ferret Play Biting Behavior

- Avoid aggressive play (pushing, rolling, wrestling).
- Avoid tug-of-war games.
- Keep fingers curled when playing with an easily excited ferret.
- Use time outs—10 to 15 minutes in a small room or pet carrier (do not use ferret's cage for time out) with no toys or towels or anything with which the ferret could play.
- When the ferret bites, make a high-pitched sound (yip, ouch). This will mimic the sound another ferret makes when play behavior gets out of hand.
- When the ferret starts biting during play, redirect it to appropriate toys such as hard rubber balls or plush toys.
- Try a gentle scruffing, and wiggle the ferret in the air while making a hissing sound (this is how a mother ferret disciplines a kit), but be mindful that the ferret may get even more excited.
- Display gentle but firm dominance over the ferret by holding it on its back for a few minutes.
- Wrap the ferret snugly in a towel or baby blanket so that it cannot get out and bite. Walk around while gently cuddling and talking to the ferret and petting when it is calm. Offer a food treat when the ferret remains calm.

believed to reflect innate dominance behavior learning.[6] Similar to other mammals, a mother ferret will tug and pull at her young as a means of discipline and control. If kits are sold to pet retailers at a young age (some kits are placed in pet shops as early as 6 weeks of age), mother-kit socialization patterns may be disrupted. This lack of maternal nurturing can lead to overly stormy play behavior, which may be perceived as aggression by new owners.

Keep in mind that the solitary pet ferret may perceive its human owner as its playmate, and nips, pokes, and attempted drags of arms or feet may be directed at him or her. Frequent handling in a quiet, subdued environment, along with behavior modification in the form of positive reinforcements, time-outs, and counterconditioning, will all go a long way toward properly socializing these belligerent kits. Remember to never incorporate physical punishment into your behavioral modification routine. This may cause a frightened or excited ferret to become even more frenzied, resulting in more intense and perhaps vicious biting. Also, ferrets may be sensitive to certain odors. Ferrets may react to sweet-smelling hand lotion or soaps by licking or nipping the wearer. Some ferrets love the smell or taste of nicotine and may react by biting the smoker's fingers. Finally, an adult ferret that suddenly becomes more aggressive and nippy should be assessed for underlying health issues such as pain or hormonal imbalances associated with adrenal disease.

Sleep Behavior

Most wild mustelidae are considered nocturnal, but wild polecats have been observed hunting during the day. Sleeping habits probably reflect habitat, territorial competition, and availability of food. Under laboratory conditions, ferrets spend over 60% of the time sleeping, with approximately 40% of total sleep time in rapid eye movement (REM) sleep.[26] This large amount of REM sleep is achieved by having a high number of REM sleep episodes rather than longer REM periods.[26] Domestic ferrets show diurnal activity in captivity and normally sleep from 12 to 16 hours in a typical day,[6] with varying sleeping patterns.

As a general rule, older ferrets demonstrate shorter, more frequent periods of activity and spend a greater part of their day sleeping. Younger ferrets, on the other hand, tend to display longer periods of activity interspersed with sleep. Regardless of age, the duration and timing of active wakefulness reflect the owner's schedule and how often the ferrets are given the opportunity to interact. Most ferrets are ready to explore and play at any time; the duration of these activities is a reflection of age.

Domestic ferrets often sleep very soundly, during which time respirations and heart rate decrease. The depth of sleep is so profound that many ferret owners mistake this deep phase of sleep for severe illness or death. Ferrets, especially older ferrets, can take several moments to awaken from sleep even with vigilant attempts at arousal. Ferret owners need to be aware of this and be patient in awakening their ferret with gentle prodding and soothing vocalizations. If deep sleep behavior becomes increasingly pronounced in duration and depth, clinical evaluation for illness, particularly hypoglycemia associated with insulinoma, is warranted.[6]

Ferrets sleep in a variety of positions, and bonded pairs or groups will pile on one another to sleep (Figure 4-15). Ferrets may sleep curled up like dogs, on their backs with all four legs sprawled out, or even hanging upside down half-way out of their hammocks. Quiet respirations are usually audible, and periodic soft whimpering sounds may be heard from the sleeping ferret.

Yawning is a normal behavior of most ferrets and is usually not of clinical concern. Ferrets just waking up from a nap will begin their wakefulness with a stretch and a yawn. It is interesting to note that scruffing the ferret (restraining the ferret by holding the skin at the nape of the neck) often elicits a yawning reflex. This may facilitate a brief oral examination. The action of scruffing causes a relaxation response and is used as a form of restraint when necessary to calm an excited ferret. The relaxation elicited by scruffing is usually consistent and is similar to the method used by the

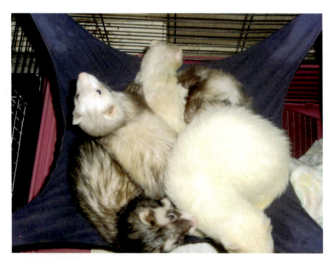

Figure 4-15
Sleep behavior. Ferrets sleep in a variety of positions, and bonded pairs or groups will pile on one another to sleep. The domestic ferret is diurnal, with the duration and timing of active wakefulness reflecting the owner's schedule and how often the ferret is given the opportunity to interact. (Courtesy Laura Powers.)

jill when disciplining young kits or moving them from one location to another.[6]

Medical Implications of Abnormal Behavior

Learning to understand the behavior of animals is a very important aspect of diagnosis in veterinary medicine. The nonemergency physical examination begins with hands-off observation of the animal for any sensory signals that give an impression of overall health status. A few minutes of observing the ferret for behavioral signs of health or illness can disclose valuable information about overall patient well-being. A healthy ferret is alert and curious about its surroundings, demonstrating attentive and exploratory behaviors, and has bright, clear eyes and a smooth, shiny hair coat. Before initiating the physical examination in any ferret, healthy or sick, it is also important to observe for temperament; behavioral signs of friendliness, fear, or potential aggression. A ferret that leans forward with interest, using its sense of smell to explore an outstretched hand, is usually a normal, friendly, inquisitive ferret.

Poorly socialized ferrets may show signs of fear such as backing up with the ears laid back and flat, and some may even give a vocal hiss. The aggressive ferret may signal its displeasure by trying to get away and/or hissing vocally, but it will not give you other warning signs—no snarl or showing of the teeth; it will bite without warning. This tends to be a fairly intense bite that breaks the skin, and the ferret may hold on despite attempts by the holder to break free.

During quiet observation the clinician can be taking the patient history. Listen to the client for behavioral clues that might aid in making a differential diagnosis. If the ferret is just lying on the examination table with a dull look in its eyes, the clinician immediately gets the impression that this ferret does not feel well. Pawing at the mouth or salivating may be a sign of nausea potentially caused by gastrointestinal discomfort secondary to gastric obstruction, gastric ulcers, or hypoglycemia secondary to insulinoma.

If clients state that their normally passive and friendly ferret has become intermittently aggressive toward cagemates, adrenal disease or pain should be ruled out. If the owner reports lethargy and difficulty in arousing the ferret from sleep, then hypoglycemia resulting from insulinoma should be considered. If the owner notices that the ferret has been standing in a hunched position with an arched back and wiggling its ears while grinding its teeth, then abdominal pain with secondary bruxism should be ruled out.

Pollakiuria and stranguria are abnormal urinary behaviors and common signs of cystitis or prostatitis, both of which may occur secondary to adrenal disease. Male ferrets with urethral calculi, severe prostatitis, or periprostatic cysts associated with adrenal disease may become obstructed and be unable to urinate. These ferrets will usually display repeated attempts to urinate, with urgency demonstrated by intense arching of the back, straining, and evidence of abdominal pain with or without vocalization. Observe the respirations to see if the ferret is showing any signs of increased respiratory rate and distress. Scratching may indicate external parasites or underlying adrenal disease.

The ferret's normal physical changes in response to seasonal changes and photoperiod, such as weight gain in the winter and weight loss in late spring, as well as seasonal shedding patterns, need to be taken into consideration if the client is concerned about weight loss or a sudden onset of increased shedding in an otherwise healthy ferret. An understanding of ferret behaviors, both normal and abnormal, therefore serves as a great aid in assessing ferret health.

Adrenal Disease

Hormonal abnormalities including elevations in plasma estrogens and androgens can occur secondary to adrenal disease. These imbalances may lead to increased sexual behavior even in neutered and spayed ferrets. These behaviors include neck gripping, mounting, and pelvic thrusting, which may be interpreted by owners of pet ferrets as an aggressive behavioral change for which they will seek veterinary counseling (Figure 4-16). As a result, any healthy ferret that is presented because of a recent onset of conspecific aggressive or sexual behavior should be assessed for adrenal disease.

Other signs of adrenal disease include bilaterally symmetric alopecia (usually beginning on the tail and then extending up over the dorsum), pruritus, vulvar swelling in ovariohysterectomized female ferrets, and prostatic enlargement and cysts in neutered male ferrets (Figure 4-17). Another less commonly reported behavioral change is the increased mothering behavior of jills associated with increased circulating levels of progesterone secondary to adrenal disease. For example, we have seen a jill with adrenal disease that showed nesting behavior by taking favorite stuffed animals and mothering them.

The underlying cause(s) of these behavioral manifestations may be clarified with a review of ferret adrenal disease physiology. In the intact ferret, gonadal estradiol or testosterone exerts a negative feedback on the hypothalamus and pituitary gland, thereby preventing excessive secretion of GnRH, LH, and FSH. It has been shown that lack of negative gonadal hormonal feedback on hypothalamic GnRH in neutered ferrets results in persistently elevated gonadotropic LH, which may induce nonneoplastic

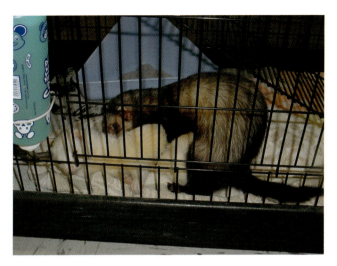

Figure 4-16
Mounting behavior. Ferret hyperadrenocorticism results in increases in plasma levels of one or more of the following sex steroids: estradiol, androstenedione, 17-alpha-hydroxyprogesterone, and dehydroepiandrosterone sulfate (DHEAS).[38] This hormonal imbalance may lead to increased sexual behavior including neck gripping, mounting, and pelvic thrusting, which may be interpreted by owners of pet ferrets as an aggressive behavioral change for which they will seek veterinary counseling. (Courtesy Peter Fisher.)

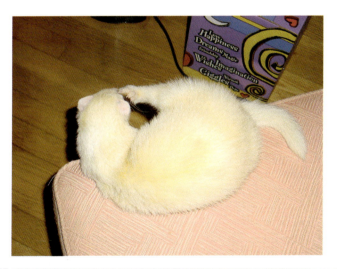

Figure 4-17
Pruritus. Pruritus can be a behavioral sign of external parasites or adrenal disease. Some ferrets with adrenal disease may manifest itching behavior as the only outward sign of this common endocrine disease. (Courtesy Peter Fisher.)

and neoplastic adrenocortical enlargement.[38] The ensuing hyperadrenocorticism may result in increases in plasma levels of estradiol, androstenedione, 17-alpha-hydroxyprogesterone, and dehydroepiandrosterone sulfate, which result in physical and behavioral changes dominated by features consistent with excessive production of these sex hormones.[38] A diagnosis of adrenal disease based on history and clinical signs can be more definitively confirmed with ultrasonography of the adrenal glands and measurement of plasma levels of androstenedione, 17-alpha-hydroxyprogesterone, and estradiol (Clinical Endocrinology Service, University of Tennessee).

Insulinoma

Insulin-secreting pancreatic islet cell tumors are among the most common neoplastic diseases affecting ferrets. Synonyms include functional islet cell tumor, pancreatic β-cell tumor, pancreatic endocrine tumor, and insulinoma. The disease affects both male and female ferrets between the ages of 2 and 8 years but is most commonly diagnosed in ferrets 4 to 5 years of age.

On histopathologic examination beta cell carcinoma is most often found, sometimes in combination with beta cell adenoma or hyperplasia. Continuous hyperinsulinemia sustains the metabolic effect of insulin; therefore hepatic gluconeogenesis and glycogenolysis are inhibited, and peripheral uptake of glucose by tissue cells is increased.[35] As the disease progresses, hypoglycemia ensues.

Insulinoma is another endocrine disease in which a history of certain behavioral changes will help the clinician narrow the differential diagnosis. The rate of development, magnitude, and duration of hypoglycemia are factors determining the severity of clinical signs. Many ferrets are presented with a history of behavioral changes including intermittent weakness and lethargy, a decrease in play and exploratory behavior, and an increase in length and depth of sleep. Ferret owners may report that the pet is no longer animated and seems dull and confused.

Signs usually progress slowly over a period of weeks to months; many owners are slow to pick up on the changes in the pet's behavior or attribute the quiet, less-responsive behavior to old age. Pawing at the mouth, teeth grinding, and hypersalivation—a result of hypoglycemia-induced nausea—are other behavioral signs that may be associated with insulinoma. Left untreated, hypoglycemia may result in seizures, coma, and death.

The definitive diagnosis of insulinoma depends on the histopathologic examination of pancreatic tissue. However, in most ferrets a diagnosis of insulinoma is made before surgery, by demonstration of hypoglycemia in association with history and clinical signs. Other causes of hypoglycemia should be ruled out, including anorexia or starvation, severe gastrointestinal disease, sepsis, neoplasia, and hepatic disease.

Behaviors Associated with Pain

Pain assessment in ferrets is often more difficult than in dogs and cats because, in general, veterinarians are less familiar with the normal behavior of ferrets.[17] Changes in behavior associated with pain can be subtle, but careful observation of the undisturbed ferret will allow the clinician to pick up on the various indicators of pain. An uncomfortable ferret will be reluctant to curl into its normal, relaxed sleeping position, may have a tucked appearance to the abdomen and a strained facial expression, and may have increased frequency and depth of respirations. The gait may be stiff, with the head elevated and extended forward. Most ferrets in pain are lethargic and anorexic.

A painful abdomen is a common sequela to ferret gastrointestinal diseases including gastric ulcers, gastrointestinal foreign bodies or trichobezoars, ECE, and *Helicobacter* infections. Owners often report that the ferret is hunched up with an arched back, immobile, or walking with a stilted gait and is grinding its teeth—all common signs of abdominal pain. A less astute owner may not recognize spasmodic teeth grinding behavior manifested in a ferret that holds its head down and rhythmically moves its facial muscles back and forth and wriggles its ears in response to painful stimuli.

Postoperative and traumatic pain are usually manifested as a reluctance to move and a facial expression demonstrating dull, half-open, noninquisitive eyes, which are overall expressions of tension. It is amazing to watch the change in behavioral attitude and facial relaxation once pain medication is administered. If possible, analgesics should be provided before painful stimulus occurs. Administering preemptive analgesia as part of the preanesthetic protocol or administering analgesics intraoperatively before discontinuing general anesthesia diminishes the wind-up effect of pain and decreases the postoperative pain caused by neuropathic and inflammatory pain.[7]

Each patient must be evaluated individually when analgesic protocols are chosen, with frequency, duration, and type of analgesic used based on clinical judgment, hematologic, and biochemical values and patient response. A return to normal attentive behavior, curling up under a towel to sleep, and a good appetite are all behavioral signs that postoperative analgesia is adequate.

References

1. Apfelbach R: Imprinting on prey odours in ferrets *(Mustela putorius F. furo L.)* and its neural correlates, *Behav Processes* 12(4):363-381, 1986.
2. Apfelbach R: Instinctive predatory behavior of the ferret *(Putorius putorius furo)* modified by chlordiazeperoxide hydrochloride (Librium), *Psychopharmacology* 59(2):179-182, 1978.
3. Bell JA: Ferret nutrition, *Vet Clin North Am Exot Anim Pract* 1:169-192, 1999.
4. Bleavins MR, Aulerich RJ: Feed consumption and food passage in mink *(Mustela vison)* and European ferret *(Mustela Putorius furo)*, *Lab Anim Sci* 31(3):268-269, 1981.
5. Bogusz L. Ferret domestication. Available at: www.practical-pet-care.com. Accessed October 26, 2004
6. Boyce SW, Zingg BM, Lightfoot TL: Behavior of *Mustela putorius furo* (the domestic ferret), *Vet Clin North Am Exot Anim Pract* 4(3):697-717, 2001.
7. Bradley T: Recognizing pain in exotic mammals, *Exotic DVM Magazine* 3(3):21-26, 2001.
8. Carroll RS, Weaver CE, Baum MJ: Evidence implicating aromatization of testosterone in the regulation of male ferret sexual behavior, *Physiol Behav* 42(5):457-460, 1988.
9. Chivers SM, Einon DF: Effects of early social experience on activity and object investigation in the ferret, *Dev Psychobiol* 15(1):75-80, 1982.
10. Clapperton BK: Scent marking behavior of the ferret, *Mustela furo L.*, *Anim Behav* 38(3):436-446, 1989.
11. Clapperton BK, Minot EO, Crump DR: An olfactory recognition system in the ferret *Mustela furo L.* (Carnivora: Mustelidae), *Anim Behav* 36(2):541-553, 1988.
12. Davis DE: The physiological analysis of aggressive behavior. In Etkin E, editor: *Social behavior and organization among vertebrates*, Chicago, 1964, University of Chicago Press.
13. Davison A, Birks JDS, Griffiths HI, et al: Hybridization of the phylogenetic relationship between polecats and domestic ferrets in Britain, *Biol Conserv* 87:155-161, 1999.
14. Donovan BT: Wheel-running during anoestrus and oestrus in the ferret, *Physiol Behav* 34(5):825-829, 1985.
15. Ehrlich A, Burns N: Exploratory behaviour of the black-footed ferret, *Can J Psychol* 12(4):235-241, 1958.
16. Etkin W: Theories of socialization and communication. In Etkin E, editor: *Social behavior and organization among vertebrates*, Chicago, 1964, University of Chicago Press.
17. Flecknell PA: Analgesia of small mammals, *Vet Clin North Am Exot Anim Pract* 4(1):47-56, 2001.
18. Fox JG, Bell JS: Growth, reproduction and breeding. In Fox JG, editor: *Biology and diseases of the ferret*, ed 2, Baltimore, 1998, Williams & Wilkins.
19. Hinde RA: *Animal behaviour: a synthesis of ethology and comparative psychology*, New York, 1970, McGraw-Hill.
20. Houpt KA: *Domestic animal behavior for veterinarians and animal scientists*, Ames, Iowa, 1991, Iowa State Press.
21. Kaufman LW: Foraging cost and meal patterns in ferrets, *Physiol Behav* 25:139-141, 1980.

22. Kelliher KR, Baum MJ: Nares occlusion eliminates heterosexual partner selection without disrupting coitus in ferrets of both sexes, *J Neurosci* 21(15):5832-5840, 2001.
23. Korhonen H: The effects of environmental enrichment in ferrets. In Smith CP, Taylor V, editors: *Environmental enrichment information resources for laboratory animals:1965-1995: birds, cats, dogs, farm animals, ferrets, rabbits, and rodents.* AWIV Resource Series No. 2, Beltsville, MD, 1995, U.S. Department of Agriculture.
24. Lazar JW, Beckhorn GD: Social play or the development of social behavior in ferrets *(Mustela putorius)*? *Am Zool* 14:405-414, 1974.
25. Leidig L: Personal communication, 2004.
26. Marks GA, Shaffery JP: A preliminary study of sleep in the ferret. *Mustela putorius furo:* a carnivore with extremely high proportion of REM sleep, *Sleep* 19(2):83-93, 1996.
27. Marler P, Hamilton WJ: *Mechanisms of animal behavior,* London, 1966, John Wiley & Sons.
28. Matulich E: Seeing is believing: ferrets' eyes and vision, *Ferrets* 1(4):26-31, 1998.
29. Medina-Vogel G, Hickling GJ, Clapperton BK: Assessing spatial activity in captive ferrets, *Mustela furo L. (Carnivora: Mustelidae)*, *NZ J Zool* 27(2):75-83, 2000.
30. Miller BJ, Anderson SH: Failure of fertilization following abbreviated copulation in the ferret *(Mustela putorius furo)*, *J Exp Zool* 249:85-89, 1989.
31. Moore DR: Late onset of hearing in the ferret, *Brain Res* 235(1-2):309-311, 1982.
32. Orcutt C: Dermatologic diseases. In Quesenberry KE, Carpenter JW, editors: *Ferrets, rabbits, and rodents: clinical medicine and surgery,* St Louis, 2003, Saunders.
33. Poole TB: The aggressive behavior of individual male polecats *(Mustela putorius, M. furo* and hybrids) towards familiar and unfamiliar opponents, *J Zool Soc Lond* 170(3):395-414, 1973.
34. Poole TB: Some behavioural differences between the European polecat, *Mustela putorius,* the ferret, *M. furo,* and their hybrids, *J Zool Soc Lond* 166:25-35, 1972.
35. Quesenberry KE, Rosenthal KL: Endocrine diseases. In Quesenberry KE, Carpenter JW, editors: *Ferrets, rabbits, and rodents: clinical medicine and surgery,* St. Louis, 2003, Saunders.
36. Ragg JR: The denning behavior of feral ferrets *(Mustela furo)* in a pastoral habitat, South Island, New Zealand, *J Zool* 246(4):443-486, 1998.
37. Schilling K: *Ferrets for dummies,* Foster City, Calif., 2000, IDG Books Worldwide.
38. Schoemaker N: *Hyperadrenocorticism in ferrets* (PhD thesis). Utrecht, Netherlands, Utrecht University, 2003.
39. Shimbo FM: *A Tao full of detours, the behavior of the domestic ferret.* Elon College, NC, 1992, Ministry of Publications.
40. Staton VW, Crowell-Davis SL: Factors associated with aggression between pairs of domestic ferrets, *J Am Vet Med Assoc* 222(12):1709-1712, 2003.
41. Stockman ER, Callaghan RS, Baum MJ: Effects of neonatal castration and testosterone on sexual partner preference in the ferret, *Physiol Behav* 34(3):409-414, 1985.
42. Stockman ER, Callaghan RS, Gallagher CA, Baum MJ: Sexual differentiation of play behavior in the ferret, *Behav Neurosci* 100(4):563-568, 1986.
43. Thompson AD: A history of the ferret, *J Hist Med* 6(4):471-480, 1951.
44. Vargas A, Anderson SH: Effects of experience and cage enrichment on predatory skills of black-footed ferrets *(Mustela nigripes)*, *J Mammol* 80(1):263-269, 1999.
45. Whary MT, Andrews PLR: Physiology of the ferret. In Fox JG, editor: *Biology and diseases of the ferret,* ed 2, Baltimore, 1998, Williams & Wilkins.

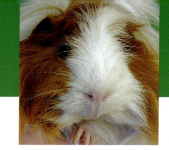

CHAPTER 5

TERESA BRADLEY BAYS

GUINEA PIG BEHAVIOR

Natural History, Behavior, and Domestication

Exactly when guinea pigs *(Cavia porcellus)* were domesticated is still unknown, but it is suspected to have happened sometime between 500 and 1000 AD. Originally from South America, guinea pigs were used for food and for religious ceremonies by the Incas. They were first introduced into Europe approximately 400 years ago.[37] In the wild they live in burrows or rock crevices in herds or in small groups of 5 to 10[43] and exhibit a definitive social hierarchy with a dominant male and female. Wild cavies are crepuscular and feed at dawn and dusk.

As with other species the process of domestication in guinea pigs has led to changes in behavior such that the domestic guinea pig is less aggressive, exhibits increased social tolerance and increased male courtship behavior, and is less attentive to its surrounding environment than its wild counterparts.[31] Guinea pigs have been used as animal models for autism in humans. The GS strain of guinea pigs, which are partially inbred, exhibit autism-like behavior patterns such as lack of response to and exploration of the environment, stereotypic motor behaviors, and poor social interaction because of cerebellar and corticocerebral abnormalities.[5]

Three original breeds were recognized: the American (or English), which has a smooth hair coat; the Abyssinian, which has a short, coarse coat with whorls or rosettes; and the Peruvian, which has long, silky hair. There are now thirteen breeds including several hairless varieties (Figure 5-1).

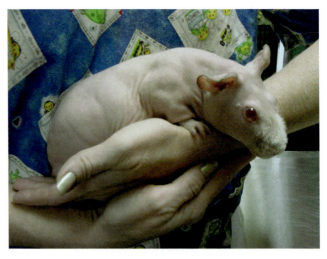

Figure 5-1
Hairless guinea pigs or "skinny" pigs are being seen more commonly as pets. (Courtesy Teresa Bradley Bays.)

Social and Antisocial Behaviors

Guinea pigs are generally nonaggressive, docile animals, and with frequent, gentle handling and petting they are extremely responsive to attention and make affectionate pets. They readily and enthusiastically respond by whistling when greeting their human companions as well as to the sound of the crinkle of a produce bag or the opening of a refrigerator door. It is not uncommon for guinea pigs to lick human companions as a sign of affection and acceptance. Also, in stressful situations (in the examination room, for instance) a guinea pig will lick its owner as if seeking comfort and familiarity (Box 5-1).

As an extremely social species, they live in the wild in small groups, seeking "safety in numbers," because more eyes help alert them to the presence of predators. They can often be seen standing or lying side by side when resting and when eating.[21] Bonding has been shown to be very important in domestic guinea pigs, and evidence of the effect of social support has been quantified by the detection of lower cortisol levels in both males and females placed in challenging situations when supported by a familiar guinea pig. Cortisol levels (as a measure of stress) are even lower when guinea pigs are challenged in the presence of a bonded mate.[26]

In a study of the effects of social stress in guinea pigs, unfamiliar males were paired and their behavior and physiological parameters measured

BOX 5-1 Common Postures of Guinea Pigs

- *Nudging or head butting*—A determined push with the head to stimulate petting or to indicate that your attention is not wanted. Angry or agitated cavies will nudge bedding, towels, and cage furniture in a show of irritation. Guinea pigs will also nudge human companions and conspecifics if they are bored, in play, and as a show of dominance.
- *Nose touching*—A greeting gesture, usually made between familiar cavies, similar to a handshake in humans or sniffing in dogs.
- *Digging*—A behavior associated with boredom, agitation, and attempts to escape.
- *Playing dead*—If extremely frightened a cavy may roll on its back and lie motionless in order to squelch a predator's instinct to attack.
- *Stretching out*—Lying on the side with rear legs stretched behind denotes relaxation and comfort.
- *Licking*—Guinea pigs will lick human and other companions in order to gain attention, to show affection, and to seek comfort.
- *Leg stiffening*—The front legs are stiffened, and they rise up in order to appear bigger and more threatening to a potential predator.
- *Standing on hind legs*—Position used to view the surrounding area or to initiate petting, attention, or feeding.
- *Alert stance*—Stretching out with head forward, watchful and ready to run if necessary.
- *Biting*—Used to show dominance, to gain attention, and to discourage unwanted attention.
- *Shudder*—A whole body shake, usually after being handled, which can indicate irritation at the handler as well as relaxation after being handled.
- *Popcorning*—A jumping for joy or leap in the air, as seen in neonates when excited or sometimes when frightened.
- *Rumba*—A swaying or swinging of the hindquarters, often performed with a purring vocalization, usually to exhibit sexual interest.

over an 8-day period. Despite the fact that visual agonistic behaviors did not appear to increase during the duration of cohabitation, physiological parameters—including weight loss, lower testosterone levels, and higher glucocorticoid and plasma catecholamine titers—indicated that the stress levels increased for the less dominant males.[41] The subordinate males behaved increasingly more passively until they finally ceased feeding and drinking.[41]

Despite the fact that guinea pigs are a precocial species that requires little maternal involvement after birth, social influences of the mother and other adults have been found to have a marked influence on behavior of the offspring.[12] In a study of social preferences in young guinea pigs it was noted that both male and female pups stayed near the mother even through the postweaning period. Littermates continued to spend time together, and periadolescent animals reaching sexual maturity did not appear to associate more with novel animals or potential breeding partners.[19] It is interesting to note, however, that male and female guinea pigs that were housed apart from the mother would then interact with her as if she were an unfamiliar female when reunited.[14]

Early social stress in guinea pig pups has been shown to create endocrine changes and changes in brain function, both of which are evidenced later by social behavioral changes. For example, several ontogenic studies have indicated that prenatal and immediate postnatal environmental and social factors affecting pregnant female guinea pigs can in turn affect how offspring will interact as adults. Stress of the mother during these periods may create a behavioral masculinity in the daughters (as evidenced by urine spraying).[28,29] Also, more infantile behavior of the males in adulthood was noted. This was probably attributable to an increase in androgens in the stressed pregnant female as well as to the effect on the endocrine system in a stress response.[25,27,29,40]

Evidence of mother-infant attachment was demonstrated when increased cortisol levels were found in lactating guinea pigs (3 days postpartum) when their pups were removed and taken out of auditory range.[15,18,39] Plasma cortisol levels also were elevated and vocalization was greater in the pups that were removed from the mother, more so in those placed alone than in those kept with their littermates.[39] The presence of an adult female guinea pig, both familiar and unfamiliar, has also been shown to decrease the hypothalamic-pituitary-adrenal response in younger guinea pigs, even though behavioral interaction did not indicate this. The presence of an unfamiliar male did not evoke the same decrease in the stress response.[14,16]

All of this research would indicate that because of the extensive social nature of guinea pigs and their obvious need for support, in captivity they tend to do better in bonded pairs or trios rather than as solitary pets (Figure 5-2). Various reports in the lay literature suggest that bonding can be accomplished except with two intact males. Suggestions for the bonding process are outlined in the next section.

Taming and the Bonding Process

Guinea pigs are generally very gentle creatures that are not prone to scratching or biting unless provoked. Each has its own personality, however, and some will bite if an unwelcome procedure such as nail trimming is performed. Care must be taken with shy, not well-socialized

Guinea Pig Behavior 211

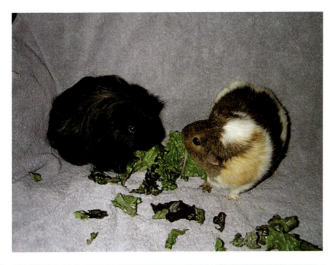

Figure 5-2
Guinea pigs are a very social species and do best if kept in pairs or trios. (Courtesy Darice Heishman.)

cavies, as they are easily stressed and may injure themselves in attempts to escape.

It is important to approach slowly and speak softly when attempting to handle a shy guinea pig that is not used to being handled. Short periods of acclimation may begin with the handler sitting with a hand inside the cage and talking in a quiet, gentle voice. This should be repeated several days in a row. As the guinea pig becomes more trusting, favored vegetable treats may be hand-fed.

Do not stress the guinea pig by chasing it around the cage before lifting, as guinea pigs that are unaccustomed to handling may run if approached from behind. Once the cavy is accustomed to a hand in its cage, you may begin to gently but firmly stroke the head and the top of the nose. Many guinea pigs like to be scratched behind the ears or petted under the chin with one finger. At this point the handler may try lifting the cavy gently and firmly by scooping the rear end as the pig is supported behind the front legs.

This process takes time, and it is best to work with shy individuals for short intervals in order to allow them to get accustomed to you without causing undue stress. An unsocialized guinea pig may also be more likely to approach a person that is no longer at predator height, so lying on the floor in a guinea pig–safe environment may be an excellent way to increase confidence and encourage handling and bonding. Once a trusting relationship is established, a daily "cuddle" session is encouraged in order to maintain it.

Intraspecies aggression can occur with two males in the presence of females. It may also be seen between cavies that have not been raised together, especially between two unaltered males. Introducing a new pig should be done slowly and carefully and with direct adult supervision. The supervisors should be prepared to separate the guinea pigs if they begin to fight. This is best accomplished by wearing leather gloves or putting tennis shoes on the hands to protect them from being bitten. A plastic dustpan or a spray bottle of water may also be used.

As with other species, introductions may be best performed in neutral territory such as in the bathtub or in a laundry basket while on a car ride, with greens and hay provided as an additional distraction. The cavies may find comfort in each other in these strange situations, creating a bond more quickly. It may also be helpful to introduce the more-dominant cavy into the established territory of the less-dominant one, giving the subordinate guinea pig a "home field" advantage. Some owners have also placed cages near each other for several weeks (not too close, so that biting or fighting cannot occur through the cage wire), after which the guinea pigs' cages are switched in order to familiarize each guinea pig with the other's scent. Castration and ovariohysterectomy may make introductions and bonding easier, as hormonal influence on behavior will be more suppressed.

Despite the risks associated with predator-prey relationships, guinea pigs can and do live in households with other pets, in some cases rather closely. It cannot be overstressed, however, that domestic pets still do what is instinctive. Therefore, close adult supervision is essential. In addition, knowing that stress can create severe physiological consequences, owners and caretakers are encouraged to examine the practice of housing different species together, as the stress that it may cause in their pets may not be readily recognizable to them.

Sensory Behaviors

Visual Behaviors

Guinea pigs have relatively small eyes compared with the size of their heads and have a prominent third eyelid tear gland that may prolapse. Cavies are nearsighted, and their eyes are placed laterally on the head, as they are in other grazing herbivorous species.

Vocalization Behaviors

Many individuals, including owners, fanciers, and researchers, have characterized guinea pig vocalizations. The most common vocalizations include short impulse sounds such as the chip, purr, and chutter and the slow, modulated, relatively long call, the whistle.[42] A list of common vocalizations as reported both in the lay literature and by researchers is included in this chapter (Box 5-2).

Auditory Behaviors

Guinea pigs have relatively good hearing, which makes them susceptible to loud noises. It is therefore important to house them in areas where noise is minimized. This is true both in the home and in the hospital environment.

Locomotor Behaviors and Activities

A diurnal (crepuscular) species, cavies are most active in the early morning and the evening and, if not disturbed, will spend most of the day quietly resting with intermittent periods of activity and nibbling on food. In one study, guinea pigs in breeding groups were videotaped to determine their level of activity in a 24-hour period and were found to be active intermittently throughout both the day and night with "no prolonged period of quiescence that would be associated with sleep."[45]

BOX 5-2 Common Vocalizations of Guinea Pigs*

- *Grunting*—Mating sound made when aroused and can sometimes be associated with hunger.
- *Chutting*—A sound made to signal curiosity.
- *Purring or gurgling*—An expression of contentment and happiness.
- *Teeth clatter, clacking, or hissing*—A chattering of teeth that denotes threat or aggression and indicates "stay away."
- *Weeping, wheeking, whistling*—A high-pitched sound denoting happiness or anticipation of a favored treat, person, or companion. Also made when cavies are hungry.
- *Squealing*—A high-pitched alert sound to signal warning of danger, pain, fear, or the need for help. Domestic cavies will also squeal when begging for food.
- *Drr*—A sound made as the pig becomes frightened or aroused.
- *Cooing*—A low, quiet sound that a sow makes to her babies to comfort them if they are frightened or that is made to reassure other adults.
- *Whining*—A sound made to signal danger, fear, or pain.

*Additional information on guinea pig vocalizations can be found in Berryman JC: Guinea pig vocalizations: their structure, causation and function, *Z Tierpsychol* 41:80-106, 1976, and Harper LV: Behavior. In Wagner JE, Manning PJ, editors: *The biology of the guinea pig*, New York, 1976, Academic Press.

When at rest guinea pigs will lie on their sides with feet extended or they will remain sternal with their feet tucked under them. If presented with the opportunity they will often seek the shelter of a towel or hide box during resting periods. They often remain still with eyes open during midday sedentary periods and may startle and jump if disturbed.

When active they ambulate by alternating all four feet as they walk, and their weight is carried evenly on all legs. Cavies walk with only the pads of the feet touching the ground. The legs are also alternated when running, but occasionally, when excited or during play, they can be seen kicking out with the rear legs as they run. With a guinea pig patient that is lame, the body weight is often shifted to compensate for the injured limb, making it difficult to assess which leg or foot is actually affected. It is therefore important to palpate and examine all four legs. If amputation of either a front or rear limb becomes a medical necessity, guinea pigs generally acclimate well postoperatively.

Head tilt, paralysis, and paresis are seen less commonly in cavies than in lagomorphs (Figure 5-3). Rule-outs, however, are similar and include trauma, infection, neoplasia, and parasites. Trauma is perhaps the most common cause. Prevention of traumatic injury necessitates care in handling and direct supervision when not in a guinea pig–safe area or when the guinea pig is being handled by young children. Pododermatitis can occur, especially in obese cavies, when bedding is not kept clean and dry. Secondary infection with *Staphylococcus aureus* is common, and it will

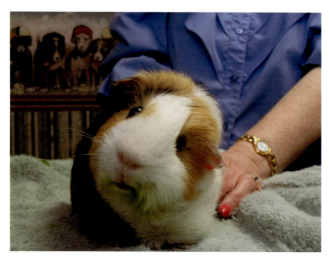

Figure 5-3
Guinea pigs can live well with a head tilt if managed carefully. (Courtesy Teresa Bradley Bays.)

Guinea Pig Behavior

cause significant pain, vocalization, and reluctance to walk. Severe untreated infections can lead to osteomyelitis of the affected limbs.

As a species guinea pigs are intelligent and playful and will often initiate play with both human and animal companions, including chase-type games. Caged guinea pigs often become obese because of overfeeding and limited exercise; therefore periods of exercise should be provided at least several times per week, preferably daily.

An increase in physical activity, as in humans and other species, may be chondroprotective, and the decrease in body mass that can be associated with increased exercise will also reduce the progression of osteoarthritis.[4] Despite the fact that it has been shown that guinea pigs respond adversely to the stress associated with change, small changes in the cage space and enclosure furniture may encourage increased motility and exercise because of increased exploratory behavior (Figure 5-4).[2]

Many owners create a guinea pig–safe area for their cavies to run in by eliminating the hazards of electric cords and dangerous items that can be eaten or chewed. Guinea pigs generally do not climb or jump, so it is not necessary to provide tops on enclosures, and small foldable portable fencing is available to create an exercise pen for cavies. Care must be taken, however, to eliminate any hazards that might be created by other household pets when these exercise pens are used. Alternatively, if these pens are used outside, it is imperative that an adult supervise the guinea pigs

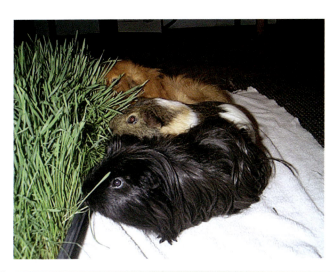

Figure 5-4
Grass can be organically grown for behavioral enrichment and to encourage exercise for guinea pigs. (Courtesy Darice Heishman.)

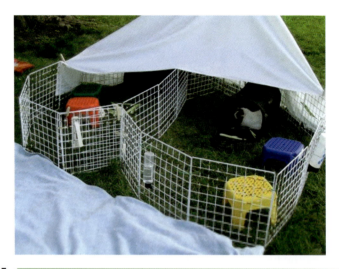

Figure 5-5
Outside pens can be easily fashioned to allow for exercise. It is imperative that shade, ventilation, and hide boxes are provided and that the guinea pigs be supervised by an adult. (Courtesy Rebecca Howell.)

to eliminate the chance that they will escape or be molested or attacked by outside pets, strays, and wildlife (Figure 5-5).

Cavies have little sense of an edge when placed on a table, counter, or bed and may readily walk off the edge and fall to the ground. When carried they will wiggle and squeal if they are not well supported and can hurt themselves in the process. Handling correctly includes grasping the trunk behind the front legs while scooping up and supporting the hindquarters with the other hand. Close supervision of children is recommended to ensure proper handling of their guinea pigs. For younger children it is best to place the guinea pig in a towel on the child's lap. Alternatively, the guinea pig may be placed on the floor in a guinea pig–safe area so the pig can be petted without carrying and therefore may feel more secure.

Grooming Behaviors

All breeds of guinea pigs have longer guard hairs with an undercoat of finer hairs. Like most small mammal species, guinea pigs tend to be meticulous groomers. However, it is important to brush longhaired species regularly to minimize matting and ingestion of hair as it is shed (Figure 5-6). Since guinea pigs are unable to vomit, prevention of trichobezoar production is important. For this reason I do not recommend bathing

Guinea Pig Behavior 217

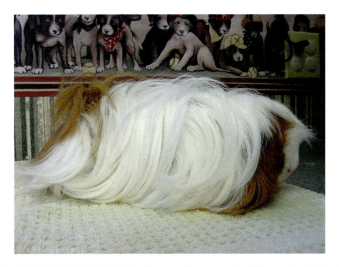

Figure 5-6
Longhaired guinea pigs should be groomed on a regular basis to prevent matting and ingestion of hair during grooming. (Photo courtesy Teresa Bradley Bays.)

guinea pigs, unless medically necessary, as the hair is shed readily after bathing. If bathing is needed, care must be taken to dry and brush the guinea pig well before self-grooming is allowed.

Cavies have sebaceous glands along the dorsum and in the anal area. The glands on the dorsal rump are often used for marking and occasionally are thought to be pathologic when "discovered" by the owner or an unknowing clinician. These glands will overproduce and create a greasy feel to the dorsum, especially in older, overweight, intact males and those with mite infestations.

Generally, little mutual grooming occurs among guinea pigs; however, mutual or self-barbering and ear nibbling can occur when a guinea pig is bored, stressed (a possible dissociative behavior), or in a situation in which a dominant pig (usually a male) barbers subordinates.[9,11] Self-barbering should be considered if only the head and neck, which cannot be reached, are unaffected. Self-barbering in rabbits has been found to be associated with low-fiber diets[20,23,24] and may also have the same cause in guinea pigs.

Barbering can be distinguished from other causes of alopecia by the fact that the hairs will be chewed near the skin and feel bristly whereas the skin beneath appears to be healthy. Stressful environments that elicit barbering may be corrected by decreasing overcrowding and providing free-choice grass hays. Hide boxes and other distractions such as cardboard boxes and paper towel rolls will also help to curb these negative behaviors. Paper towel rolls should be cut in half lengthwise so smaller cavies do not get stuck in them.

Alopecia in guinea pigs can have many other causes. Hormonally induced alopecia created by functional ovarian cysts will result in bilaterally symmetric hair loss in the flank regions. Late gestation sows may also lose hair because of hormonal influence. Guinea pigs will pull and chew hair at sites of pain, including on the limbs and the abdomen. If the hair and skin are otherwise normal and alopecia is noted dorsally, laterally, or in the flank area, it is wise to palpate for masses or pain in the abdomen.

Dermatophytosis and ectoparasites may also result in alopecia. Occasionally pathologic conditions of the skin such as a serious mite infestation can lead to severe seborrhea and a secondary overproduction of secretions from glands in the skin (Figure 5-7). Often these cavies will have rough hair coats, appear unkempt, and be too uncomfortable, in too much pain, and too pruritic to groom. They often squeal, panic, and run when touched. Pruritus may be so severe that the guinea pig will begin to seize as it scratches and can often be seen scratching again as it comes out of the seizure. In some cases, especially in overweight males, the penis can become surrounded and even constricted by a combination of these secretions and shed hair (Figure 5-8). Therefore, careful examination of the penis should be performed in all male guinea pigs during physical examination, especially if mites are suspected.

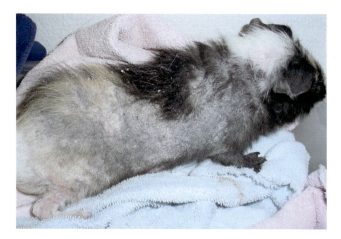

Figure 5-7

Dermatologic problems are common in cavies, and mites can cause alopecia, seborrhea, pruritus, and even seizures. (Courtesy Teresa Lightfoot.)

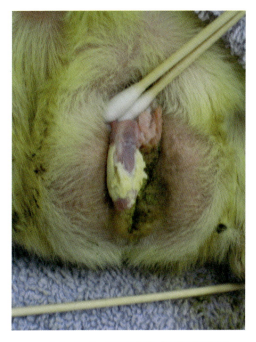

Figure 5-8
It is common for older males with mites to have a lot of sebum and hair trapped around the penis, as epilation and sebum production is increased and grooming is decreased because of pruritus. (Courtesy Teresa Bradley Bays.)

Eating Behaviors

Members of the Caviidae family, guinea pigs are herbivorous rodents that have monophyodont dentition (no primary teeth) with four incisors, no canine teeth, four premolars, and twelve molars (1/1, 0/0, 1/1, 3/3).[33] Because guinea pigs are hystricomorphic rodents, both their incisors and their cheek teeth are open rooted and continue to grow throughout life. The incisors of guinea pigs are white and not pigmented yellow as they often are in other rodents, and in normal occlusion the maxillary incisors are shorter than and overlap rostral to the mandibular incisors.

Cavies tend to be messy eaters and enjoy mixing food and water in their mouths. An oral examination with an otoscope should be performed whenever a guinea pig is presented for examination. This is somewhat hindered by a greenish mush of food that is ever present in the oral cavity. If particulate food matter is not detected in the mouth, however, the guinea pig has likely been off feed for some time.

220 Exotic Pet Behavior

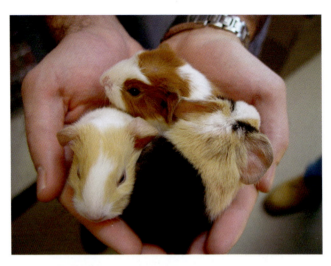

Figure 5-9
Guinea pigs are a precocial species and therefore are born fully haired with their eyes open. These babies are just 20 hours old. (Courtesy Jöerg Mayer.)

As a precocial species, guinea pigs are fully haired when born and are able to eat solid foods within hours of birth (Figure 5-9). They are monogastric herbivores, and juveniles will imprint on a food item in the first few days, after which they are often reluctant to change to other food items.[21,37] It is therefore important to provide a variety of food items right from birth in order to prevent imprinting on a few food items so that a balanced, varied diet will be accepted later on. Pairing a juvenile with an adult may facilitate a food change, as the juvenile will often mimic the adult and accept a new food more readily.

Addition of new foods should be made gradually, with only a small amount provided over the first few days to weeks. It is best to add only one new food at a time so that adverse reactions (such as diarrhea) to a particular food may be noted. Often it will take a week or more for a new item to be accepted. Cavies may refuse to eat or drink if there are any changes in texture, color, shape, or taste of the food or if the water is fouled. For this reason it is not recommended to add supplements to the water, as they may discourage the guinea pig from drinking enough water.

A limited quantity of fresh pellets made specifically for this species (containing additional vitamin C) such as Cavy Cuisine (Oxbow Pet Products, Murdock, NE) should be provided. Timothy-based pellets are preferred for adults, although juvenile cavies should be fed alfalfa-based pellets. The addition of seeds and treats to the pellets may create problems,

Guinea Pig Behavior   221

as a guinea pig may selectively eat only favored items, which will decrease the nutritional completeness of the diet. In my experience, gastrointestinal stasis and obstruction have been noted in both guinea pigs and rabbits that were provided with a new treat-pellet mix and ate the Canadian trapper peas to the exclusion of all other food items.[3]

Guinea pigs are a crepuscular species, and when maintained under controlled day-night light cycles and fed ad libitum they will exhibit increased eating activity at the beginning and at the end of the light period.[22] Because of an extremely high metabolic rate, guinea pigs need to be eating almost continuously, and the reason for any decrease in the amount eaten should be assessed immediately. Supportive care of the ill, painful, or stressed guinea pig includes providing oral nutritional supplementation. Oxbow Pet Products has a diet that is nutritionally complete for herbivores and is easily syringe-fed (Critical Care) (Figure 5-10). In an emergency, when veterinary care is not immediately available, a mixture of canned pumpkin and garden vegetable baby food can be syringe-fed until a nutritionally complete diet for syringe-feeding is available.

Access to free choice timothy or other grass hay is imperative. Dark-green leafy vegetables should be available twice per day when guinea pigs are most active, usually at twilight and before sunrise.[9] The addition of hay and greens to the diet provides a needed distraction and stimulation for these naturally grazing animals. Hay and greens also help to maintain

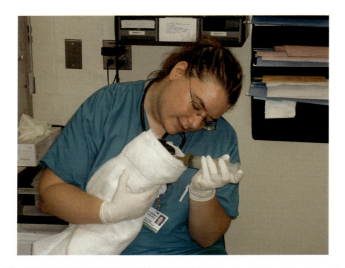

Figure 5-10
Sick guinea pigs should be syringe-fed a nutritionally complete supplement such as Oxbow Pet Products' Critical Care. (Courtesy Oxbow Pet Products, taken at Tufts University School of Veterinary Medicine.)

proper nutritional balance, healthy teeth, and normal gastrointestinal function.

Guinea pigs are one of a few species that require a dietary source of vitamin C. Vitamin C deficiency (scurvy) will occur if a daily supply of dietary vitamin C is not provided. Subacute ascorbic acid deficiency leads to general unthriftiness and immune suppression, which may be evidenced by poor hair coat, dull eyes and demeanor, chronic mite infestation, mandibular deformity leading to malocclusion, weight loss, anorexia, diarrhea, lameness, predisposition to infection, and delayed wound healing. Signs of advanced scurvy include unsteady, painful locomotion, hemorrhage from gums, swelling of joints, and emaciation.

Care has to be taken not to chronically oversupplement guinea pigs with vitamin C, as recent research has found an association between ascorbic acid oversupplementation and a worsening of the severity of spontaneous knee osteoarthritis.[31] Oversupplementation with vitamin C can also cause ocular changes including ossification of the ciliary body.*

Vegetables and fruits that are high in vitamin C include parsley, red and green peppers, kale, beet greens, spinach, chicory, broccoli, tomatoes, cabbage, kiwi fruit, and oranges. Spinach, kale, and cabbage are also high in oxalates, which may contribute to calculi formation in guinea pigs, and therefore, should be fed sparingly.[7]

One quarter of an orange per day can be given to guinea pigs to help provide adequate vitamin C. As with any new food item the orange may not be readily recognized as a food item or accepted, and it may take up to 4 weeks for a new food to be recognized as such and eaten. Provide a fresh slice of orange each day until it is readily eaten. Offer some of the orange with the peel and some without. Also, providing the orange or other new food item in the morning before giving any other favored fruit or vegetable treats makes it more likely to be eaten.

Liquid vitamin C supplements that can be added to the water are not recommended. They may change the color and taste of the water and necessitate cleaning the water bottle daily with hot soapy water in order to decrease the buildup of bacterial slime on the inner surface of the bottle. Vitamin C tablets can be crushed and put into solution of a fruit flavored drink or water and given orally via syringe or dropper. Chewable vitamin C tablets for children can be divided and are palatable to many guinea pigs. However, vitamin C tablets that can be fed daily are available specifically for guinea pigs from Oxbow Pet Products (GTN-50C).

Normal water intake is approximately 100 mL/kg. Guinea pigs are notorious for putting masticated food up in the tip of a sipper bottle, which may lead to clogging and bacterial contamination. Cavies will often defecate in food and water bowls. It is therefore important to clean water bottles and water and food bowls daily with hot soapy water in order to keep them fresh and to minimize bacterial contamination. Typically guinea pigs will stand up on the edge of bowls and crocks to eat, making it necessary to provide stable heavy containers to minimize tipping.

Elimination Behaviors

Cavies are monogastric herbivores with a large cecum that contains about 60% to 70% of the gastrointestinal contents. Gastrointestinal transit time is approximately 20 hours, but as guinea pigs are coprophagic the total transit time for the cecals is up to 66 hours.[37]

When kept in enclosures, guinea pigs have been shown to use the periphery of the cage more than the center of the cage[45] and will usually urinate and defecate in approximately the same place(s) each day, in areas on the periphery. Healthy guinea pigs produce large quantities of stool and urine, necessitating daily changes of soiled bedding and at least weekly replacement of all of the bedding. It is not uncommon for them to defecate in food and water containers.

Because of their extremely high metabolic rate healthy guinea pigs defecate almost continuously. Feces tend to be dark green or brown, firm, cylindric pellets. Defecation is a relatively passive process and guinea pigs rarely strain to defecate. Soft cecal feces are ingested directly from the anus (cecotropes) throughout the day.[38]

Lack of stool production, which is usually secondary to anorexia and gastrointestinal stasis, is unfortunately often misinterpreted by clients and veterinarians as constipation and therefore mistreated. Specifically, enemas should never be given to a guinea pig or other small mammal unless radiographs indicate obstipation or other treatments have been unsuccessful.[3]

Predominantly gram-positive bacteria are present in the gastrointestinal tract, and the flora is sensitive to sudden changes in diet, including changes in food brand, which may precipitate gastrointestinal stasis and anorexia. Stasis can also occur if antibiotics used are that are of the gram-positive spectrum including oral amoxicillin, lincomycin, erythromycin, and streptomycin; use of such antibiotics often creates a fatal enterotoxemia.

Any change in the quantity or consistency of stool should be monitored carefully, and clients should be counseled to seek veterinary care if it persists for more than 12 hours. Older, obese guinea pigs, especially males, may get loose feces trapped in the perianal folds, which necessitates weekly gentle cleaning with a moistened cotton swab, along with manual expression. This may occur because of the presence of additional fatty folds in this area, loss of muscle tone,[20] and the inability of the guinea pig to groom the perianal area because of obesity. For this reason, every physical examination should include a check of the perianal folds regardless of the reason for presentation.

Urine can range from creamy white to thick and yellow with a turbid consistency. As in all herbivores the urine will have an alkaline pH and may normally contain many crystals.[21] Urination is a relatively passive process in which guinea pigs will just barely squat and raise their heads slightly. It is my experience that a guinea pig may urinate if it is stressed, nervous, or frightened. As with other species, pollakiuria, stranguria, and oliguria can be seen with cystitis, cystic calculi or other uroliths, cystic ovaries, pyometra, hydrometra, and metritis. Other signs of urinary tract disease include anorexia, hematuria, dysuria, and a huddled, hunched posture. Stranguria in guinea pigs is evidenced by an exaggerated lifting of the bottom and may be accompanied by grunting sounds and a strained facial expression. Porphyrin staining of the urine can occur with stress, with ingestion of certain legumes, and when taking certain antibiotics. Clients often mistake this brownish- or orangish-colored urine for hematuria.

Reproductive Behaviors

Male Reproductive Behaviors

Males reach puberty at 10 to 12 weeks of age but will exhibit mounting behavior as early as 1 month and will ejaculate as early as 2 months of age. Courtship behaviors of males include circling the female, sniffing and licking the female, swinging movements of the rump (known as the "rumba"), with or without a purring vocalization, and mounting.[6]

During mating, copulation time is short and ejaculation occurs immediately. Several hours after breeding, a rubbery or waxy copulatory plug of coagulated ejaculate may be seen in the cage.[21] The copulatory plug has been shown to completely block the spermatozoa of males that mate with females secondarily. In one study a second mating by males with colored coats did not affect the coat colors of pups from female albino guinea pigs previously mated to albino males.[34]

Sexual behavior of males toward their mother and their female siblings has been shown to be suppressed in continuous housing situations.[17] However, juvenile male guinea pigs (35 days old) that were removed from their mothers for a 1- to 2-day period were found to exhibit sexual behaviors toward their mother when reunited.[15] Castration and ovariohysterectomy should nevertheless be performed if siblings of varied gender are to remain in family groups to eliminate the chance of inbreeding.

Female Reproductive Behaviors and Parental Care

Sexual maturity in female guinea pigs occurs as early as 4 to 6 weeks of age, and sows are nonseasonally polyestrous, cycling every 15 to 17 days (range, 13 to 21 days) with spontaneous ovulation. During proestrus the sow will experience an increase in activity, will chase cagemates while making a guttural sound, and will often exhibit a swaying of the hindquarters (the rumba). Estrus lasts approximately 6 to 11 hours; the sow will exhibit lordosis by elevating the rump, and the vulva will dilate. Sows have a membrane over the vagina that opens for 2 days during estrus and at about 26 days into gestation to prepare for parturition.[44]

Gestation is 59 to 72 days, with an average of 68 days. Within 2 days of parturition a separation of the pubis and the ischium of up to $1\frac{1}{5}$ inches (apporoximately 3 cm) occurs. Relaxin causes the fibrocartilage of the pubic symphysis to break down. Sows should be bred before 6 months of age to prevent complications in farrowing that can occur because of fusion of the pelvic symphysis as the suture line mineralizes. Also, with age an accumulation of fat in the pelvic area can cause difficulty at parturition.

Females do not exhibit nest-building behavior before giving birth.[21] They may experience bilateral alopecia of flanks and back, and the abdomen can double in size during the 59- to 72-day gestation period. Quickening can be noted approximately 1 week before parturition. Prepartum eclampsia or toxemia can occur late in gestation. If the late-term sow becomes lethargic and anorexic, immediate cesarean section is warranted in order to preempt seizures, coma, and death.

Litter size is usually 2 to 4 but has been documented from 1 to 13. Gestation may be shorter in primiparous sows and those with small litters.[37] Sows carrying only one fetus may not show until late in gestation. Sows will readily eat the placenta after parturition, and in an uncomplicated farrowing little straining is noted as the birth of each pup occurs relatively quickly, with approximately 5 minutes between births and less than 30 minutes for the entire birthing process.

Dystocia is a relatively common problem in guinea pigs and can occur because of fusion of the pubic symphysis, obesity, and large fetal size. Straining, vocalizations, anxiousness, and biting at the abdomen may indicate dystocia. If the sow is noted to be straining for longer than 30 minutes, appears depressed, or exhibits a hemorrhagic or greenish discolored vaginal discharge, veterinary advice should be sought immediately, as an emergency caesarean section is warranted.

A fertile postpartum estrus occurs from 2 to 24 hours after parturition. The boar should be separated before parturition and remain away until the pups are weaned and separated at about 15 to 21 days.

Pups need sow's milk for up to 5 days but will nurse for up to 3 weeks even though they are also eating solid foods. The female generally stands or sits up as the pups nurse from her, and the pups push up under the abdomen to reach the mammary glands. Nursing sows will readily "aunt" or foster babies from another litter and are protective of one another's pups. An inexperienced sow, however, may cannibalize or reject her young if stressed or disturbed during the periparturient period. Neonates may not nurse for up to 12 hours after parturition,[9] and the sow and litter should not be disturbed during this time.

Neonatal Behavior

As stated previously, newborn cavies are born with their eyes open and are fully haired. They are active, alert, and grooming soon after birth. They will nurse several times throughout the day and will show an interest in solid food within the first 24 hours. Pups that do not receive sow's milk within the first 3 to 4 days after birth rarely survive.[10] As with other species, it is necessary for sows to lick the anogenital region of the young in order to stimulate defecation and urination for the first 7 to 14 days.[21] Pups will also eat the sow's feces, which helps to populate their gastrointestinal tract with a proper balance of bacterial flora.[38]

Neonates will begin to eat solid food within the first few days, and food preferences are developed early; therefore it is best to provide a variety of foods in these important first weeks to months of life (Figure 5-11). When excited or frightened the babies may jump up in the air in a movement referred to as "popcorning."

Behavioral Enrichment

Life for guinea pigs can be made more interesting by catering to their behavioral and instinctual needs. As stated previously (in the discussion of locomotor behaviors and activities), providing time outside of the cage is important in order to increase exercise and mental stimulation. Many owners use portable folding pens either indoors or outdoors; however, with a little imagination and supervision a guinea pig–safe area can easily be created. A small plastic swimming pool with a newspaper or bed sheet lining makes a novel enclosure, and when laced with greens, hay, and carrots becomes a welcome change to caged living (Figure 5-12). Converting a room (or a small area of a room) into a play area can be easily accomplished by providing a series of connected cardboard boxes, plastic or PVC tubes, or towels or sheets draped to create tunnels and caves.

Guinea Pig Behavior 227

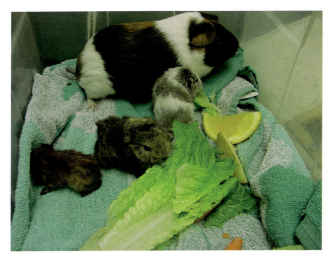

Figure 5-11
Guinea pigs will begin to eat solid food within the first 1 or 2 days after birth. Food preferences develop early, so a variety of food items should be offered at a young age to increase acceptance. (Courtesy Teresa Bradley Bays.)

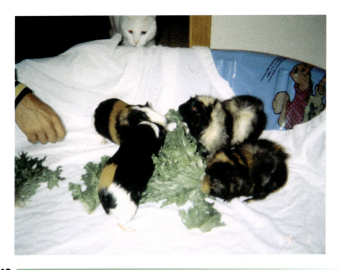

Figure 5-12
Placing guinea pigs in a plastic baby pool will help to provide exercise and enrichment. An adult should supervise them, especially if other household pets are nearby. (Courtesy Teresa Bradley Bays.)

Medical Implications of Abnormal Behavior

Healthy guinea pigs are active, inquisitive, and curious about their environment. They have both bright eyes and a shiny coat, and the eyes and nose are free of discharge. Cavies that are ill are inactive and lethargic, with dull, unfocused eyes and dull, rough hair coats (Figure 5-13). They eat and defecate less or not at all. Immediate veterinary care is necessary when these signs of sickness are noted.

Except when anorectic, guinea pigs will always have food in the oral cavity or pharynx, so care must be taken to gently swab out the mouth when they are anesthetized so this "green slime" will not be aspirated. Also, salivary and respiratory secretions tend to be copious and thick in guinea pigs, and some practitioners use anticholinergics such as glycopyrrolate (Baxter Healthcare, Deerfield, IL.).

An examination of the oral cavity of every guinea pig patient is recommended in order to check the teeth and verify that the guinea pig has been eating. A complete examination with the patient under anesthesia is imperative if dental pathology is suspected. This procedure should be referred to a veterinarian who has the proper small mammal speculums and dental equipment. Skull radiographs taken with the guinea pig under anesthesia are also recommended to assess tooth roots and to check for maxillary and mandibular osteomyelitis.

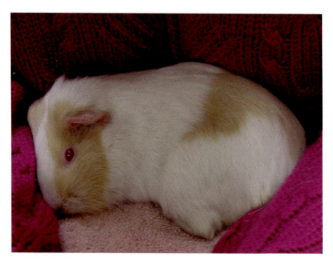

Figure 5-13
Seriously ill guinea pigs do not respond to their environment, have glazed eyes, and are very lethargic. This photo of a recently acquired cavy was taken in the examination room. The owner thought it was just a "mellow" guinea pig. (Courtesy Teresa Bradley Bays.)

> **BOX 5-3** **Clinical Signs of Dental and Orofacial Problems in Guinea Pigs**
>
> Anorexia
> Weight loss
> Hypersalivation
> Perioral dermatitis
> Dermatitis of the chin or neck area
> Lack of grooming
> Staining on the forelimbs
> Pawing at the mouth
> Grinding of teeth
> Restricted jaw movement
> Lumps or masses around the face and jaw
> Discomfort on palpation of the cheek teeth
> Discomfort on palpation of the ventral mandible
> Exophthalmos
> Ocular or nasal discharge
> Polydipsia
> Changes in quantity and consistency of fecal droppings
> Dysphagia
> Preferential chewing on one side of the mouth
> Exhibiting interest in food without eating it
> Picking up, then dropping food items
> Avoiding preferred food items

Dental and orofacial problems in guinea pigs may be evidenced by clinical and behavioral changes that range from subtle to obvious (Box 5-3). More obvious clinical signs of pathology may include anorexia, weight loss, hypersalivation, and lumps or masses around the face and jaw. More subtly, dysphagia may create preferential chewing on one side of the mouth or exhibiting interest in a food item without its consumption, as evidenced by picking up and then dropping food items.[3] Changes in food preferences such as avoiding preferred food items might also indicate oral pathology. Early detection of orofacial problems depends on the ability of the owner and the clinician to recognize these often minor behavioral changes.

The upper arcade of cheek teeth (molars and premolars) naturally slants toward the buccal surface; therefore elongated spikes and spurs can cause trauma and abscessation of this area. The lower arcade of cheek teeth slants toward the center of the mouth, so elongation of the teeth secondary to malocclusion may cause trauma to or even entrapment of the tongue.

Malocclusion, as in other species, can be the result of a genetic predisposition or of trauma, infection, or poor diet. As stated previously, vitamin C deficiency may cause a decrease in collagen formation, resulting in tooth movement. Diets without high-fiber grass hays and greens do not encourage the lateral grinding movement that is natural for this species and that helps to keep the teeth from overgrowing. A lack of natural sunlight in cavies housed indoors can create decreased production of vitamin D_3, which affects calcium metabolism and has been implicated as a cause of malocclusion in rabbits.[8]

Antibiotic-associated endotoxemia will result in an overgrowth of *Clostridium difficile*, and clinical signs will include diarrhea, anorexia, dehydration, and hypothermia. If a guinea pig is presented with these signs, it is important to ascertain whether the patient has been prescribed antibiotics with a primarily gram-positive spectrum by another unknowing veterinarian or if perhaps the owner treated the guinea pig with drugs left over from another pet.

Normal weights for females range from 700 to 900 g (25 to 32 oz), and weights for males range from 900 to 1200 g (32 to 42 oz). Unfortunately obesity is a relatively common problem for domestic guinea pigs. Obesity, as in other species, can lead to or exacerbate medical problems including osteoarthritis, problems with locomotion, and difficulty grooming (Figure 5-14). Counseling owners on proper diet and exercise and recognizing

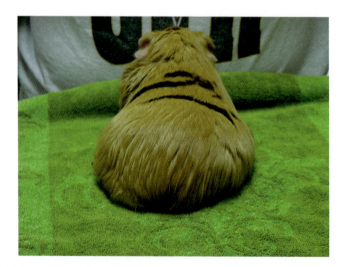

Figure 5-14
Obesity because of too much food and not enough exercise is becoming a more common problem in guinea pigs. Pododermatitis leading to open lesions and osteomyelitis are common sequelae of obesity. (Courtesy Teresa Bradley Bays.)

how obesity can affect daily activities and well-being is an important aspect of providing veterinary care to guinea pigs.

Fecal impaction of the anus can occur and is often seen in geriatric guinea pigs, more frequently in overweight males in my experience. Again, this may be a result of loss of muscle tone or the inability to eat cecotropes from the anus,[37] possibly associated with obesity, osteoarthritis, or discospondylosis. Congealed ejaculum in boars may also create a proteinaceous urethral obstruction that may result in urethritis.[36]

Cystic ovaries are common in females and occur in about 76% between the ages of 2 to 4 years.[30] Because this can be a painful and recurrent condition that may lead to secondary gastrointestinal stasis, prophylactic ovariohysterectomy should be discussed with owners when guinea pig pets are young. Pregnancy toxemia, also known as *pregnancy ketosis,* can be seen in obese, usually primiparous sows in the last 2 weeks of gestation or in the first postpartum week. Signs occur quickly, and the sow will become anorectic and stop drinking. She will become prostrate and dyspneic within 24 hours due to hypoglycemia and ketonemia. Because obesity and fasting can lead to this metabolic state, overweight males can also succumb.

Guinea pigs are extremely susceptible to heat stress and if kept outdoors can succumb in temperatures as low as 70° to 75°F (21° to 24°C).[36] Clinical signs include hypersalivation, tachypnea, pale mucous membranes, and increased rectal temperature. Prognosis even with supportive care is guarded, and coma and death are common sequelae.

Hospitalization, Stress, and the Sick Guinea Pig

Both outpatient and inpatient guinea pigs should be handled carefully when in the hospital. A towel or mat should be placed on the examination table to provide traction and warmth in order to decrease stress in guinea pig patients. Visually observe behavior, mobility, and alertness while collecting dietary and environmental history and assessing clinical complaints. Greens, hay, and carrots should be provided in the examination room (after oral examination with an otoscope has been performed). This is another way a clinician can assess the overall health of the cavy as well as calm a nervous patient. Approach the guinea pig patient slowly and quietly from eye level. Talking quietly about what you are doing as you do it also seems to keep guinea pig patients calmer.

Guinea pigs feel more secure when hospitalized if provided with a hide box, shelter, or towel to burrow into and under for sleeping as well as to retreat to if startled. These simulate the burrows that are often used in the wild for shelter and safety. Solid plastic igloos are not recommended, as they do not provide ventilation and a shy guinea pig may spend all of its time in the igloo, sitting in its own urine and feces. It is important to keep guinea pigs in a quiet area of the hospital away from cats, barking dogs, and other loud noises.

Because guinea pigs are unable to vomit, it is not necessary or recommended to fast them for more than 1 hour before surgery. I usually encourage them to eat and drink right up to the time of surgery and, it is hoped, soon after they recover from anesthesia. As previously stated, the oral cavity usually contains a green sludge, and this should be carefully removed when anesthetic induction has been accomplished. Postoperative supportive care includes syringe-feeding Critical Care (Oxbow Pet Products, Murdock, Neb.) until the guinea pig is eating well on its own. After gastrointestinal surgery, however, a short fast of 12 to 15 hours is recommended.

Preoperative, perioperative, and postoperative analgesics are imperative to decrease postoperative stress and pain in this delicate prey species. Preoperative and postoperative use of gastrointestinal motility enhancers as well as warmed fluids and analgesics as needed is recommended in order to maintain gastrointestinal function, which may be compromised secondary to anesthesia, pain, fear, stress, and illness.

For nail trimming and examination of the ventrum and the feet, the guinea pig should be held in the C position, with the holder grasping under the front feet with one hand and cupping the rump with the other (Figure 5-15). If the guinea pig begins to squirm, a minor alteration in the C position often makes the patient feel more secure.

As stated previously (see the discussion of social and antisocial behaviors) guinea pigs tend to be susceptible to stressful situations and do not accept change well, often going off feed and losing weight in response to new or different situations such as a new cage or other environmental changes. Sick guinea pigs stress easily and do not tolerate much in the way of handling, so excess handling should be avoided if they are nervous, frightened, or ill. It is important to limit diagnostic procedures and to minimize handling in severely debilitated guinea pigs while providing the necessary supportive care.

Guinea pigs that are socialized and well-adapted to their environment tend to have a much better prognosis regardless of the disease. The decrease in stress and subsequent stress-induced physiologic response seem to provide and increased tolerance for surgery and hospitalization. These patients also appear to respond better and faster to treatment when handled, stroked, and talked to gently by the veterinary staff at times other than when being handled for treatment.[3]

As practitioners, we often insist on separating hospitalized and postsurgical patients from other pets. As stated previously, however (see the

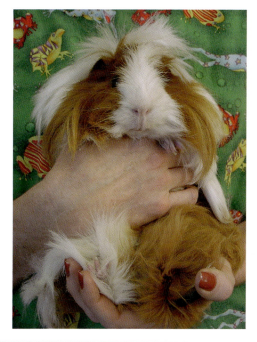

Figure 5-15
Guinea pigs should be well supported when held. This photo demonstrates the C position, in which the rump is cupped with one hand and the other hand is placed beneath the front legs. Examinations, nail trims, and other procedures can be easily performed using this position. (Courtesy Teresa Bradley Bays.)

discussion of social and antisocial behavior), the stress associated with separating bonded pairs and trios is sufficient enough that it may lead to impaired healing and secondary physiologic compromise. It is therefore recommended to place bonded guinea pigs back together as soon as possible (i.e., once the patient is standing and eating postoperatively).

Guinea pigs that are normally passive may bite when afraid and may squeal and struggle to escape. If startled or scared they may run quickly in circles and stampede while squealing, and it is not uncommon for them to hurt themselves or trample young if they are underfoot during this stampeding.[9] Because of the tendency to stampede in a circular fashion, providing square or rectangular cages or pens is recommended.

Cavies tend to panic when frightened and may freeze with the head elevated slightly and eyes bulging or legs drawn in as the pig presses against objects. Guinea pigs are one of the species that exhibit tonic immobility when faced with a predator-prey confrontation whereby innate fear creates a temporary state of profound and reversible motor inhibition.[35] Guinea pigs also may make explosive attempts to escape[37] if frightened or in reaction to an unexpected noise or other stimulus. Care must be taken to protect them from falls or injury in the hospital environment.

Guinea pigs that are isolated in a new environment initially respond by vocalizing and running around; with increased time they will enter a passive stage in which they will crouch with eyes closed and exhibit extensive piloerection and an increase in rectal temperature.[13] This "stress-induced sickness behavior" was shown not to occur if the pigs were with their mother in the new environment.[13]

Behaviors Associated with Pain

As with any prey species, early recognition of pain is extremely important, as pain can produce secondary physiologic changes that can be life threatening. These changes include decreased peripheral circulation, decreased body temperature, gastrointestinal stasis, shock, and even death. Signs of pain in a guinea pig can range from subtle to obvious behavioral changes (Box 5-4) and are more easily recognized when the practitioner is familiar with how a guinea pig would behave under similar circumstances when not in pain.[3]

BOX 5-4 Clinical Signs of Pain in Guinea Pigs*

Anorexia
Production of fewer, smaller, or no fecal pellets
Polydipsia (especially with gastrointestinal pain)
Subnormal body temperature
Ears and limbs that are cool to the touch
Splinting/stinting on palpation of affected area
Rapid, shallow breathing
Chewing over affected area
Strained facial expression with bulging eyes
Pressing of abdomen to the floor or table
Dull unfocused eyes and/or half-closed lids
Standing with head extended
Squealing during handling or touching of affected area
Aggression in a normally mild-mannered guinea pig
Immobility
Lethargy and lack of resistance to handling and procedures
Pale mucous membranes

*These are signs that can be seen with any disease process, but if associated with disease or procedures that have pain as a component, then pain should be managed.

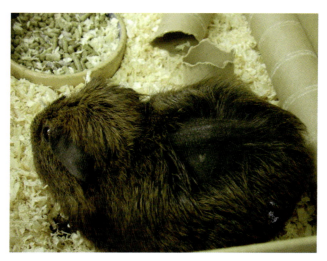

Figure 5-16

Alopecia can occur in guinea pigs from self-barbering or mutual barbering, secondary to parasites, or as a result of hormonal imbalance such as occurs with ovarian cysts or during pseudopregnancy. Alopecia also is seen during late stages of pregnancy. Guinea pigs may pull hair at sites of pain as well. (Courtesy Jörg Mayer.)

Guinea pigs in pain may have eyes that appear dull and unfocused (sometimes with lids partially closed) or fixed and bulging in a strained expression. They will often stand quietly with head extended, and breathing may be rapid and shallow. Also, polydipsia is commonly noted in small mammal herbivores experiencing gastrointestinal or other abdominal pain.[3]

Cavies may chew at the abdomen or other affected body part, which will create areas of alopecia and even excoriations from self-trauma (Figure 5-16). They also may stop eating and defecating and appear reluctant to move. A normally mild-mannered guinea pig that is in pain may bite, jump, squeal, or run when touched. A nervous, flighty cavy may become lethargic and allow handling without a struggle.

Managing pain in all species has become a priority in veterinary medicine, and for guinea pigs and other prey species that easily succumb to the stress associated with pain, the necessity for appropriate analgesics cannot be overemphasized. As in other species, when pain is managed in guinea pig patients they tend to recover more quickly from trauma, illness, and surgery, eat sooner, and are less prone to suffer from the effects of gastrointestinal stasis, which can be life threatening.

Guinea Pigs and Euthanasia

Like many other types of pets that have become popular since the 1990s, guinea pigs are becoming more commonplace in shelters and at rescue groups. Unfortunately, this also means that many are being euthanized, as it is often more difficult to find homes for them. For this reason it is best to counsel clients to adopt rather than to buy pet guinea pigs. If it becomes necessary to euthanize a guinea pig patient that is suffering, I prefer to anesthetize them first in an anesthetic chamber using isoflurane (Isoflo, Abbott Laboratories, North Chicago, IL). Euthanasia solution is then administered via intracardiac injection.

References

1. Berryman JC: Guinea pig vocalizations: their structure, causation and function, *Z Tierpsychol* 41:80-106, 1976.
2. Birmelin I: Behavior of pet animals, *Dtsch Tierarztl Wochenschr* 97(6):243-247, 1990.
3. Bradley TA: Normal behavior and the clinical implications of abnormal behavior in guinea pigs, *Vet Clin North Am Exot Anim Pract* 4(3):681-696, 2001.
4. Brismar BH, Lei W, Hjerpe A, Svensson O: The effect of body mass and physical activity on the development of guinea pig osteoarthrosis, *Acta Orthop Scand* 74(4):442-448, 2003.
5. Caston J, Yon E, Mellier D, Godfrey HP, et al: An animal model of autism: behavioural studies in the GS guinea pig, *Eur J Neurosci* 10(8):2677-2684, 1998.
6. Cohn DWH, Tokumaru RS, Ades C: Female novelty and the courtship behavior of guinea pigs *(Cavia porcellus)*, *Braz J Med Biol Res* 37(6):847-851, 2004.
7. Gelatt KN: *Veterinary ophthalmology*, ed 3, Philadelphia, 1999, Lippincott, Williams & Wilkins.
8. Harcourt-Brown F: Dental disease. In *Textbook of rabbit medicine*, Woburn, MA, 2002, Read Educational and Professional Publishing.
9. Harkness JE: *A practitioner's guide to domestic rodents*, Lakewood, Colo., 1993, American Animal Hospital Association (AAHA).
10. Harkness JE, Wagner JE: *The biology and medicine of rabbits and rodents*, ed 4, Baltimore, 1995, Williams & Wilkins.
11. Harper LV: Behavior. In Wagner JE, Manning PJ, editors: *The biology of the guinea pig*, New York, 1976, Academic Press.
12. Hennessy MB: Enduring maternal influences in a precocial rodent, *Dev Psychobiol* 42(3):225-236, 2003.
13. Hennessy MB, Deak T, Schiml-Webb PA, et al; Responses of guinea pig pups during isolation in a novel environment may represent stress-induced sickness behaviors, *Physiol Behav* 81(1):5-13, 2004.
14. Hennessy MB, Maken DS, Graves FC: Presence of mother and unfamiliar female alters levels of testosterone, progesterone, cortisol, adrenocorticotropin, and behavior in maturing guinea pigs, *Horm Behav* 42(1):42-52, 2002.
15. Hennessy MB, Mazzei SJ, McInturf SM: The fate of filial attachment in juvenile guinea pigs housed apart from the mother, *Dev Psychobiol* 29:641-651, 1996.

16. Hennessy MB, O'Leary SK, Hawke JL, Wilson SE: Social influences on cortisol and behavioral responses of preweaned, periadolescent, and adult guinea pigs, *Physiol Behav* 1:76(2):305-314, 2002.
17. Hennessy MB, Reed J, Wilson SE, Pitstick L: Sexual interactions of maturing male guinea pigs with their mothers, sisters, and unfamiliar adult females in the home cage, *Dev Psychobiol* 42(1):91-96, 2003.
18. Hennessy MB, Sharp K: Voluntary and involuntary maternal separation in guinea pig pups with mothers required to forage, *Dev Psychobiol* 23(8):783-796, 1990.
19. Hennessy MB, Young TL, O'Leary SK, Maken DS: Social preferences of developing guinea pigs *(Cavia porcellus)* from the preweaning to the periadolescent periods, *J Comp Psychol* 117(4):406-413, 2003.
20. Hillyer EV: Dermatologic diseases. In Hillyer EV, Quesenberry KE, editors: *Ferrets, rabbits, and rodents: clinical medicine and surgery,* Philadelphia, 1997, Saunders.
21. Hillyer EV, Quesenberry KE, Donnelly TM: Biology, husbandry, and clinical techniques of guinea pigs and chinchillas. In Hillyer EV, Quesenberry KE, editors: *Ferrets, rabbits, and rodents: clinical medicine and surgery,* Philadelphia, 1997, Saunders.
22. Horton BJ, West CE, Turley SD: Diurnal variation in the feeding pattern of guinea pigs, *Nutr Metab* 18(5-6):294-301, 1975.
23. Jenkins JR: Skin disorders of the rabbit, *J Small Exot Anim Med* 1:64-65, 1991.
24. Jenkins JR: Skin disorders of the rabbit, *Vet Clin North Am Exot Anim Pract* 4:543-563, 2001.
25. Kaiser S, Heeman K, Straub RH, Sachser N: The social environment affects behaviour and androgens, but not cortisol in pregnant female guinea pigs, *Psychoneuroendocrinology* 28(1):67-83, 2003.
26. Kaiser S, Kirtzeck M, Hornschuh G, Sachser N: Sex-specific difference in social support—a study in female guinea pigs, *Physiol Behav* 79(2):297-303, 2003.
27. Kaiser S, Kruijver FP, Straub RH, et al: Early social stress in male guinea-pigs changes social behavior, autonomic and neuroendocrine functions, *J Neuroendocrinol* 15(8):761-769, 2003.
28. Kaiser S, Kruijver FP, Swabb DF, Sachser N: Early social stress in female guinea pigs induces a masculinization in adult behavior and corresponding changes in brain and neuroendocrine function, *Behav Brain Res* 15:144(1-2):199-210, 2003.
29. Kaiser S, Sachser N: The social environment during pregnancy and lactation affects the female offsprings' endocrine status and behaviour in guinea pigs, *Physiol Behav* 63(3):361-366, 1998.
30. Keller LSF, Griffith JW, Long CM: Reproductive failure associated with cystic rete ovarii in guinea pigs, *J Vet Pathol* 24:335-339, 1987.
31. Kraus VB, Huebner JL, Stabler T, et al: Ascorbic acid increases the severity of spontaneous knee osteoarthritis in a guinea pig model, *Arthritis Rheum* 50(6):1822-1831, 2004.
32. Kunzl C, Sachser N: The behavioral endocrinology of domestication: a comparison between the domestic guinea pig *(Cavia aperea f. porcellus)* and wild ancestor, the cavy *(Cavia aperea), Horm Behav* 35(10):28-37, 1999.
33. Legendre LF: Oral disorders of exotic rodents, *Vet Clin North Am Exot Anim Pract,* 6(3):601-628, 2003.
34. Martan J, Shepherd BA: The role of the copulatory plug in reproduction of the guinea pig, *J Exp Zool* 196(1):79-84, 1976.

35. Olsen CK, Hogg S, Lapiz MD: Tonic immobility in guinea pigs: a behavioral response for detecting an anxiolytic-like effect? *Behav Pharmacol* 13(4):261-269, 2002.
36. O'Rourke DP: Disease problems in guinea pigs. In Quesenberry KE, Carpenter JW, editors: *Ferrets, rabbits, and rodents: clinical medicine and surgery*, ed 2, Philadelphia, 2003, Saunders.
37. Quesenberry KE, Donnelly TM, Hillyer EV: Biology, husbandry, and clinical techniques of guinea pigs and chinchillas. In Quesenberry KE, Carpenter JW, editors: *Ferrets, rabbits, and rodents: clinical medicine and surgery*, ed 2, Philadelphia, 2003, Saunders.
38. Richardson VCG: *Diseases of domestic guinea pigs*, London, 1992, Blackwell Scientific.
39. Ritchey RL, Hennessy MB: Cortisol and behavioral responses to separation in mother and infant guinea pigs, *Behav Neurol Biol* 48(1):1-12, 1987.
40. Sachser N: Of domestic and wild guinea pigs: studies in sociophysiology, domestication, and social evolution, *Naturwissenschaften* 85(7):307-317, 1998.
41. Sachser N, Lick C: Social stress in guinea pigs, *Physiol Behav* 46(2):137-144, 1989.
42. Suta D, Kvasnak E, Popelar J, Syka J: Representation of species-specific vocalizations in the inferior colliculus of the guinea pig, *J Neurophysiol* 90(6):3794-3808, 2003.
43. Walker ER: *Mammals of the world*, vol II, ed 3, Baltimore, 1975, Johns Hopkins University Press.
44. Weir BJ: Reproductive characteristics of hystricomorph rodents, *Symp Zool Soc London* 34:265-301, 1974.
45. White WJ, Balk MW, Lang CM: Use of cage space by guinea pigs, *Lab Anim* 23(3):208-214, 1989.

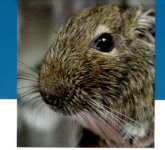

CHAPTER 6

ELIZABETH I. EVANS

Small Rodent Behavior: Mice, Rats, Gerbils, and Hamsters

Introduction

Animals in the order Rodentia are generally thought of as small, nocturnal, ground-dwelling animals that chew or gnaw constantly. Actually rodents vary greatly in size and habitat preference, but they all have continuously growing incisors and tend to be nocturnally active.[2,3,13,16] The constant need to chew can be endearing, as it makes them very busy and entertaining animals. It may also be somewhat unfortunate in pets, as it drives them to chew on their living quarters, often destroying their primary enclosure. This nocturnal behavior may also be annoying if these pets live in the bedrooms of their owners. But if we remain cognizant of normal rodent behaviors and provide appropriate caging, small rodents make great pets. Although many rodent species are kept as pets, only mice, rats, gerbils, and hamsters are discussed in this chapter.

The common house mouse *(Mus musculas)*, from which the pet mouse is derived, is native to Asia, India, and Europe, and the Norway or brown rat *(Rattus norvegicus)* originated in Asia. Both of these species have now been introduced almost worldwide and have adapted to life in close proximity to humans. They have become an integral part of the world's food chain and have many characteristics and behaviors that help them survive in large numbers. In addition, they have learned to eat almost anything they can find.

Gerbils *(Meriones unguiculatus)* are native to Mongolia, China, and Manchuria and were first brought to the United States as research animals. In their native home, they live in a wide variety of desert habitats. The golden, or Syrian, hamster is native to southeast Europe and northwest Syria and was domesticated and brought to the United States as a research animal. Chinese hamsters are a separate species *(Cricatus griseus)* (with a lower chromosome number) and are native to eastern China. There are other species of hamsters, but these are the two most commonly seen as pets and in research.

Many behaviors are found in all of these species in captivity. Unless otherwise noted, the following information applies to all applicable of these rodent species. The emphasis is on behaviors that vary appreciably from those typical of mammals.

Sensory Behaviors

Because these rodents are nocturnal and live on or in the ground, vision is their least-developed special sense, and rats, at least, are known to be colorblind.[13] The rodent's hearing is fairly well developed, and they appear to be able to sense ground vibrations.

The rodent's sense of smell is very well developed. Individuals of all four species initially investigate changes in their environment with their sense of smell. These rodents frequently hold their heads up in the air and sniff to identify the source of odors. If an odor is unknown, they may flare their nostrils and sniff faster, while moving around the cage to better determine the source of the odor. If they recognize a threat, they may try to hide or escape. When these rodents are manually restrained, they constantly smell their handlers and the environment and will struggle to get away if disturbed. For this reason it is important that veterinary personnel remember to wash their hands, change gloves, and wear clean lab coats when working with rodents. This is especially true in a veterinary hospital setting, in which the staff may handle predator species such as dogs and cats before handling the rodent.

Mice and rats do not have any grossly obvious scent-marking glands, but they may occasionally rub their faces and whiskers on their environment to mark their territory. This is seen more often in the males of these species.

Gerbils have a large ventral midline sebaceous gland that they often vigorously rub on substrates or surfaces in their cages (Figure 6-1). They slide on the belly or rub the abdomen on a vertical surface in an effort to mark territory. Male gerbils housed in social groups, with or without females, exhibit this behavior, with the most activity being evident in more dominant males housed with reproductively active females.[10] This gland may actually enlarge and be mistaken by an owner or unknowing clinician for a tumor or abscess. Occasionally these glands may "plug," forming a cystlike structure that is easily opened either when the gerbil is grooming or by rubbing it with a warm, moist gauze sponge.[2,13,16] In lactating female gerbils, studies have shown that removal of this ventral scent

Small Rodent Behavior 241

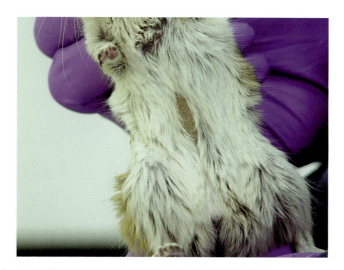

Figure 6-1
This is the ventral scent gland of a male gerbil. (Courtesy Kathleen Pritchett.)

gland caused retarded development of the nursing pups, indicating that the gland may have some form of brood patch function.[6]

Hamsters have bilateral scent glands on their flanks that are more developed in males (Figure 6-2).[2,3,13,16] When hamsters mark their territory, they often throw themselves on their sides, then quickly rub the flank area on the substrate. They also will stand next to a surface and rub the flank, appearing to be "wiggling" the hips. These glands are commonly mistaken for tumors or abscesses, especially in actively breeding animals, when they are usually surrounded by wet fur.

Communicative Behaviors

Generally gerbils are vocally quiet animals, whereas mice, rats, and hamsters often produce a wide range of sounds. However, most rodent species can be vocal when they are in pain or frightened with no means of escape.

Mice and rats produce similar vocalizations and often make clucking-type noises in the back of their throats, with or without other audible sounds, and occasionally while also grinding their teeth. If the animals are hungry or actively seeking food, these sounds may continue intermittently until they start eating. Female mice and rats are often heard making similar soft clucking noises while caring for their pups or grooming quietly in the cage. If mice and rats become agitated or frightened, their vocalizations become louder and sound more like squeaks or squeals. Generally,

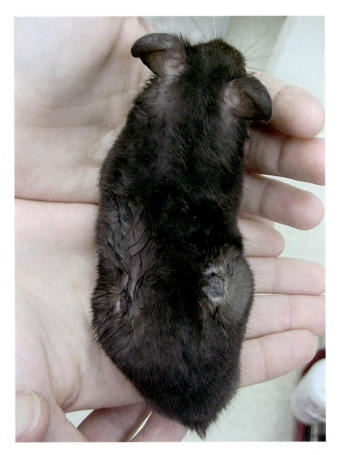

Figure 6-2
This photo depicts the flank (hip) scent glands of a male hamster. These glands can be mistaken as pathologic by owners and unknowing veterinarians and are more evident when the hair coat is unthrifty or if alopecia is present. (Courtesy Dan Johnson.)

if a mouse or rat in pain is left alone, it remains very quiet. If it is handled or lifted by the base of the tail, however, the vocalizations can become quite loud, and the animal will also struggle to get away and may bite.[3]

Hamsters often "chortle" in their throats while they are alone in their cages, are interacting in a group, or are handled by a human. If they are not accustomed to being handled or are roughly handled by a stranger, they can "gritch" quite loudly, often simultaneously baring their teeth. If a hamster is disturbed while sleeping, it usually immediately rolls to its back, bares its teeth, and gritches quite loudly for several seconds, often continuing for many more seconds after being left alone.[13] When the "threat" is over or they have been released into the cage, hamsters often continue vocalizing, gradually decreasing in volume to quiet "chortling" noises in the throat, while they pace around, settling back into a resting position. During this post-stress period, they can still be very easily and quickly aroused to a full "attack mode" with very little additional stimulation.

Hamsters in pain may remain very quiet in their bedding if the cause of the pain is located in one of the extremities. If they have abdominal, thoracic, or cranial pain, they may either remain quiet and tucked tightly into the bedding, or they may be very restless or pace around the cage quietly "chortling".

Although gerbils are not generally very vocal, they occasionally "chortle" quietly in their throats. But in the face of a potential threat, gerbils are more likely to stand on their hind legs and thump quickly with their hind feet than to vocalize.[2,13] This thumping may occur more frequently when gerbils are housed in cages with floors that accentuate the noise or cause significant vibrations. If in pain, gerbils do occasionally squeak or squeal when restrained and may attempt to bite if they cannot get away.

Social and Antisocial Behaviors

In general, rodents are highly social animals. However, when rodents are confined in cages, there are limits to the number of individuals that can coexist peacefully. It is important that each animal have an adequate amount of space and the opportunity to perform species-typical behaviors.[7] For rodents, two important and normal behaviors are chewing and hiding or burrowing. Therefore appropriate and adequate hard substrates for chewing and various types of nest boxes or bedding material should be provided to ensure normal social behaviors in caged rodents.[3,7]

Most mice can coexist quite peacefully, even in rather cramped quarters, with only a few exceptions. Males of some strains of mice (such as BALB/c) are quite aggressive, inflicting rather serious fight wounds on the tail or near the base of the tail, when confined together.[3,13] In the laboratory, male mice have been reported to exhibit physiologic and behavioral stress along with increased aggression when housed in continuous light.[17] Pet mice are generally not particularly aggressive toward one another, and males can often live in groups of two or maybe three in a large aquarium or cage. However, if someone wants to keep a group of mice as pets, it is recommended to purchase only females or to raise the males together from puberty, which can occur as early as 50 to 60 days of age (depending on the strain of mouse). Because mice are usually prolific breeders, it is recommended to keep single-gender groups to reduce antisocial behaviors such as fighting or cannibalism of pups.[3,13]

Mice and rats in compatible groups usually nest together and often pile on top of one another, usually in a corner of their enclosure (Figure 6-3). If there are any outcasts in the cage, they usually sleep separately from the group and may sleep in a more alert posture to allow them to easily monitor activity in the rest of the cage. In groups of adult mice and rats, hierarchies are often created, with the dominant animal easily identified. Especially in mice, the dominant animal can often be seen chewing the hair off other animals in the cage, a practice known as *barbering*.[13,16] If areas of alopecia are devoid of parasites or signs of other medical causes such as seborrhea and excoriations barbering should be considered as a probable cause.[3]

Although mice usually tolerate being handled, they are more prone to biting their owners than are rats. In fact, if mice are not accustomed to handling or believe they cannot escape, they are very likely to bite (Figure 6-4). If they do not break the skin when they bite, they usually pinch very hard and often hang on without letting go.

Rats are generally very social, regardless of their gender, and usually acclimate to crowded cages much better than mice. In cages, male rats occasionally have slight tiffs that may include vocalization and jumping at each other. This rarely results in injury to either individual and appears to be quickly forgotten. It is generally easier to introduce adult rats to a group than it is to introduce adult mice to one another.

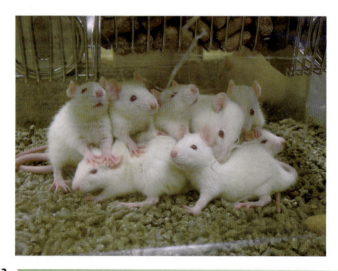

Figure 6-3
These juvenile rats are exhibiting normal "piled-on" social and sleeping behavior. (Courtesy Teresa Bradley Bays.)

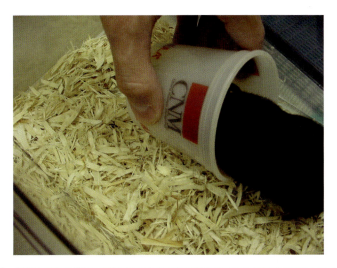

Figure 6-4
Hamsters and other rodents can often be coaxed into cups to facilitate capture and restraint without the handler being bitten. (Courtesy Dan Johnson.)

Of all the typical rodent species, rats and gerbils are the least likely to bite their owners, unless they are in pain. They are very tolerant of handling and even appear to show signs of affection for their owners. In my experience both rats and gerbils have responded to their spoken name and to the arrival of their owners.

Gerbils are a highly social and interactive species. They live well in pairs or small groups, especially if introduced to one another before puberty, and generally show signs of aggression only if in extremely overcrowded conditions. Barbering may also occur in gerbils, most often around the face and base of the tail. Unlike other rodents, gerbils are not truly nocturnal, as they are easily awakened and can remain quite active during the day. This, in combination with the lack of biting tendencies, makes gerbils ideal interactive pets, although they may be active during the night.[13]

Hamsters are often described as vicious animals, but if attention is paid to normal hamster behavior it can be better understood how we contribute to or cause that image. In general, hamsters lead more structured lives than the other common rodent pets and can therefore become more easily stressed in overcrowded conditions or when confined in a cage that is too small. Even when hamsters are living in a group, it is not uncommon for them to act as if they are living alone. They usually designate specific areas of their environment for separate activities (e.g., sleeping, eating, elimination) and use their extensive cheek pouches to move materials around the cage on a regular basis.[3,13] Chinese, or dwarf, hamsters do not appear to be as easily stressed but do exhibit behaviors similar to those of the golden, or Syrian, hamster. All hamsters prefer having one or more hiding places per individual in a single cage.

When sleeping, hamsters tuck their head entirely under their abdomen, making them completely oblivious to their surroundings, regardless of whether they are sleeping inside a nest or on a solid surface. Their heads are so covered that they cannot smell or hear anything that is approaching them. Therefore, when they are disturbed or touched while sleeping, they are quite startled and usually respond by rolling onto the back, baring the teeth, and "gritching" loudly in an effort to intimidate the intruder. If the intruder is another hamster, a fight may ensue in which serious injuries may be inflicted. However, if the hamsters have grown up together or have a large enough space, this type of confrontation is relatively rare and is much less likely to result in injury. If an owner or a clinician causes or persists in handling the hamster in this startled state, a serious bite is usually the result. However, if instead of immediately touching or grabbing the sleeping hamster, the owner or clinician taps loudly on the cage, jiggles the cage, or creates other appropriate disturbances to awaken the hamster, biting can be avoided, as the hamster is much less stressed if handled when already awake and alert.

Female hamsters can be extremely aggressive when caring for pups, and this aggression can be directed at other hamsters in the cage or at the owner.[16] Newborn hamsters should not be disturbed for at least 3 to 4 days after birth to reduce the chance of cannibalism that may occur when a potential threat is perceived by the mother. Whenever possible, pregnant females should be housed in separate cages without males, to decrease the likelihood of maternal cannibalism. Even with all of these precautions, however, cannibalism by mother hamsters is still a strong possibility if they are stressed.[13]

Reproductive Behaviors

Male Reproductive Behaviors

Breeding behavior in all of these rodent species occurs mostly at night. Male rodents are increasingly territorial when housed with or able to smell females in estrus. Since estrous cycles occur more than once a week, it is best to house only one male in a cage with three to five female mice or rats. During this time, male mice may be a little more stressed and, therefore, may be more likely to bite their owners, even when housed only with females. Male rats may appear more anxious or active when housed with multiple breeding females but generally are not more inclined to bite.

Male rodents have open inguinal canals and can pull their testes into their abdominal cavity, especially when stressed or frightened. Therefore, the presence or absence of a scrotum should not be used to determine gender of a rodent. Instead, the anogenital distance is used to sex these species. Males have the longest distance between the anus and the genital opening, and their external genitalia has a circular opening rather than a slit.*

Gerbils are usually bred in pairs, which can remain together throughout life. The male is not inclined to be aggressive when breeding or after the babies are born and does not need to be removed from the primary cage at any time.

Male hamsters are not usually more aggressive when housed with females in estrus. The concern is that the female hamster may be more aggressive and may harm the male. Therefore, after breeding occurs in hamsters, the male is usually removed for his protection and to help reduce the incidence of maternal cannibalism.

Female Reproductive Behaviors

As rodents are an important part of the food chain, many behaviors exist to help ensure breeding success. Mice, rats, gerbils, and hamsters deliver litters of altricial pups (i.e., no hair or teeth, eyes closed) that require maternal care for approximately 3 weeks.[1,13] Most of these animals breed easily and repeatedly in captivity, although gerbils do not usually breed as frequently as the other three species. Estrous cycles occur approximately every 4 to 8 days, depending on the species and strain, and generally continue throughout the year if temperatures are appropriate. Postpartum estrous cycles are usually fertile in mice and rats (and occasionally in hamsters and gerbils), although implantation is delayed, thereby increasing the length of the subsequent gestation.[3,4,12,13] This is often the explanation for a second litter of pups after a male has been removed from the cage after delivery of the first litter.

Female mice living in single-gender groups tend to become pseudopregnant for several weeks at a time in order to conserve metabolic energy.[1,4] When a male is introduced to the group, most of the females will be in estrus within approximately 72 hours, often breeding with that male the third night after the introduction.[1,4] However, if that male is removed from the cage within the first 4 days after fertilization (approximately 7 days

---

*References 1,2,3,5,13,16.

after the original introduction into the group), and a different male is placed into the cage, many of the females may spontaneously abort (with no overt clinical signs) and enter estrus to breed with the new male approximately 72 hours later. This phenomenon may also occur in female rats and hamsters under similar circumstances. In gerbils the presence of strange males and females can block implantation, as can physical separation of newly mated monogamous pairs, but only if the female is not lactating.[9,11]

An early behavioral sign of estrus in the female rat is quivering of the ear when the head or back is gently stroked. In addition, female rats will also exhibit characteristic lordosis (ventral curvature of the lumbar spine) with digital stimulation of the pelvic area.[1]

Rodent semen contains a great deal of dissolved protein that thickens when deposited in the female's vagina. This forms what is called a *copulating* or *mating plug*, which helps to seal the sperm inside the female reproductive tract to increase the likelihood of fertilization. This plug may be seen either in the entrance to the female tract or in the bedding after it falls out of the female. Although breeders look for these plugs, it is important to remember that they only document the act of mating and they do not indicate that fertilization (or pregnancy) has occurred.[1,2,13]

Female hamsters have a thick, opaque, stringy, postovulatory discharge that is normal but is often mistaken for vaginitis. The presence of this discharge can be used to determine receptivity for breeding 3 days later.[5] A female hamster may be slightly more irritable at approximately this point in her estrous cycle, so this behavior may contribute to the overall image of an aggressive animal, especially as the estrous cycle is so short. However, at peak estrus, female hamsters demonstrate lordosis almost immediately after introduction of a male.[5]

Gestation in rodents is relatively short, with hamsters having the shortest—approximately 16 days. Gerbil gestation is approximately 25 days, and for rats and mice it is approximately 20 to 23 days, depending on the strain. Following a postpartum estrus, gestation is generally increased by approximately 3 to 5 days as implantation is delayed because of the onset of lactation. Gerbil postpartum gestations are delayed only if three or more young are nursed.[9] Hamsters may begin reproductive activity at a very early age, perhaps as early as 1 month of age, so weaning should be done as quickly as possible if prevention of additional litters is desired.[5]

One unique characteristic of almost all mice, and often of rats, is that females are capable of lactation even if they have not been pregnant. In order to determine the biologic mother of a litter, it is necessary to separate pregnant females one to a cage before delivery because once the first litter is born, all females in the cage will demonstrate equal maternal behavior within just a few hours. Virgin females can lactate within 24 hours of exposure to newborn pups, making it relatively easy to cross-foster pups for various reasons. This trait definitely increases the survival rate of pups in the wild when a mother might succumb to a predator. When more than one litter is present in a cage, all litters become co-mingled shortly after birth, even if multiple nests are maintained in the cage. Mothers are frequently seen carrying pups from one nest to another and have no preference for their biologic pups over other pups in the enclosure.

Even though most rodents are very good mothers, cannibalism is a common problem.[1,2,5,13] Hamsters are the species most likely to cannibalize their young, especially if two females are housed together or the male is left with the mother after the pups are born. First litters are the most likely to be cannibalized in all rodent species, and highly inbred females are also more likely to cannibalize their young. If this happens, changes can be made for subsequent litters to decrease the chance of cannibalism. Isolation of the mother from other females and removal of the male before parturition may help. Placing the cage in a quiet area away from as many potential causes of stress as possible and providing a solid hiding place for the pups may also help to control cannibalism. In addition, the mother and pups should not be disturbed for up to a week after their birth. Removing the male before parturition will ensure that no postpartum breeding occurs, which may also decrease cannibalism, especially in a female's first litter. Although ultimately this reduces the number of possible litters per female per year, it provides a physiologic rest that may keep the female healthy for a longer period of time.

Nervous mothers often prefer solid nest boxes rather than elaborate nests built out of bedding material. These can be provided very inexpensively in the form of cardboard boxes with a small opening. Baking soda or other small cans (with sharp edges removed), toilet paper or paper towel rolls, or similar objects can also be used. Cardboard objects will probably eventually be chewed up to become part of the bedding. If provided less than a week before delivery, however, they will often last as a nest for the first 1 or 2 weeks after the pups are delivered. The purpose of these nest boxes is to provide a dark, quiet space in which the pups can be hidden from view. Handling the nest, even to gently pick up a nest box to look inside, may be enough to convince the mother rodent that a threat is present and increase the chances of cannibalism.

In all of these species, females that breed continually may have thin hair in their interscapular area if the males chew on the female's hair while mating. Sometimes female hamsters will have abrasions of the skin if they struggle during mating.

Eating Behaviors

The most obvious eating behavior of all rodents is their continuous need to chew. As nocturnal species, food and water consumption occurs mostly during the night. Mice, rats, gerbils, and hamsters locate food by sniffing, grasp food with their mouths, sit on their haunches to eat, use their elbows to grasp food, and manipulate their food with their front feet as they are eating, even if the food is too large to be held in their paws.[18] They will also stick their incisors through any opening to gnaw on anything they can reach that is outside their primary enclosure. This intense need to chew may result in the incisors getting caught, broken, or misaligned. Hamsters have a more rounded muzzle, so they are not always capable of eating through traditional metal feeders or chewing between the wires of a standard cage.

If fed with a bowl, it is not uncommon for mice and rats to move their bedding around enough that the food bowl gets covered. But, despite popular thought, they do not generally hide food with the intent of storing it for later use. If fresh vegetables or fruits are fed, the cage should be checked carefully and any leftovers removed before they spoil, as mice and rats will eat the spoiled food, which could result in gastrointestinal upset.

Gerbils are efficient desert animals and therefore do not have a large daily requirement for water, but supplemental water should be provided at all times.[13,16] Unlike other species, they do not often play with their water bottles, so owners may not be able to tell that they are drinking any water at all. If they are fed any fresh moisture-containing food as a treat, gerbils may indeed not need to drink any supplemental water. Therefore, if a gerbil is observed drinking large quantities of water or if the water bottle volume appears to be dropping quickly without evidence of a leak, the gerbil may have a medical condition such as renal disease.

Many of the diets sold for gerbils are seed mixtures, often containing large numbers of sunflower seeds. Gerbils and other rodents preferentially eat sunflower seeds almost as quickly as their bowl is filled. If the owner continues to provide sunflower seeds, the rodent may eat them exclusively, thus producing an oily hair coat suggestive of nutritional deficiency.

Hamsters have very large cheek pouches that extend back to the shoulder area. They are also hoarders, so when their food bowl is filled, hamsters will use their cheek pouches to transport all the food to another location, where it is buried under bedding. If owners are not aware of this hoarding behavior, hamsters will empty the food bowl every time it is filled. And with even the little dampness normally found in a cage, the food will often spoil or sprout, causing diarrhea if the hamster eats the spoiled food.[2,3,5,13,16]

Small Rodent Behavior

Cheek pouches are also used by hamsters to carry bedding materials and babies. If a lactating hamster is stressed, she will often put her entire litter into her pouches to protect them. If the perceived threat does not quickly dissipate, the babies may suffocate in her cheek pouches.[3] The cheek pouch is an immunologically privileged site whereby there is no lymphatic tissue present, so bedding or other material can stay in the cheek pouches for a very long time, even months, without a significant risk of infection.[13]

Elimination Behaviors

These species do not generally reserve a specific area for defecation, and fecal pellets are normally found throughout the cage and the bedding material. All rodents practice coprophagia, but it is not required for nutritional reasons and it is not prevented when rodents are housed on wire floors.[12] Rodents may randomly pick up fecal pellets from the cage and eat them, or they may eat feces directly from the anus.

Mice, rats, and gerbils urinate at random in their cages, although not usually in their sleeping areas. Gerbils, being desert animals, do not urinate large volumes, and it is usually hard to find wet litter in their cage. This lack of urine volume not only keeps the cage dry but prevents a buildup of odor, so it is not necessary to clean gerbil cages as often as those of other rodent species. Because gerbils often build elaborate nests with their bedding materials, it may not be necessary to remove the nest when cleaning but simply to scoop out and replace the bedding unrelated to the nest.

Hamsters, on the other hand, usually designate a specific corner of the cage as their "potty corner" and routinely urinate in that exact same spot.[13] Their urine is concentrated and opaque in appearance because of high protein and mucus content. Because of the volume and chemical content, hamster urine is more odorous than that of other rodents and also more destructive to metal cages. Urine deposition results in lime deposits in the urine corner of the hamster's cage.

Locomotor Behaviors and Activities

Most locomotive behavior occurs at night, as rodents are generally nocturnal. They spend considerable time exploring their enclosures and will climb over every available surface. It is not uncommon for them to also spend considerable time burrowing in their bedding or attempting to dig into the bottom of the cage (Figure 6-5). Gerbils are especially persistent diggers and will spend hours every night scratching at the corners and edges of their cage, often aggressively scattering their bedding in many

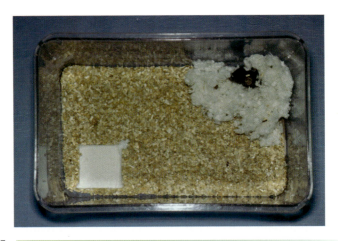

Figure 6-5
This mouse is sitting in a nest that it made from a compressed cotton pad like the one in the opposite corner. Similar nests can be made from paper towels or other materials. (Courtesy Kathleen Pritchett.)

directions and over long distances. Hamsters are well known for their ability to escape cages, as they can squeeze out of very small spaces and actively seek opportunities to do so. If a weld on a wire cage is broken, hamsters will continue to chew in that area, making an opening large enough for them to escape (Figure 6-6).[13,16]

Most rodents are cognizant of heights and will climb or intentionally jump to move to various levels in their cages. They will also back away from edges that are very high. Hamsters, however, do not always exhibit the same behavior and often fall off ledges and tables and may even knock themselves unconscious when they fall.

Mice, rats, gerbils, and hamsters commonly sit up on their hind legs, especially when manipulating food materials. It is in this position that a gerbil will thump, often making it difficult to tell that it is actually moving.

Rats and mice have very long, flexible, hairless tails, which they frequently wrap around their bodies as they move or sleep. They often wrap their tails around their owners' fingers as they are held, but they are not truly prehensile in nature. Their tails are very strong and can be grasped at the base to lift an animal out of its cage and quickly place it on a solid surface. Even though their tails are fairly strong, rats and mice should not be dangled by their tails as they may struggle, thereby causing damage to the tissue. Their tails stabilize their posture and provide support as mice and rats sit to eat or stretch up in the air to investigate an odor or sound.

Small Rodent Behavior 253

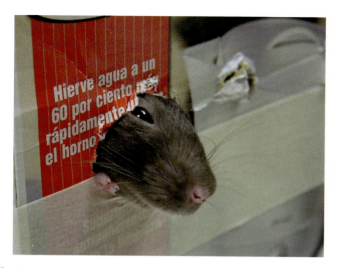

Figure 6-6
Rats and other rodents love to chew and should be provided with cardboard and other appropriate materials on which to chew. (Courtesy Jörg Mayer.)

Gerbils have long, haired tails that are not very flexible and usually stick straight out behind them. Their tails are not very strong and are easily broken if caught in a cage door or grabbed by an owner. Lifting a gerbil by the base of the tail is not recommended, as a degloving of the skin of the tail can occur. This is known as "tail slip" in lay terms (Figure 6-7).[2,13,16] Gerbil tails can be amputated if necessary, using surgical techniques appropriate for dogs and cats. Hamsters have very short, stubby tails that are barely visible and are usually covered with very thin hair. The tail helps to stabilize their posture when sitting.

Rodents are prone to tumors, especially as they age, and rats and mice commonly have mammary tumors (see Medical Implications of Abnormal Behavior). Because mice and rats have extensive mammary glands, often extending into the flank and axillary regions,[3] these tumors may adversely affect the ability of the animal to walk normally. Tumors in the axillary or inguinal areas may cause one limb to remain elevated, making it difficult for the animal to move normally around the cage.

Grooming Behaviors

All healthy rodents spend time grooming and occasionally will groom conspecifics in the same cage. Grooming behavior normally starts on the face with the animal licking one or both of its front paws and then rubbing the paws over the face. Once the face is completed, the animal will then

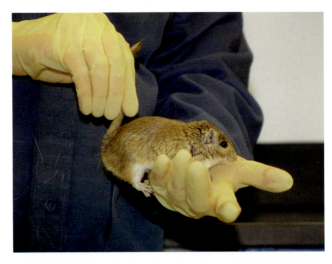

Figure 6-7
This photo demonstrates the proper hold on the tail to prevent tail slip during restraint of a gerbil. (Courtesy Kathleen Pritchett.)

groom up over the ears and on to the back of the head, although there may be periodic interruptions in the process. Grooming then moves to either the abdomen or the flanks, usually ending with the base of the tail and finally the tail itself.[12] This process does not normally make the fur look wet, even though the animals repeatedly lick the fur. If fur does appear to be greasy, it is most often because of excessive humidity in the primary enclosure, which may then cause individuals to groom excessively.

Grooming is frequently observed immediately after a rodent has been handled by the owner or shortly after a cage is cleaned. It can also sometimes be observed after two animals have confronted each other, even if there was no contact between the two individuals. Mothers groom their pups frequently, and breeding pairs occasionally groom each other. It is not uncommon for a dominant individual, regardless of gender, to use grooming to help establish dominance in the group. Sometimes this dominance grooming may include fur barbering, often creating areas of alopecia with or without abrasions of the skin. These areas of alopecia are most commonly seen around the head and neck and occasionally down the back.

The harderian gland is a deep gland of the nictitating membrane, or third eyelid.[1,3,12,13] Its secretions are routinely groomed into the fur as rodents start on the face and gradually move out to the rest of the body. Normally the gland's secretions are not visible on the fur, but if an animal is prevented from grooming, secretions may begin to accumulate around the edge of the eyes or at the opening of the nares, often described by the owner as a "bloody nose." These secretions are rich in lipids and porphyrin pigments that fluoresce under ultraviolet light, so they can be easily differentiated from blood with the use of a UV lamp.

Evidence also suggests that cold temperatures stimulate self-grooming in gerbils and that the harderian secretions help to protect against cold and wetness and darken the hair coat to increase heat absorption.[14] Routine grooming schedules can be interrupted when rodents are transported, are constantly handled, or suffer from chronic stress or illness, including malocclusion of the teeth.[12] With some of these conditions, animals may also appear to be lethargic, so the appearance of a "bloody nose" may seem to point to a disease process instead of an interruption in grooming (Figure 6-8). Unless the history suggests exposure to a disease or clinical signs of disease are present, it is best to leave these individuals alone in the home cage for at least 24 hours to see if they resume normal grooming behavior. If grooming is resumed, it is not uncommon to see a reddish-brown band of color across the head, especially on white or albino animals, as the harderian pigments are worked into the fur in the normal grooming pattern.[2,16]

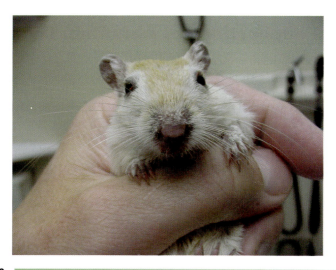

Figure 6-8

Often described by clients as a "bloody nose," this gerbil has harderian gland (porphyrin) secretion on its face that has not yet been groomed away, indicating a sick or stressed animal. Note the porphyrin secretion visible on hairs superior to the medial canthus of the eye and below the nares. (Courtesy Dan Johnson.)

Temperature Sensitivity

Rodents have difficulty regulating body temperature, as they have no sweat glands and cannot pant.[1] Mice, rats, and gerbils are prone to heat stress, especially if the relative humidity is above 70% in their primary enclosure. But they can tolerate temperatures that are quite cool as long as they have bedding into which they can burrow or are living in a social group. The recommended temperature for housing rodents is 64° to 79°F (18° to 26°C) with a relative humidity of 30% to 70%.[7]

Hamsters can go into a physiologic state of torpor when exposed to temperatures below approximately 60°F (approximately 16°C). This condition may also be stimulated by an ongoing lack of food or extremely short light cycles. This can happen in pet hamsters when the owners go away on vacation and turn down the thermostat. This condition is not a true hibernation as they do not generally store up fat before lowering their body temperature, but their heart and respiratory rates do decrease significantly.[3,13] If they do not "wake up" and eat and drink every few days, they will die from this condition. However, when found in this state of torpor, it is very easy to miss any possible signs of life and assume they are already dead. Hamsters that are cool to the touch should be gently warmed and given fluids (by subcutaneous or intraperitoneal injection) to see if they will revive before it is assumed they are dead.

Medical Implications of Abnormal Behaviors

Alopecia is not uncommon in rodents. After checking for common mammalian causes, including external parasites such as mites, consider that it may be normal dominance or barbering behavior. If animals can chew somewhere in the cage that causes them to rub their muzzles while they chew, they may have vertical lines of alopecia along each side of the muzzle or a horizontal line of alopecia above and/or below the muzzle (Figure 6-9). Periodic scratching that does not cause skin lesions is a common behavior in these animals that burrow and live underground.

Epilepsy (epileptiform fits) does occur in gerbils but may sometimes be confused with their normal thumping behavior. Treatment for epilepsy is not generally effective in gerbils, so owners should be advised not to breed affected animals. Seizures may be triggered by fright, stress, or illness, so the owner should be advised to keep the epileptic gerbil in a relatively calm location in the house.[13,16]

The presence of a porphyrin discharge around the eyes or the nares often indicates a sick rodent but may also be indicative of an interruption in normal grooming behaviors (see Grooming Behaviors). Careful examination of the animal may reveal other clinical signs of disease, which

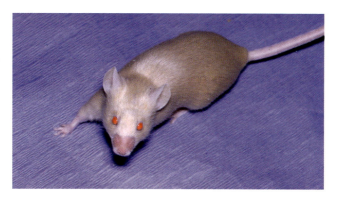

Figure 6-9
The alopecia around the nose of this mouse is a result of eating through or chewing on metal bars, a common behavior of mice and other rodents in captivity. (Courtesy Kathleen Pritchett.)

would indicate that the lack of grooming has a medical cause. If no overt signs of disease are present, consider leaving the animal alone in its cage for at least 24 hours to allow resumption of normal grooming behavior.

Owners are often concerned about hamster cheek pouches that are full for extended periods of time. If babies are present in the cheek pouches, it is imperative to place the cage in a quiet location and leave the female alone so she will feel safe enough to remove the babies and return them to the nest. Any other materials may remain in the cheek pouches for an extended period of time without causing a medical problem. Occasionally, if a hamster is provided soft chewing substrates, a splinter may penetrate the cheek wall and require removal and localized treatment. But because the cheek pouch is an immunologically privileged site, treatment or removal of material from the pouch is rarely necessary.

Rodents in general are quite prone to tumors, and rats and mice are especially prone to mammary tumors (see Locomotor Behaviors and Activities). Gerbils develop tumors of the genital system and of the skin, and hamsters most commonly develop lymphosarcomas.[15] If the tumors are on the ventral surface and continue to grow, they may become abraded from continual friction on the floor of the cage, thus increasing the likelihood of secondary infections. In addition, as the tumors increase as a percentage of the animal's body weight, it may become impossible for the animal to ambulate at all. Studies have shown that, in general, solid tumors in excess of 10% of the animal's normal body weight (or other conditions causing a similar increase in body fluid or ascites) do produce significant distress and probably concurrent pain, so euthanasia should be considered if surgery is not an option.[19]

Behaviors Associated with Pain

Small rodents are prey species, so they often do not exhibit overt signs of pain as may be seen with other species.[12] Add to that their small body size, nocturnal activity, and burrowing habits, and it can often be very difficult for an owner to determine if a rodent is sick or in pain. Therefore one has to learn to look for subtle changes in behavior that might indicate pain or an underlying medical condition.

The first sign most commonly seen in rodents that are sick or in pain is a rough hair coat or piloerection.[3] Instead of appearing sleek and shiny, the hair coat appears to stick out and looks spiky. An owner may notice a difference in the appearance without being able to identify the specific change. As a practitioner it is important to understand that a bonded owner may note that the animal "just doesn't look right" and that this recognition of subtle behavioral changes should not be overlooked or underestimated.

Another common nonspecific sign of pain or illness is a hunched posture (Figure 6-10). There appears to be a slight increase in the arch of the back in the area of the caudal thoracic and cranial lumbar vertebrae. This occurs with either abdominal or thoracic pain and may be difficult to identify without considerable prior experience observing normal rodents.[3]

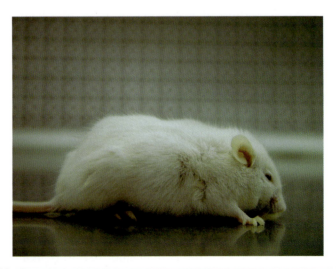

Figure 6-10
A slightly hunched posture and rough hair coat are evident in this sick mouse. (Courtesy Kathleen Pritchett.)

If the pain progresses, the hunched back becomes more prominent and begins to affect movement, causing the animal to take shorter steps when moving. Often the hunched posture is associated with pacing or restlessness, especially during the day when the nocturnal animal should be sleeping. If the animal can sleep, it is often stretched out on one side, rather than in the normal tucked position usually seen in rodents. In a social group setting, the individual in pain frequently removes itself from the group and may even sleep separately on the floor of the cage rather than in the pile or nest with the rest of the cagemates.

Food consumption is not usually closely monitored in small rodents, but anorexia may be another sign associated with pain, especially with conditions of the head or abdomen.[12] Small rodents do not generally produce copious amounts of saliva, but the chin may be wet, especially if there are lesions in the mouth such as those seen with malocclusion of the incisor teeth. Animals attempting to either groom themselves or rub at lesions of the mouth will often cause saliva to create matted fur on the inside (medial) surface of the front foot, another indication of an underlying problem.

Rodents are also notorious for exhibiting avoidance behaviors when they are in pain. Individuals living on wire floors will simply stop moving around if they get a foot caught and will adopt a posture that allows them to be as comfortable as possible without making it obvious that they cannot move. For this reason, it is important to carefully examine an animal that does not appear to be moving around the cage in a normal fashion. Animals that normally enjoy interaction with their owners may avoid being touched or may turn specific areas of the body (such as the tail, a foot, or the mouth) away from the owner's attempt to handle or pet them. This would indicate a specific area of the body that should be carefully examined, probably with the animal under anesthesia.

Small rodents in pain rarely vocalize unless they are physically handled or restrained (Figures 6-11 and 6-12). When they do vocalize, it may be accompanied by some degree of aggression toward their cagemates or humans.[3] Mice and hamsters will almost always attempt to bite if they are in pain. Rats and gerbils are more likely to bite when in pain than when they are healthy, but not all rats and gerbils bite even when evidence of extreme pain is present.

In summary, it is critical to respond when small rodents exhibit a behavior change for reasons that are not immediately obvious. The most subtle change in behavior or level of aggression may be an indication of an underlying medical condition, even if no lesions are obvious. Hopefully the owner of the pet rodent can accurately describe any changes seen so that a complete picture may be put together to help make an appropriate diagnosis.

260 Exotic Pet Behavior

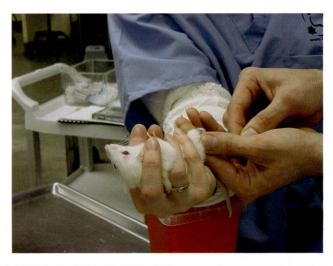

Figure 6-11
Rats are extremely tolerant of handling, even for potentially painful or stressful situations such as blood collection. (Courtesy Teresa Bradley Bays.)

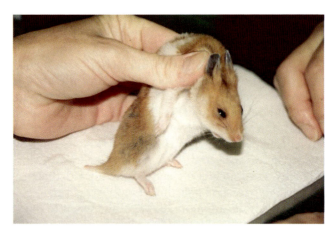

Figure 6-12
Hamsters can be restrained by scruffing the skin of the neck. As much of the loose skin as possible must be grasped so that they cannot turn their heads to bite the holder. (Courtesy Teresa Lightfoot.)

References

1. Baker HJ, Lindsey JR, Weisbroth SH, editors: *The laboratory rat: biology and diseases*, San Diego, 1979, Academic Press.
2. Ballard B, Cheek R, editors: *Exotic animal medicine for the veterinary technician*, Ames, Iowa, 2003, Iowa State Press.
3. Evans EI, Maltby CJ, editors: *Technical laboratory animal management*, Kansas City, 1989, mtm associates.
4. Foster HL, Small JD, Fox JG, editors: *The mouse in biomedical research: normative biology, immunology, and husbandry*, San Diego, 1983, Academic Press.
5. Hoosier GL Jr, McPherson CW, editors: *Laboratory hamsters*, Orlando, 1987, Academic Press.
6. Kittrell EM, Gregg BR, Thiessen DD: Brood patch function for the ventral scent gland of the female Mongolian gerbil, Meriones unguiculatus, *Dev Psychobiol* 15(3):197-202, 1982.
7. National Research Council (NRC): *Guide for the care and use of laboratory animals*, Washington, DC, 1996, National Academy Press.
8. Norris ML: Disruption of pair bonding induces pregnancy failure in newly mated mongolian gerbils *(Meriones unguiculatus)*, *J Reprod Fertil* 75(1):43-47, 1985.
9. Norris ML, Adams CE: Mating post partum and length of gestation in the Mongolian gerbil *(Meriones unguiculatus)*, *Lab Anim* 15(2):189-191, 1981.
10. Pendergrass M, Thiessen D, Friend P: Ventral marking in the male Mongolian gerbil reflects present and future reproductive investments, *Percept Mot Skills* 69(2):3553-3567, 1989.
11. Rohrback C: Investigation of the Bruce effect in the Mongolian gerbil *(Meriones unguiculatus)*, *J Reprod Fertil* 65(2):411-417, 1982.
12. Schulte MS, Rupley AE: Exotic pet management for the technician, *Vet Clin North Am Exot Anim Pract* 7:206-221, 2004.
13. Sirois M: *Laboratory animal medicine: principles and procedures*, St. Louis, 2005, Mosby.
14. Thiessen DD: Body temperature and grooming in the Mongolian gerbil, *Ann N Y Acad Sci* 525:27-39, 1988.
15. Toft J II: Neoplasia, commonly observed spontaneous neoplasms in rabbits, rats, guinea pigs, hamsters, and gerbils, *Semin Avian Exot Pet Med* 1:80-92, 1992.
16. Tully TN, Mitchell MA: *A technician's guide to exotic animal care*, Lakewood, 2001, AAHA Press.
17. Van der Meer E, Van Loo PL, Baumans V: Short-term effects of a disturbed light-dark cycle and environmental enrichment on aggression and stress-related parameters in male mice, *Lab Anim* 38(4):376-383, 2004.
18. Whishaw IQ, Sarna JR, Pellis SM: Evidence for rodent-common and species-typical limb and digit use in eating, derived from a comparative analysis of ten rodent species, *Behav Brain Res* 96(1-2):79-91, 1998.
19. Workman P, Balmain A, Hickman JA, et al: UKCCCR guidelines for the welfare of animals in experimental neoplasia, *ILAR J* 31(3), 1989.

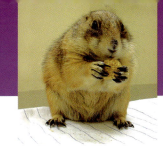

CHAPTER 7

DAN H. JOHNSON

Miscellaneous Small Mammal Behavior

Chinchillas

Natural History and Behavior

The family Chinchillidae is made up of three genera consisting of six species. Two species of chinchilla are recognized: *Chinchilla brevicaudata* and *Chinchilla lanigera*. The species kept in captivity is *C. lanigera*; the status of this species in the wild is considered to be highly endangered, and the species is listed in Appendix I of the CITES treaty.

C. lanigera is native to the Andes mountain ranges of Northern Chile. These chinchillas live in crevices and holes among the rocks on the relatively barren slopes at elevations of 3000 to 5000 m (900 to 16,000 ft).[24]

Chinchillas are primarily crepuscular and nocturnal but can also be active in the daytime[45] and do not hibernate.[24] They sit erect to eat, using their forepaws. Their natural diet of grasses, cactus fruit, leaves, and bark is fibrous and low in energy. Chinchillas live in colonies of up to 100 individuals and are naturally very social creatures. They may live up to 10 and even 20 years.

Sensory Behaviors

Chinchillas have large ears and enormous auditory bullae. The behavioral hearing range of chinchillas resembles that of humans,[8,22] so they are often used in hearing research (Figure 7-1). Chinchillas are sensitive to noise and startle easily. In spite of this, chinchillas acclimate to familiar sounds and will sleep during their daytime resting period, even with the stimulus of people in the environment. Chinchillas will quickly rouse if disturbed by unfamiliar sounds, however, and when so alerted to potential danger, they stand on their hind limbs and may react with a warning cry.

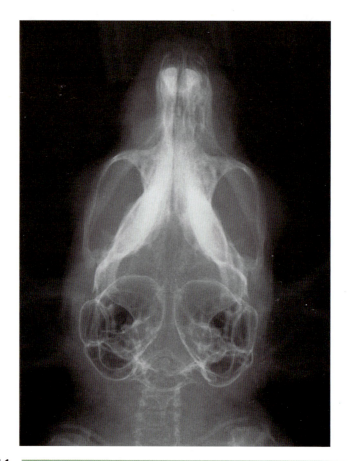

Figure 7-1

Chinchillas are primarily crepuscular and nocturnal. Accordingly, they have large ears and auditory bullae. The hearing range of chinchillas is similar to that of humans, so they are often used in hearing research. (Courtesy Dan Johnson.)

Chinchillas are largely nocturnal and use their vibrissae to find their way in darkness.[24] Their eyes are large and black with a vertical, slit pupil. Chinchillas are sensitive to light and should ideally get 12 hours of darkness per night and undisturbed rest during the daytime. Chinchillas are sensitive to heat above 26° C (80° F).[8] This may be one reason that they tend to dislike being held.

Chinchillas will use their mouths to explore their environment. They are curious about their surroundings, and will investigate the entire home. They normally chew on the cage and furnishings. Potential hazards (e.g., electrical cords) need to be addressed before chinchillas are allowed to exercise outside of their cage. A chinchilla may give a trial bite to the handler's finger. This is normal exploratory behavior but can be painful nonetheless.

Communicative Behaviors

Chinchillas are generally quiet. Normal communication among members of a group is by soft, high-pitched grunting noises.[52] Chinchillas "bark" if they are angry or defensive and "honk" for attention (e.g., if lonely or wanting a treat). Their warning cry is a whistling sound.[50]

Social and Antisocial Behaviors

Chinchillas are generally social and can be housed as pairs, single-sex groups, or polygynous units (one male per two to six females).[38] Social groupings are preferred in captivity; however, single housing may be necessary to prevent aggression. Aggression is most common during initial introduction and breeding (Figure 7-2). If pet chinchillas are singly housed, they need substantial human interaction for social enrichment.

Chinchillas can be territorial and will aggressively defend against intruders (Figure 7-3). Anecdotally, female chinchillas are more territorial

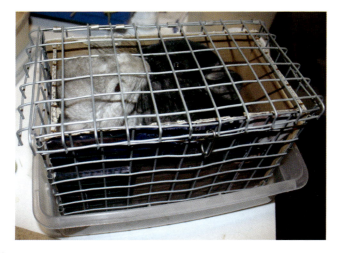

Figure 7-2
One method of introduction involves applying camphor to each chinchilla and then confining both in a very small cage for a short period. The new pair is then introduced into new living quarters that neither has occupied before and allowed to dust bathe and groom. After this process, fighting between the two is less likely. (Courtesy CLAWS, Inc., Kindra D. Mammone.)

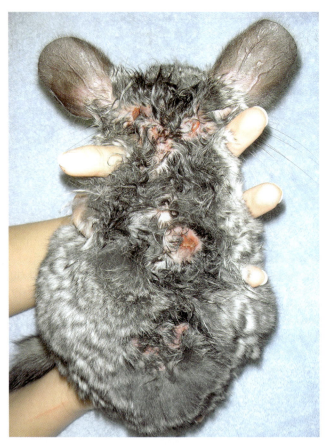

Figure 7-3
Chinchillas can be territorial and aggressive toward intruders. The aggressor will typically pin down the victim and bite it on the neck and back, inflicting wounds like the ones shown here. (Courtesy Dan Johnson.)

than males, and some may defend their territory by positioning themselves vertically on the cage and spraying urine in an upward stream, directed at the intruder. Some males also attempt to engage in this behavior.

When new chinchillas are introduced, barking, chasing, and biting are common. Chinchillas are capable of inflicting severe and fatal injuries on one another. When attempting to kill another chinchilla, the aggressor typically gets on top of the victim, pins it down, and bites it on the back and the neck. New introductions should be attempted only after caging animals near each other for at least 1 week. When pairing chinchillas for breeding, the female should be placed into the male's cage so that she is in new territory.

An alternative method involves closely confining the two chinchillas to a cage sufficiently small enough so that they are barely able to turn around, in order to prevent fighting via crowding. This is commonly referred to as the "smoosh" method by laypersons and fanciers.[50] A strong-smelling substance (e.g., camphor) is first applied to both chinchillas, and they are smooshed together for approximately 15 minutes. Then both chinchillas are placed in a new, larger cage (one that is neutral territory for both of them) containing two dust baths. Both chinchillas will typically begin to bathe immediately, in a furious attempt to remove the odor-causing substance. By the time they are clean the pair will no longer tend to fight.[50] Always provide small houses for each chinchilla to escape to that can be defended to prevent attacks (see Female Reproductive Behaviors).

The majority of chinchillas are tractable and nonaggressive toward humans. Young chinchillas tend to be easier to tame than older ones. They will usually come and sit to be petted for a short time, but even friendly chinchillas will resist being held. Chinchillas are a prey species and do not generally mix well with other pets. Loud noise, traffic, and commotion cause them stress. It is recommended that chinchillas be kept in a room apart from the daily activities of a household or veterinary practice. Chinchillas do not handle change well. Whenever possible, situations that disrupt their normal routine (e.g., moving, travel, car rides) should be avoided. Prolonged stress can result in anorexia, gastrointestinal stasis, impaired sleep cycle, fur-chewing, secondary infections, and death.

Reproductive Behaviors

Male Reproductive Behaviors

Chinchillas usually reach sexual maturity at approximately 8 months of age. Occasionally accidental breedings occur in chinchillas as young as 2 to 3 months. Young kits should be separated from opposite-sex parents and siblings by 8 to 10 weeks. Males can be housed with several females. Chinchilla males tend to be smaller than females.

Adult male chinchillas sometimes develop paraphimosis caused by a ring of matted fur trapped around the penis inside the prepuce. This condition, known as "fur ring," occurs most commonly in breeding males but can occur in nonbreeding males as well. Treatment is gentle removal using lubrication and anesthesia if necessary. Routinely check all males by everting and inspecting the penis at regular intervals. If a male is seen to be continually cleaning, he needs to be checked for a hair ring. Males may also routinely clean their penises as a form of masturbation.

Fighting will occur between two males if they are housed in the same cage with a female, and it may also occur if they are in close proximity to females in heat. Males can remain with the female during gestation and parturition and will participate in the care of the young.

Female Reproductive Behaviors

Female chinchillas are the dominant sex. They are generally larger than and display higher levels of aggression than males. Threats are expressed by growling, chattering teeth, and spraying urine. Chinchillas are polyestrous and are capable of breeding throughout the year in captivity. An estrus plug may be noted in females during heat, and this is expelled before mating.

When putting a pair of chinchillas together for breeding, always put the female into the male's cage. A female in heat may be aggressive toward the male, and placing her into his territory will lessen this tendency. If she attacks the male he will generally not try to defend himself and may be killed. To reduce this possibility, provide numerous small hiding places that can be defended. These are small spaces in which only one chinchilla can fit, turn around, and face outward to fend off attacks. Examples include large coffee cans that are bent partially shut and commercially available covered dust baths. Nulliparous females may refuse to mate during their first estrus.

A female may initially reject a male's advances and then later accept him. Mating usually occurs several times during the night. A loss of some fur from the female is normal during mating, but excessive fur slip may indicate the need to separate the pair. Mated females will have an ejaculatory plug in their vaginal opening (Figure 7-4). This will be expelled within days of breeding, and although it is much larger than the estrus plug, it is rarely found.

Females are seasonally polyestrous from November to May.[24,38] A vaginal closure membrane is open during estrus, making the opening between the urethral papilla and anus slightly moist and easily visualized.[24] The estrous cycle for chinchillas is approximately 28 days, and a postpartum estrus occurs. Gestation is 105 to 115 days, 110 days average. Parturition generally occurs at night or in the early morning, and litter size averages two to three; however, chinchillas can have up to six kits. Females do not usually make a nest.[24]

Chinchillas deliver one uterine horn at a time, and the two horns can go up to an hour between deliveries. The strenuous phase of labor usually lasts 1 to 2 hours or less. During that time the female writhes and stretches, and she may vocalize as if in pain.[50] The female will continually lick her vent as each fetus emerges, and she will normally help to deliver each baby using her teeth. Therefore, breach or difficult labor may result in fetal

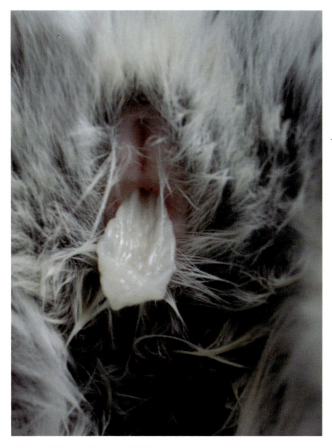

Figure 7-4
An ejaculatory plug may be noted at the vaginal orifice in mated females and is usually expelled within a few days of breeding. (Courtesy CLAWS, Inc., Kindra D. Mammone.)

trauma. Minor laceration, amputation, or death of the newborn may result. The mother's face may therefore be bloody after labor. Chinchillas are placentophagic, and dystocia is uncommon[58]; however, cesarean section should be undertaken if more than 4 hours of unproductive labor is observed.[24] After labor the female should be palpated to be sure no feti have been retained; mummified fetuses are relatively common.

Females have two pair of lateral thoracic and one pair of inguinal mammary glands (Figure 7-5). Chinchillas sit on top of their babies to nurse them and keep them warm (Figure 7-6). Kits tend to develop a preference for one teat and may become territorial over it. They are capable

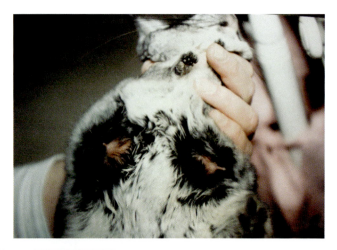

Figure 7-5
Female chinchillas have two pairs of lateral thoracic (one of which is shown here) and one pair of inguinal mammary glands. (Courtesy Dan Johnson.)

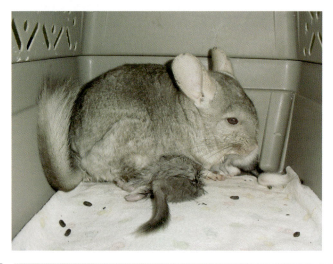

Figure 7-6
Chinchillas nurse their young while standing over them. (Courtesy Dan Johnson.)

of fighting and inflicting injury or even death to one another from the time they are born. For litters of three or more, rotating kits out of the cage may be necessary in order to prevent sibling rivalries. To reduce the risk of mastitis and uterine infections, females and their kits should not be allowed to dust bathe for the first 10 days after parturition.

Newborn chinchillas are born fully furred with a complete set of teeth, and their eyes will open within 24 hours.[38] They are very vocal, and they normally make a continuous whimpering sound[50] and can be very aggressive toward one another.[38] This behavior is normal and does not indicate a problem. Weaning can occur as early as 6 weeks of age, although lactation can last up to 8 weeks. The kits are able to eat solids from birth.[24] Both male and female chinchillas tend to their young, and a group of chinchillas may communally raise their young. In the pet trade, chinchillas are separated from their mothers at 7 to 8 weeks of age; if orphaned they can be weaned at as early as 3 weeks.[38] They are usually sold at 3 to 6 months of age.

Eating Behaviors

Chinchillas are monogastric hindgut fermenting herbivores. They are also reported to eat insects on occasion.[28] Chinchillas normally sit upright on their haunches to eat, and hold food with their forefeet. They mainly eat at night, ingesting more than 70% of their daily intake during the evening.[58] Gastrointestinal transit time is 12 to 15 hours.[58] Chinchillas are coprophagic, and, like other small herbivores, chinchillas do not regurgitate or vomit.

Chinchillas need a high-fiber, low-energy diet in order to prevent enteric problems and prolonged mastication of the high-fiber food maintains the integrity of their open-rooted teeth. A tough, fibrous diet, however, requires a high volume intake. Pet chinchillas should be offered high-quality grass hay (e.g., western timothy grass) free choice and a small amount (1 to 2 tablespoons) of commercial chinchilla pellets daily. Breeding chinchillas may require free-choice hay and pellets.

An adult chinchilla should consume approximately 1 ounce of chinchilla pellets, one teaspoon of vegetables, and free choice hay each day.[38] Dietary changes should be made gradually, as abrupt changes in diet can result in anorexia and gastrointestinal stasis. Treat foods should be fed sparingly, and those containing high starches and sugars avoided. Dark green leafy vegetables can be fed instead of other, less-appropriate treats.

Elimination Behaviors

Chinchillas tend to urinate in the same place but do not practice site-specific elimination for feces. They produce very little odor. Fecal pellets dry quickly and are easy to clean up, and chinchillas produce relatively little urine. Fecal excretion occurs mainly at night, when most of the food is ingested.[58] Cecotropes are consumed in the mornings.[23]

Male and female chinchillas will attempt to urinate on intruders; females are more accurate at a close range (see Social and Antisocial Behaviors). Targeted urination can be aimed at the clinician attempting to remove the animal from a carrier or the hospital cage. Lack of fecal pellet production and reduction of fecal pellet size are major indicators of anorexia and gastrointestinal stasis. Lack of feces is often misdiagnosed as constipation by clients and veterinarians alike.

Locomotor Behaviors and Activities

Chinchillas are most active in the evening and in partial light conditions. This is when the most accurate assessment of their behavior can be made. Chinchillas are also very athletic and agile. They like to jump and climb and so should be provided with multilevel cages.[24] They can jump over 6 feet high (one of our clients has watched her chinchilla jump to the top of her refrigerator from a dead standstill on several occasions). They have no fear of heights, and their active nature frequently leads to injuries, especially of the caudal extremities. They tend to get their delicate legs caught in cage wire, air conditioning return vents, and so on. The radius, ulna and/or tibia are the bones most often affected. Most fractures respond well to either splinting or external fixation. If amputation becomes necessary, chinchillas respond well if analgesics are used judiciously.

Chinchillas will run on running wheels for exercise. To prevent injury the running wheel should be solid, without wire rungs or cross bars. Chinchillas may run on running wheels to excess, and removal of the wheel may be necessary in order to prevent weight loss. Although chinchillas normally sleep upright, sleeping in lateral and dorsal recumbency is completely normal. They will also squeeze into tiny spaces and crevices to sleep (even upside down).

Fearful chinchillas cower in the corner of a cage, dart for cover, and can wedge themselves into unbelievably small spaces for protection. A relatively shy species, they should be provided with places to hide such as PVC pipe and cardboard boxes. Chinchillas should be confined when not observed. If chinchillas are allowed to roam freely, care must be taken to prevent accidents including electrocution, burns, drowning, toxicity, dietary overload with fruits or treats, and injuries.

Grooming Behaviors

Known for their soft, dense hair coat, chinchillas have approximately 60 hairs per follicle, which are loosely attached.[24] Like other small mammals, they are fastidious groomers. Lack of grooming usually indicates medical problems.

As previously noted, a predator defense mechanism in chinchillas is to lose large patches of fur to free themselves in the event of a struggle, and gentle handling is necessary in order to prevent this loss, known as "fur slip"(Figure 7-7). If this should happen during an examination, clients should be warned that it could take up to 6 to 8 weeks for this hair to grow back and several more months before the hair will appear completely normal.[58]

Adult males are susceptible to accumulations of fur inside the prepuce. So-called "hair rings" or "fur rings" can result in constricting damage to the penis and can be fatal if they become severe (Figure 7-8). These constrictions may occur repeatedly in stud males in a breeding situation.[45] Males routinely groom their penises and also masturbate in the same manner (see Male Reproductive Behaviors). Both males and females will groom, care for, and clean their young. Chinchillas are fastidiously clean and have little odor. Fur chewing is abnormal and may have many causes (see Medical Implications of Abnormal Behaviors).

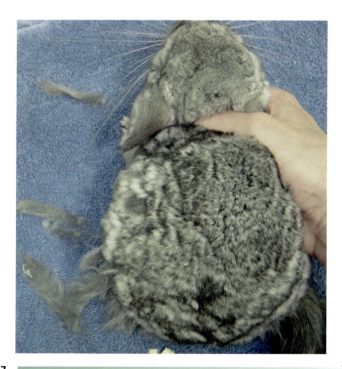

Figure 7-7
If roughly handled, chinchillas will readily shed hair as a defense mechanism. This process is commonly known as "fur slip." (Courtesy Dan Johnson.)

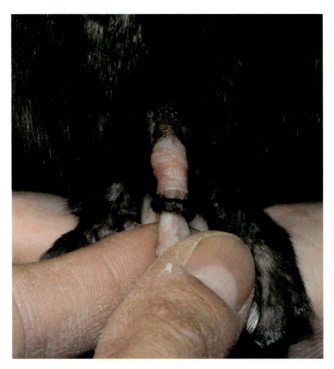

Figure 7-8
Male chinchillas are prone to developing hair rings within the prepuce. If left untreated, a hair ring can result in constricting injury to the penis and substantial discomfort to the patient. Male chinchillas must be routinely checked to remove hair accumulation around the penis. (Courtesy CLAWS, Inc., Kindra D. Mammone.)

Chinchillas require dust bathing in Fuller's earth every 24 to 72 hours (Figure 7-9). If the animal does not have access to a dust bath, the fur will become matted with oily secretions. Unlimited access to dust baths has led to conjunctivitis and dry skin. The dust bath should be provided in a dishpan or aquarium outside of the chinchilla's enclosure so that it is not overused or defecated in. The recommended exposure to the dust bath is approximately 5 minutes per day. Excess hair may be removed by brushing with a canine "slicker" brush. Their nails do not generally require trimming, and ectoparasites are uncommon but can be treated as in other small mammalian herbivores.

Medical Implications of Abnormal Behaviors

Like most small exotic mammals, chinchillas are stoic and do not display abnormal behaviors until disease is relatively advanced. Sick chinchillas

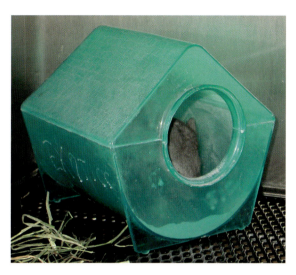

Figure 7-9
Dust bathing is an important part of the grooming process for chinchillas. They should be allowed to dust bathe for approximately 5 minutes each day. (Courtesy Dan Johnson.)

are less active and less vocal than their healthy counterparts. They exhibit dyspnea only when respiratory disease is severe. Because chinchillas are obligate nasal breathers, dyspnea is an advanced presentation of respiratory compromise. Illness from any cause may result in depression, anorexia, and weight loss. Sick chinchillas generally groom less, have an unkempt appearance, and may have a soiled vent when ill.

Anorexia is a common presenting complaint for chinchillas. It is most often associated with gastrointestinal disease (ileus, enterotoxemia, and bloat), dental malocclusion, elongation of tooth roots, and pneumonia; however, any severe illness or stress can be responsible. Anorexia and gastrointestinal stasis will rapidly lead to decreased fecal output, both in quantity and size of fecal pellets. Appetite and fecal output are harder to measure in a multiple-chinchilla enclosure, and this may further delay the identification of anorexia.

Gastrointestinal stasis, as in other herbivorous species, is a common presentation and usually secondary to other disease, illness, or pain. Signs include lethargy, anorexia, decreased or no fecal pellets, distended abdomen, and bruxism. Treatment includes supportive care such as subcutaneous and oral fluids, anti-gas medications, analgesics, motility stimulants, and antibiotics if appropriate. Syringe feeding with Oxbow Pet Products (Oxbow Pet Products, Murdock, NE) Critical Care will also help to stimulate gastrointestinal motility.

Hypersalivation and anorexia are common signs of dental malocclusion in chinchillas (Figure 7-10). Affected animals may go to food and

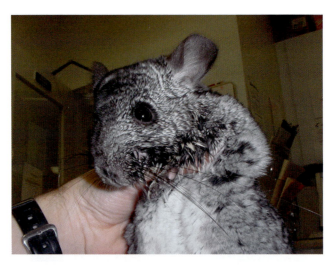

Figure 7-10
Hypersalivation is commonly associated with dental disease in chinchillas. Other possible causes include overheating and gastrointestinal disease. (Courtesy Dan Johnson.)

pick it up but have extreme difficulty eating. They may drop the food item, and then repeat the process many times, indicating a desire to eat but an inability to do so. Also called "slobbers," the clinical signs of malocclusion or dental infection may include wet chin, face, chest, and forepaws; weight loss; dysphagia; halitosis; and loss of appetite. Sedation is usually necessary for a thorough dental examination and treatment. It is imperative that the clinician have the proper dental specula for small mammals to ensure safe, complete, oral examination. Use of a rigid endoscope is recommended, as visualization of all tooth surfaces is limited without one. Tooth root elongation, a relatively common problem, may be evident only on skull radiographs.[24]

Hypersalivation can also be associated with heat stress. Chinchillas originate from the dry, cool, Andes mountain region of South America. Prolonged exposure to temperatures above 80° F (26° C) can result in heat stress and even death.[58] High humidity adds to heat stress. Symptoms of overheating include hypersalivation (wet chin, paws, and chest), recumbency, panting, cyanosis, hyperthermia, and death. Gastrointestinal stasis and anorexia are very common after an episode of hyperthermia.

Fur chewing may result from stress caused by noise (e.g., a dog barking, construction, home repairs), overcrowding, hormonal imbalance, excessive handling, or drastic changes in routine. Affected animals will chew from their shoulders backward and may also barber their cagemates. Fur chewing may also have a hereditary component. In the chinchilla fur industry, fur chewing has an incidence as high as 15% to 20%. It generally develops in both genders at 6 to 8 months of age.[62] Chinchillas with fur-chewing behaviors also have been shown to have adrenal and skin histopathologic changes consistent with hyperadrenocorticism.[62]

Fur-slip (see Grooming Behaviors) may result from rough handling or from the chinchilla's struggles to get away when being examined. The chinchilla can be restrained by gently but firmly grasping the base of the tail while supporting the rest of the body with the other hand. The client should be prewarned that fur slip can occur during the examination and handling for procedures.

Repetitive movements such as racing back and forth on the bottom of the cage may be a sign that the cage is too small or does not have enough perching platforms for jumping behavior. Epiphora or blepharospasm may indicate corneal abrasion, ocular foreign body, conjunctivitis, or tooth root problems (Figure 7-11).

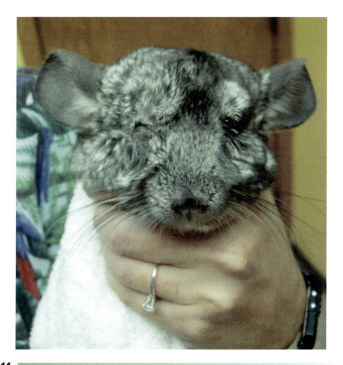

Figure 7-11
Ocular swelling, conjunctivitis, epiphora, and "winking" behaviors are commonly associated with dental disease in chinchillas. Diseased maxillary cheek teeth can cause these symptoms. Other causes include ocular foreign bodies (e.g., chinchilla bath dust) and infection. (Courtesy Dan Johnson.)

Chinchillas are extremely sensitive to perceived threats. Loud noises and sudden changes in the normal routine are stressful. The visual contact, noises, and odors associated with predatory species will cause stress; therefore chinchillas should not be caged near dogs, cats, ferrets, or large birds. Birds and cats should never be allowed up onto a chinchilla's cage to sit or perch. Minor veterinary procedures such as blood collection can usually be accomplished with manual restraint (e.g., wrapping in a towel and holding at the base of the tail with the rest of the body supported).

Chinchillas can easily become stressed or overheated, however, and anesthesia is recommended for painful or lengthy procedures. Pain control before, during, and after surgery, using multimodal pain therapy, is paramount. Under normal circumstances skin sutures are avoided and subcutaneous and subcuticular sutures are preferred because chinchillas tend to chew on sutures.

Behaviors Associated with Pain/Euthanasia

Chinchillas experiencing pain will tend to huddle in a corner and refuse to eat. Bruxism may occur. They may stop grooming and develop a poor hair coat. They will usually sit in a hunched position with all four legs tucked under the body. Drooling and slow or exaggerated chewing movements are often signs of dental disease and oral pain. If a chinchilla is not eating due to pain, it will be underweight and its fecal production will be diminished.

If euthanasia becomes necessary, chinchillas should be anesthetized in an anesthetic chamber before intravenous or intracardiac injection of euthanasia solution.

How Behavior Relates to Captivity

Chinchillas have many qualities that make them desirable as pets. They are long lived, active, clean, and odorless. Although chinchillas are reasonably easy to feed and maintain, clients will need guidance in order to avoid husbandry problems that can lead to illness. As with most exotic pets, chinchilla diseases are usually the result of errors in husbandry.

Chinchillas normally spend much of the day chewing. In addition to a high-fiber, low-energy diet, chinchillas need many items to chew on for enrichment, including rough cement perches designed for birds, pumice stones, lava, and items made of wood.

Chinchillas are easy to handle, and they rarely bite; however, they are active and move very quickly. Hold the patient gently around the thorax with one hand and cradle the rump with the other hand. Alternatively, as previously described, the tail can be held at the base as long as the body is supported. If the dense fur is handled roughly, "fur slip" may result.

Chinchillas are social by nature and are generally housed in small groups. They can be kept as individual pets, but social interaction is very important and needs to be provided by the owner. Without this interaction, abnormal behavior is likely to develop. Very large cages are preferred. Two females that are raised together or a mother-daughter pair will get along fine. Intact males in the same cage may fight. Injuries resulting from aggression can be minimized by offering adequate cover that can be defended (see description of hide boxes under Female Reproductive Behaviors).

Chinchillas are creatures of habit and prefer a routine. Setting up a cage in a family area is fine if the area is normally calm, but chinchillas may do better in another room of the home if a lot of noise and chaos are present. Chinchillas are sensitive to heat above 26° C (80° F) and relative humidity above 40%. Do not put them in direct sunlight. Chinchillas need 12 hours of darkness each night when they are active and undisturbed rest during the daytime.

Chinchillas' normal response to any threat is to run away. If they cannot get away, they experience undue stress, and illness or death may result. Provide sufficient hiding places for chinchillas. Keep them separate from dogs, cats, ferrets, birds, and any other animal a chinchilla may perceive as a threat. Eliminate noises, odors, and visual contact with potential predators.

Acknowledgments

The author wishes to thank Kindra Mammone (CLAWS, Inc.), for her assistance in preparing the chinchilla section and for the photos indicated.

Client Education Handout: Chinchilla (Chinchilla lanigera)

Biologic Facts
- Chinchillas are native to the Andes in Chile. Their natural environment is rocky, cool, and dry.
- Their natural diet is fibrous and low in energy: grasses, cactus fruit, leaves, and bark
- Their teeth continue to grow throughout life: the incisors chisel and cut food, and the cheek teeth grind it until it can be swallowed.
- Chinchillas usually reach sexual maturity at 8 months of age; however, breeding as young as 2 to 3 months occasionally occurs.
- Females are generally larger than males.
- Gestation is 110 days, and litter size is usually two or three young.
- Chinchillas can live 10 to 20 years.
- Chinchillas are very clean and have little odor.

Behavior
- Chinchillas are agile and able to jump great distances.
- They are primarily nocturnal but are also active in the daytime.
- Chinchillas are highly social. They do best in pairs or small groups, but single pets are fine as long as they get plenty of human interaction. Single housing should be reserved for chinchillas that are aggressive toward cagemates.
- Chinchillas are generally "pettable" animals; however, most prefer not to be held. "Fur slip" will occur (a defense mechanism) if chinchillas are forced to struggle. Handle them gently, supporting the whole body, in order to prevent loss of fur.
- Females in heat can be very aggressive toward others.

Diet
- Chinchillas need a high-fiber, low-energy diet.
- A fibrous diet requires continuous grazing and a lot of chewing. This helps to maintain healthy teeth and digestive function.
- Offer high-quality grass hay (e.g., western timothy) free choice and a small amount (1 to 2 Tbsp) of commercial chinchilla pellets daily.
- Small amounts of fruit or greens can be offered as treats. Avoid breads, cereals, and nuts.
- Changes in diet should be made gradually.

Housing
- Chinchillas require a large, multi-level cage. Exercise is necessary to avoid abnormal behaviors (e.g., fur chewing), promote general health, and prevent gastrointestinal stasis and obesity.
- A metal cage is necessary, because chinchillas chew on everything in their environment. To reduce the risk of toxicity, use cages without paint or coatings.
- To prevent foot and limb injury, the wire mesh should be small (15 mm × 15 mm; 0.6 in × 0.6 in), and part of the cage floor should be solid.
- Chinchillas naturally rest during the daytime. Provide them a room away from daytime activity and noise.
- High temperatures and humidity must be avoided. Optimal environmental temperature is 10° to 16° C (50° to 68° F) and should not exceed 26° C (80° F). Relative humidity should be 40% or less. Avoid direct sunlight.
- A dust bath should be offered for 5 to 10 minutes every 1 to 3 days using commercially available chinchilla dust (Fuller's earth).
- A solid-constructed (not wire) exercise wheel and a hide box should be provided.

Common Medical Conditions Requiring Veterinary Attention
- Heat stress: risk if exposed to direct sunlight, high temperature, and humidity
- Dental disease: malocclusion, molar abscessation, cheek teeth, and incisor overgrowth
- Limb trauma: entrapped feet and legs
- Gastrointestinal disease: bloat, diarrhea, bacterial overgrowth; often caused by improper diet, stress, and other illnesses, not eating, decreased or no fecal pellets.
- Respiratory infection: bacterial pneumonia, nasal infections (discharge from eyes or nose and/or difficulty breathing)
- Fur ring: accumulation of hair around the penis can cause injury; check males regularly, and keep area clean
- Dystocia: difficult labor, incomplete labor; may require surgery
- Fetal trauma: mothers may injure babies when helping to deliver them

Preventive Care
- Twice yearly complete physical examinations*
- Fecal examination for parasites
- Complete blood count and chemistry panel as recommended by veterinarian
- Skull radiographs to aid in the early detection of dental disease

*Locate a veterinarian who obtains continuing education about exotic pets and who has experience with chinchillas.

Fennec Foxes

Natural History and Behavior

The fennec fox *(Fennecus zerda* or *Vulpes zerda)* lives in the Sahara desert region of North Africa, from Morocco and Niger to Egypt and Sudan. Two reports of sightings have been recorded from the Middle East, one from Kuwait and the other from the Sinai.[59] In these desert and subdesert habitats fennecs are usually found in sandy areas, where they occupy a permanent den several meters long that they dig themselves. Fennec foxes are the smallest canid, weighing 1 to 1.5 kg (2 to 3 lb) and are primarily nocturnal. Their omnivorous diet includes plant material, small rodents, birds, eggs, lizards, and insects.[52]

Fennec foxes exhibit many unique physiologic adaptations to desert life. Fennec metabolism functions at only 67% of the rate predicted for an animal its size.[47] Similarly, resting heart rate is only 118 beats per minute (bpm), 40% lower than would be expected, and the respiratory rate at rest is 23 breaths per minute. Their normal body temperature is 38.2° C (100.8° F). Fennec foxes shiver when the ambient temperature drops below 20° C (68° F).[49]

As air temperature rises, the fennec radiates body heat by dilating blood vessels in its feet and large, vascular ears. Fennec foxes start to pant only when the temperature exceeds 35° C (95° F), and the jaws open to a full pant only at 38° C (100° F).[49] They reduce water loss by not sweating until body temperature rises to 40.9° C (105.6° F), and when they pant fennecs curl the tongue to minimize the loss of saliva.[47] Panting rates of up to 690 breaths per minute have been observed.[49]

Sensory Behaviors

Fennec foxes are nervous and distrustful by nature. They are shy and wary of strangers. They generally cannot tolerate the chaos and confusion that domestic dogs can. Fennec foxes are easily alarmed by strange or loud noises and run from sudden movements such as opening doors. Fearful behavior includes cowering, running away, and hiding. Therefore they may not make the best candidates for captive pets and in certain situations can become aggressive.

Fennec foxes are largely dependent on hearing for predation. They have exceedingly large tympanic bullae and the biggest ears relative to body size in the canid family, measuring up to 15 cm (6 in) in length and constituting 20% of the body surface area (Figure 7-12).[47] Fennec foxes are mostly nocturnal and have a well-developed tapetum lucidum.

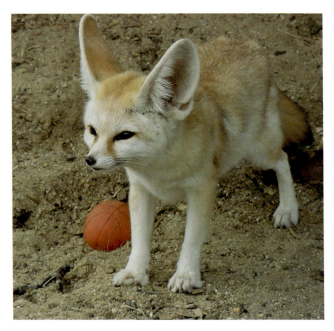

Figure 7-12
Fennec foxes are largely nocturnal, and their hearing is well developed. They have extremely large auditory bullae. Fennecs have the largest ears relative to body size of any canid, and their vascular pinnae assist in regulating body heat. (Courtesy Dan Johnson.)

Communicative Behaviors

As with other canids, scent-marking appears to play a prominent role in chemical communication among fennec foxes. They have paired anal sacs on both sides of the anus that coat feces with scent and can be evacuated voluntarily. The caudal gland is a black spot that is covered with bristles and is located proximally on the tail (Figure 7-13). Glands are located between the toes, as well. Fennec foxes will also urine-mark their territory.

Fennec foxes are generally quiet and do not draw attention to themselves. However, they use a variety of vocalizations to communicate. They will whine, growl, snarl, and bark in the same manner and context as small domestic dogs. The ears are held sideways if the animal is angry or upset, and backward with aggression or biting. Squeaking occurs as part of a greeting ceremony directed toward other foxes or human keepers. They emit a similar scream when they are happy or excited (e.g., when carrying a favorite toy and running with it). Fennec foxes will also emit a scream if they are distressed (e.g., if stared at intensely or if cornered or

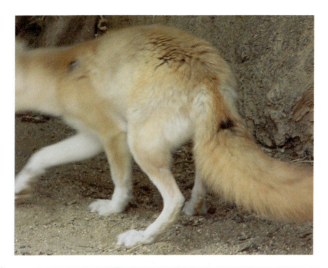

Figure 7-13
The caudal gland sits in a patch of dark hair at the base of the tail. Its function is unknown, but it may be involved with chemical communication. (Courtesy Dan Johnson.)

threatened). A howl-scream may accompany reproductive activities. When they are content, purring may be observed. This behavior is unique to fennec foxes and kit foxes.[1,59]

Social and Antisocial Behaviors

Fennec foxes are more social than other fox species. Although they hunt alone in the wild, fennec foxes live in colonies of up to 10 individuals. Their basic social unit is a mated pair and their offspring (Figure 7-14). In the wild, fennec foxes commonly sleep and rest while lying in contact with or on top of one another. A group of fennec foxes may engage in play behavior such as mock fighting and chasing games. Fights are accompanied by screaming, hip slamming, and pushing with extended forelimbs.

Fennec foxes can be taught to retrieve, which provides exercise. They often entertain themselves by throwing, stalking, and pouncing on small dog and cat toys. When approached by a keeper or another member of their group a fennec fox normally cowers and lies on its side, yelping, wagging its tail, and grimacing in a typical canine greeting display, just as in the wild (Figure 7-15). Although fennec foxes are mostly nocturnal, they are also active during the day and enjoy basking in the sun (Figure 7-16). Those that are hand-raised and imprinted on humans are generally tame and more suitable as pets than parent-raised babies.

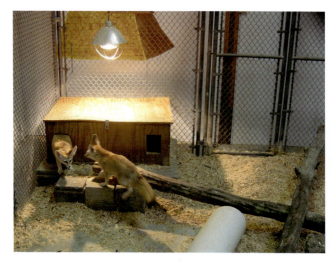

Figure 7-14
Fennecs are more social than other foxes. The ideal social grouping is a mated pair; however, a solitary fox may be kept as long as it is provided companionship by people, dogs, or cats. (Courtesy Dan Johnson.)

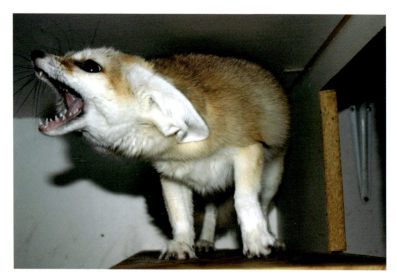

Figure 7-15
This photo illustrates a defensive aggressive posture for fennec foxes. A similar greeting display of fennec foxes is typical of canines and includes cowering, grimacing, exposing the underbelly, yelping, and tail wagging, usually while lying on its side. (Courtesy CLAWS, Inc., Kindra D. Mammone.)

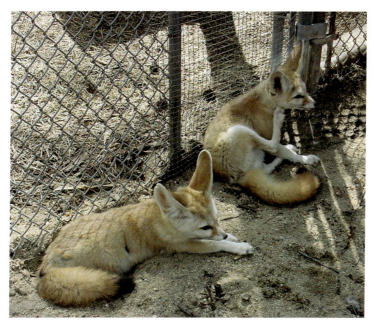

Figure 7-16
Although fennec foxes are nocturnal, they may be active during the day and appear to enjoy basking in the sun. (Courtesy Dan Johnson.)

Captive fennec foxes are extremely predatory by nature. Fennec foxes are capable of killing animals much larger than themselves, and they will attempt to take down "prey" many times their size (e.g., fawn, rabbit).[50,59] They tolerate predator species (e.g., dog, adult cat, and skunk), but they should not be trusted with other animals. They can and will inflict a painful bite.

Reproductive Behaviors

Fennec foxes are unusual among wild canids in that the female, referred to as the "vixen," is seasonally polyestrous.[1,59] If the first litter is lost, a second may be produced $2\frac{1}{2}$ to 3 months later. Breeding pairs are monogamous and will peacefully coexist year round. In captivity, mating occurs during January and February. The male, referred to as the "reynard," will urine-mark his territory during this period, and the female may develop dorsolateral alopecia.[20,32] Females stay in heat for 1 to 2 days. Mating is accompanied by vocalization and concludes with a copulatory tie that lasts up to 2 hours. The gestation period for fennec foxes ranges from 49 to 63 days (average is 51 days).

Fennec foxes are very nervous and aggressive during breeding and rearing. Breeding pens must be large and supplied with adequate hiding places to provide the parents with privacy and security. If the parents are disturbed, the mother may attempt to move the litter or cannibalize them. To prevent neonatal deaths, avoid disturbances until the kits reach 3 to 4 weeks of age and provide supplemental heat in the den.

There are usually two to five offspring in a litter. Kits open their eyes at 12 to 14 days. The fennec male remains with his mate after she gives birth, feeding her and protecting the den. The female does not allow him to interact with the kits until they are 5 to 6 weeks old. Parent-raised offspring are weaned by 8 to 10 weeks of age. Carrying, grooming, and nursing of the young continue until this time. Wild fennec foxes stay with their family until they are at least 1 year old.

Kits are sometimes pulled at 10 to 12 days and hand-raised with a fox milk replacer. Solid food may be introduced to hand-raised kits at approximately 1 month, and weaning can occur as early as 6 weeks. Fennec foxes attain adult size and sexual maturity by 9 to 11 months. Their lifespan is 12 to 16 years.

Male Reproductive Behaviors

Males are in rut for 4 to 6 weeks. During the breeding season males become extremely aggressive and mark their territory with urine. Males remain with their mates after the young are born and defend them but do not enter the maternal den. Male breeding behavior including mounting the female may be the cause of flank alopecia on females during breeding season.

Female Reproductive Behaviors

Females are in heat for approximately 2 days. During courtship the female flags her tail horizontally to one side. For successful breeding the female must be allowed uninterrupted visual, auditory, and olfactory contact with other fennecs, indicating the degree of their social nature.[59] The young are born in late winter to early spring, and the female becomes aggressive and defends her nest site during this time.

Experimentally, contraception in fennec fox females has been achieved by using the gonadotropin-releasing hormone (GnRH) analogue deslorelin.[5]

Eating Behaviors

The fennec fox has the same dental formula as the domestic dog (I3/3, C1/1, PM4/4, M2/3). Compared with other vulpines, their canines are reduced and their teeth are sharply cuspidate, which may facilitate insectivory.[59] The diet of fennecs in the wild includes plant material, fruits, small rodents (gerbils, jerboas), birds, eggs, lizards, and insects (locusts). Digging for plant roots (tubers, bulbs) is an important source of moisture.

In captivity, Mazuri Exotic Canine Diet (Mazuri Exotic Canine Diet #5M52, Mazuri/Purina Mills, St. Louis, MO) is widely used for this species. Other food items include high-quality dry dog or cat food, canned dog or cat food, vegetables, fruits, pinkie mice, rodents, eggs, gut-loaded crickets, and mealworms. Live insects or rodents can be provided as enrichment. Raw meat and rodents impart an unpleasant odor to the urine. Owners may attempt to feed fruit and vegetables exclusively in an effort to reduce urine or fecal odor or make fennecs "more tame." This should be discouraged, as malnutrition can be a potential sequela.

Laboratory studies suggest that fennec foxes can survive indefinitely without access to free water,[52,59] however, they will drink freely if water is available. Fresh water should be provided at all times.

Fennec foxes kill prey using a neck bite and normally eat prey beginning at the head.[3] They tend to carry bits of food away from the bowl to a quiet area to be consumed, then return for more and repeat the process until the bowl is empty. They will sometimes attempt to bury food, even in plain sight such as in the middle of the floor or on a couch or a bed. Fennec foxes obtain some of their food in the wild by digging, so pronounced scratching and raking occurs at the time of eating in captivity. In a group setting, food jealousy is common. Skirmishes for food among fennecs normally escalate into back-arched threat displays and fighting. Fennecs should be fed in the evening when they are most active.

Elimination Behaviors

Fennec foxes practice site-specific defecation in the wild. If a suitable substrate is provided, they will eliminate in a shallow depression they have scraped with their feet, and cover the spot by pushing litter with the nose or hind feet.[3,59] They may learn to use a litter box in captivity; however, attempts to train them are met with varying success. Because of their digging habits, a covered litter box with regular clay litter is recommended. Avoid clumping litter, as this will stick to their fur and nose. Anecdotal reports suggest that fennec foxes will also soil the house as a sign of displeasure or unhappiness.

Locomotor Behaviors

The soles of a fennec fox's feet are covered with fur, protecting them from heat and enabling them to run in loose sand. They dig so rapidly that they have earned a reputation for being able to sink into the earth, although digging can lead to eye injuries. Fennec foxes are able to jump 60 to 70 cm (2 to 2.5 ft) high from a standing position and can leap 120 cm (4 ft) horizontally.[47] They are extremely agile and fast moving. Their heavily furred tail (sometimes referred to as a "sweep") helps the fox to change direction quickly and keeps the fox's nose and feet warm when it curls up to sleep.

Grooming Behaviors

Fennec foxes are fastidiously clean, and unlike other foxes they have no odor. If bathing is necessary, provide a warm environment afterward in order to prevent chilling.

Dorsolateral alopecia often occurs in females at the time of breeding (Figure 7-17). Bilaterally symmetric patches of alopecia with scale and hyperpigmentation can also appear on the flanks. The cause is uncertain. Differentials include mounting trauma from a male and endocrine effects, but the condition could also signify undiagnosed skin pathology.

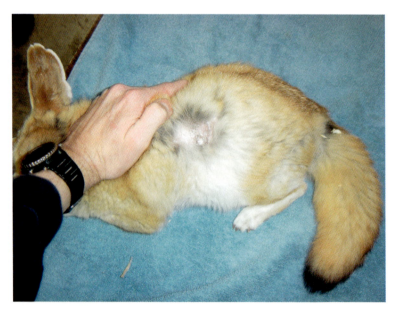

Figure 7-17
Alopecia may appear bilaterally on the flanks of females at the time of breeding. Lesions may be erythematous, lichenified, and hyperpigmented. The cause is not known. These so-called "love handles" may occur as a result of hormonal effects, trauma from mounting by the male, or other pathology. (Courtesy Dan Johnson.)

Medical Implications of Abnormal Behaviors

Healthy fennec foxes are alert, with bright eyes and upright ears. They move quickly with the head held high. Fennec foxes with illness or injury will be withdrawn and tend to seek a quiet, dark, isolated area (e.g., in a closet, under the bed, behind the couch). The ears may droop, the eyes may look dull, and the coat may appear unkempt. A sick fennec fox generally carries its head lower than its shoulders and moves more slowly than normal.

Fennec foxes are similar to other canines in their susceptibility to trauma and disease. Therefore most companion animal practitioners readily recognize disease symptoms in fennecs. Lameness, anorexia, or reluctance to move should raise suspicions that something is wrong.

Foxes (including the fennec) differ from other canines in their response to canine adenovirus (CAV-1). In foxes CAV-1 manifests primarily as "fox encephalitis" and results in central nervous system (CNS) signs and alterations in behavior. Other viral diseases causing CNS signs in foxes include canine distemper and rabies. Fennec foxes are susceptible to heart and liver disease, and CNS symptoms and behavioral changes can result from these diseases, as well. Other common medical conditions seen in fennec foxes are listed below.

- Trauma (bite wounds, fractures)
- Neonatal death (nervous mothering)
- Eye injuries
- Ear and skin infections
- Flea infestation
- Neoplasia
- Renal disease
- Liver disease
- Cardiomyopathy
- Pneumonia

Behaviors Associated with Pain

Fennec foxes are stoic with a strong instinct for self-preservation, and they generally do not vocalize in response to pain. Rather, they tend to become less vocal and less visible so as not to draw attention to themselves. Fennec fox vocalizations associated with pain should not be confused with the normal yelping and screaming associated with greeting displays, play behavior, or breeding.

How Behavior Relates to Captivity

Fennec foxes should be kenneled while unsupervised. A large, multilevel ferret or cat cage with shelves makes a suitable crate. They can easily climb out of fenced enclosures (Figure 7-18). If fennec foxes are kept outdoors, cages should be designed so that occupants cannot dig out or otherwise escape. The enclosure should be placed in a low humidity, well-ventilated environment. They have a strong instinct to dig and should be provided a soft cage substrate for burrowing. Dusty cage substrates should be avoided. Putting a collar with a bell on it may help owners to avoid accidentally stepping on the fox and aid in locating it when it is free in the house.

Fennec foxes can be trained to walk on a harness or leash but are unreliable and can slip out of these if they are startled. If a fennec escapes, recapture is difficult. Transport in a carrier or kennel is strongly

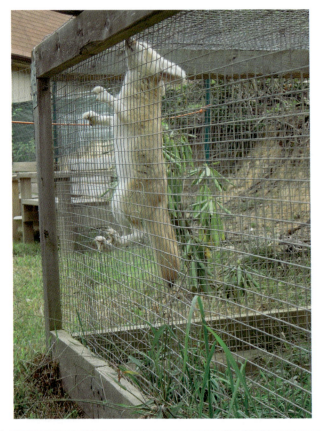

Figure 7-18
Fennec foxes are capable of climbing and digging out of fenced enclosures. Fencing material needs to be extended across the top and bottom of fenced pens if they are intended to house fennecs. (Courtesy Dan Johnson.)

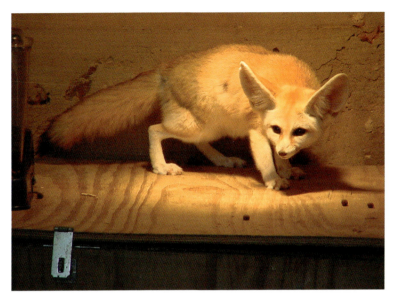

Figure 7-19
Fennecs are more easily frightened by new situations than are domestic dogs. They tend to be shy, quickly retreating at the first sign of a perceived threat. (Courtesy Dan Johnson.)

recommended. They are able to jump up onto countertops and get into cabinets. Baby latches may be necessary in order to protect them from poisons and other household hazards. Fennec foxes may be illegal in some states.

Fennecs are unusual among foxes in that they are highly social. They need the socialization and companionship of other fennecs or people, dogs, and cats as surrogates. The ideal social grouping for fennec foxes is a mated pair. Owners must be cautioned that a fennec fox will attack other animals it perceives as prey. Conversely, the fennec is small and may be unsuitable as a companion for large breed dogs (Figure 7-19). Fennec foxes usually have little odor, although they have anal sacs similar to those in domestic dogs that are not routinely removed.

Acknowledgments

The author gratefully acknowledges the assistance of the following wildlife educators in the development of this section on fennec foxes: Dora Turner, Noah's Landing, Coats, NC, and Kindra Mammone, CLAWS, Inc., Chapel Hill, NC.

Client Education Handout: Fennec Fox *(Fennecus zerda)*

Biologic Facts
- The smallest of the wild canids
- Live 12 to 16 years
- Sexual maturity at 9 to 11 months
- Very agile; can jump high and far; dig rapidly
- Adapted to desert life, heat tolerant, and very effective at conserving body water

Behaviors
- More social than other fox species
- Live in colonies of up to 10 individuals in the wild
- Need the companionship of people, dogs, cats, or other foxes
- Will normally cower, lie on its side, yelp loudly, and wag the tail in a submissive manner as a greeting
- Can be taught to fetch, which provides exercise
- Are shy and will usually retreat to safety when strangers visit
- Putting a collar with a bell on the fox may help owners to avoid accidentally stepping on the fox and aid in locating it when it is free in the house
- Can be leash or harness trained, but a crate is recommended
- Can be litter box trained; a covered litter box with regular clay litter is best
- Are primarily nocturnal but are active during the day and enjoy basking in the sun

Housing
- Should be kenneled while unsupervised
- Need a large, multilevel ferret or cat cage with shelves
- Can easily climb or dig out of fenced enclosures unless pens are constructed to prevent escape
- Require a low-humidity, well-ventilated environment
- Have a strong instinct to dig and should be provided a soft cage substrate for burrowing
- Dusty cage substrates should be avoided
- Live insects and rodents should be provided as enrichment and to supplement the diet

Diet
- Fennecs in the wild are omnivorous.
- A diet designed for foxes (e.g., Mazuri Exotic Canine Diet, Purina Mills) is recommended.
- Other food items include high-quality dry dog or cat food, canned dog or cat food, vegetables, fruits, pinkie mice, rodents, eggs, crickets, and mealworms.
- Fresh water should be provided at all times.

Problems Requiring Veterinary Attention
- Trauma (bite wounds, fractures)
- Neonatal death (nervous mothering)
- Eye injuries, discharges from eyes or nose
- Ear and skin infections
- Flea infestation, dandruff, itchiness
- Not eating
- Decreased stool production or diarrhea
- Lumps or bumps on skin or felt in the abdomen
- Changes in the urination habits or excessive drinking
- Yellow tinge to the skin
- Coughing or difficulty breathing

Preventive Care
- Twice yearly physical examinations* and fecal examination for internal parasites
- Rabies vaccination (IMRAB [Merial])
- Canine distemper virus, adenovirus and parvovirus vaccination (Recombitek [Merial])
- Flea control (Advantage [Bayer])
- Canine heartworm preventative
- Discuss diet and husbandry

*Check state and local regulations regarding the maintenance of fennec foxes in captivity. Locate a veterinarian who obtains continuing education about exotic pets and who has experience with fennec foxes.

Hedgehogs

Natural History and Behavior

The species of hedgehog that has been traditionally available in the pet trade is *Atelerix albiventris*, commonly called the *African pygmy hedgehog*. This species is native to West and Central Africa,[52] and was the pet hedgehog most often encountered in the United States. Since the cessation of importation, however, many captive-raised hedgehogs are the result of cross-breeding with another species of the same genus, *Atelerix algirus*. However, at least 12 different species of hedgehogs of African or Asian origin exist and are occasionally presented to the practitioner. The temperaments of these vary, and in particular *Hemiechinus auritus* (the long-eared Egyptian hedgehog) has been noted by some to be aggressive. These species differ considerably from the larger European hedgehog, *Erinaceus europaeus*, which is not commonly seen in the United States. However, abundant literature is available, especially in Britain, regarding the care, rehabilitation, and biology of the European hedgehog. It is not known to what extent this information can be extrapolated to African species, and the practitioner should use caution in assuming specific correlations.

Hedgehogs are monogastric omnivores, consuming a variety of invertebrates, frogs, lizards, snakes, mice, eggs, fruit, and fungi. They are generally solitary and nocturnal, and they inhabit a wide range of habitats including grassland, scrub, savanna, and suburban environments. Hedgehogs live in brush piles, rock crevices, and burrows and are able to climb, dig, and swim. Hedgehogs have a fairly small home range with a radius of 100 to 300 meters (109 to 330 yards).[27,63]

African hedgehogs may become dormant during periods of prolonged environmental stress (such as cold or excessive heat), but they do not truly hibernate, as do the European hedgehogs, which live in a more temperate climate. Dormancy can last for weeks but is not a continuous state; the animal wakes periodically and emerges at intervals. While dormant the animal remains sensitive to sound and touch in the area of the head, but it remains so sluggish that it cannot respond to an attack. Metabolism, heart rate, and respiratory rate decrease, whereas synthesis of endogenous heparin increases, preventing the formation of thrombi. Decreased metabolic rate also renders the hedgehog more susceptible to infection. Pet hedgehogs should therefore be prevented from hibernating or going into dormancy.[43] African pygmy hedgehogs do not appear to have a physiologic need for dormancy. Maintaining them at warm temperatures and providing a consistent and ample food source will prevent dormancy.

Hedgehogs exhibit a unique behavior known as "self-anointing" or "anting." Substances that cause self-anointing behavior are typically novel or irritating. The object is licked or chewed until thick, frothy saliva accumulates. The saliva (and presumably the chemical trigger) is then carefully placed onto the spines of both sides of the body using the tongue. Self-anointing may serve to attract mates or as a defense mechanism.[7] African hedgehogs have been documented to spread toad venom on their spines, making the prick of their spines more painful and the spines more irritating to handle.[6] The self-anointing process may continue for up to 20 minutes and has been observed in hedgehogs as young as 15 days of age.

When threatened, hedgehogs curl up into a ball, extend their spines, puff up, and emit a high-pitched hissing sound. This behavior can facilitate the administration of injections subcutaneously or intramuscularly in hedgehogs without sedation. A concern with this technique is that a thick layer of fat is present over the dorsal spinous surface, and injections must be sufficiently deep to penetrate through to the subcutaneous and/or muscular tissue.[43]

The spines of hedgehogs are modified hairs made of keratin. They are not barbed and usually do not cause injury to handlers. However, the spines do have sharp tips that can penetrate soft skin, which could cause the handler to drop the hedgehog; care should therefore be exercised, when lifting the animal, to do so over a protected area. Occasionally, penetration of a spine through the skin of a handler will cause an allergic reaction or infection.

Sensory Behaviors

Hearing appears to be very acute in pygmy hedgehogs, especially in the ultrasonic range.[29] They will jump, recoil, or curl up in response to sudden noises and do not habituate to them. Hedgehogs usually exhibit a continuous sniffing as they explore their environment, which some research has suggested is involved in echolocation.[63] Hedgehogs use their sense of smell to find food and are capable of detecting prey that is buried. Cedar and pine bedding are not recommended for hedgehogs because of the strong odor of these materials.

Hedgehog eyesight is not particularly acute, and their color recognition is poorly developed; however, bright lights will stimulate a fear response. Loss of vision is common in captive hedgehogs, with one or both eyes being damaged and requiring enucleation. It is not known whether this is a result of an inherent tendency for ocular prolapse or whether the fact that close observation of captive hedgehogs' eyes is so seldom accomplished that ocular disease is not noted until it is advanced.[64] Regardless of the cause, hedgehogs in captivity do amazingly well with one or both eyes enucleated, providing the position of the food and other elements of the enclosure are not altered.

Hedgehogs have a well-developed sense of touch through their vibrissae and spines, but tactile sensitivity of the toes is poorly developed. Hedgehogs may be sensitive to changes in balance and orientation. Motion sickness has been reported, and car rides and excessive handling are usually responsible. Research regarding hedgehog sensory anatomy and physiology is limited and is largely restricted to verification of taxonomic associations.[7]

Hedgehogs may exhibit a flehmen* response, indicating intense interest and attentiveness to a smell or taste. An individual exhibiting the response will hold its head high, with the mouth slightly opened. The upper lip will be curled up, and the tongue will be extended.

Communicative Behaviors

Hedgehogs communicate through a variety of vocalizations such as chattering, snorting, hissing, and soft growling. Under normal circumstances hedgehogs emit grunting and snuffling noises. When they are anxious or threatened, hedgehogs let out a noise similar to the hissing of a snake. If severely distressed, hedgehogs can emit a loud scream. Vocalization is relatively uncommon except between mothers and offspring and during courtship.[29]

Puffing, sniffing, and coughing are threatening sounds made if the hedgehog is disturbed or annoyed. The sniffing sounds are clear and sharp and should not be confused with rales or other respiratory symptoms. Some hedgehogs may scream if they become impatient for their food. Hedgehogs display alarm by erecting the spines over the forehead or curling up entirely.

Social and Antisocial Behaviors

African pygmy hedgehogs are primarily solitary and territorial as adults. Small groups may be found in the wild but may represent an adult female and her subadult young. Fighting is rarely observed, but individuals may react aggressively toward one another with hissing, snorting, and head butting. Captive hedgehogs are best maintained in separate cages. Youngsters should be transferred to their own cages as soon as they are independent of their mother. It is therefore acceptable for hedgehogs to be kept as solitary pets.

---

*Flehmen—a curling of the lips that facilitates transfer of chemicals to the vomeronasal organ and is seen in ungulates, felids, and many other mammals to smell urine in order to detect reproductive and physiologic status or to determine how long ago another animal passed by.

When distrustful or wary the hedgehog will erect spines on its forehead in a visor-like fashion. If afraid, hedgehogs roll up completely. Babies learn to roll up in defensive posture at 7 to 14 days of age. Laying the spines flat all over the body indicates a lack of fear. Hedgehogs are most tolerant of handling if they are handled while they are very young, and adult hedgehogs are generally more wary of and less interactive with humans than juveniles.

African pygmy hedgehogs are normally shy and reclusive; therefore a hiding place such as a hollow log or flowerpot should be in the enclosure in order to provide cover. Hedgehogs may be trained to be active during the day by gradually feeding them later and later until they are fed early in the morning and again in the middle of the day. This does not appear to have any ill effects and has the added advantage of keeping them active when they are most likely to get close attention from their caretakers.

Socialized hedgehogs may exhibit behaviors to obtain the attention of their owners. They may also paw at their owners to get attention. In one author's experience[63] a hedgehog was observed to scratch at a doorway with its forefeet to show that it wanted to be let in the door. African pygmy hedgehogs occasionally bite as a result of fear, defensiveness, or hunger.

Reproductive Behaviors

Male Reproductive Behaviors

Hedgehogs are polygamous, and males play no role in the care of their young. Hedgehog males will begin courtship behavior almost immediately after encountering a female; actively enticing the female to mate by hissing, squeaking, nudging her, and running in circles around her. Courtship and mating may continue for up to several days and be very noisy.[34] The male should be removed if the female becomes aggressive. Reintroduction can be attempted after a suitable break. The male hedgehog should be removed from the enclosure after breeding has occurred. His presence may stress the female and lead to cannibalism of the young by either adult.

Female Reproductive Behaviors and Parental Care

African pygmy hedgehog females are capable of breeding at a very early age. Females react to males during courtship with hissing and snorting in a manner almost identical to a territorial or threat display. Females are spontaneous ovulators.[2] During mating the female flattens out her spines and stretches out her rear limbs. After copulation a seminal plug from the male will seal her vagina. Gravid females will not permit further copulation.

Hedgehog mothers are attentive to their offspring, aggressively licking their newborns after parturition. They will carry the babies in their mouths and place them on the teats to suckle.[63] Females normally eat their afterbirth. The female hedgehog may cannibalize, kill, or abandon her newborn young if she is disturbed or stressed. Therefore, the male must be removed before parturition, and the mother should not be disturbed for 5 to 10 days postpartum. Females may be at increased risk for cannibalizing their young if the cage is too small or if they are bred too young. Providing two nest boxes (one for nesting, the other as a refuge), and a spacious cage may help to prevent cannibalism. Sexual maturity can occur as early as 60 to 70 days, but breeding before 6 to 8 months is not recommended.

Care of the young is always the sole responsibility of the mother. Hedgehogs nurse for 5 to 7 weeks (Figure 7-20). Juvenile hedgehogs will normally remain with the mother for some time before leaving the nest. During this time they may accompany her on her evening rounds, learning how to forage on their own. Spines are present just under the skin at birth and will emerge and harden within hours after birth. These white "nest spines" are normally shed at approximately 1 month, at which time per-

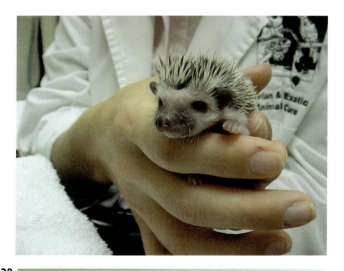

Figure 7-20
Baby African pygmy hedgehogs nurse for 5 to 7 weeks and are independent by 2 months of age. (Courtesy Dan Johnson.)

manent spines appear (Figure 7-21). Young hedgehogs are independent by 1½ to 2 months.

Eating Behaviors

Hedgehogs feed primarily at ground level but are excellent climbers and swimmers. They feed predominantly at night, covering significant distances in the wild in search of food they find in nooks and crannies, in leaf litter, and in the top layers of soil. Hunting behavior can be encouraged in captivity by hiding food and prey items in the bedding material. Providing a limited number of crickets and other insects that have been gut-loaded with a calcium fortified diet encourages exercise through foraging.[37] Hedgehogs will readily dig in carpet, dirt, and potted plants if these are encountered. They will also forage in the house for spiders and insects if they are allowed to roam freely.[34]

African hedgehogs have been observed to feed on extremely venomous animals such as vipers, cobras, scorpions, bees, toxic beetles, and spiders, and it has been postulated that they are resistant to the toxic effects of multiple toxins and venoms. Their resistance to adder venom, for example, can be up to 40 times that of laboratory mice. Hedgehogs are able to consume the beetle toxin cantharidin in quantities equivalent to 3000 times the dose toxic to humans.[27]

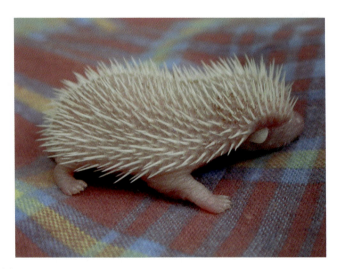

Figure 7-21
White "nest spines" emerge just after birth and are shed at approximately 1 month of age when permanent spines appear. (Courtesy Joerg Mayer.)

It should be noted that research has shown that hedgehogs' digestive tracts contain multiple chitinases, and so it is likely that a higher percentage of fiber than is normally fed (when dog and cat foods are used as the primary food source) should be provided.[19] Those fed free-choice cat food are prone to cystic calculi.[37] Therefore an insectivore diet should be provided in an amount that will be consumed before dawn.[34,37]

Elimination Behaviors

Hedgehogs tend to eliminate indiscriminately throughout their environment, although some animals can be trained to use a litter box within their enclosure. The best cage bedding and litter is shredded recycled paper or recycled newspaper products; however, the fiber type may get stuck in the animal's spines. Approximately 10 cm (4 in) of bedding is an ideal depth. Change bedding frequently to reduce odor and to avoid contact dermatitis from urine and fecal contamination. Avoid cedar and pine shavings, which can be irritating. Cat litter and soil should also be avoided. Avoid using cloth or towels as bedding materials, as these may be ingested or strings from them may cause strangulation of limbs.

Locomotor Behaviors and Activities

Hedgehogs normally spend much of the day hidden under cage furnishings. They feed and explore during the night and may spend hours running on a running wheel. They are prone to injury of the feet and legs from wire cage enclosures, running wheels, air return vents, and so on. Specialized, solid exercise wheels are recommended for hedgehogs. Hedgehogs, however, have a tendency to defecate as they use the wheel.[37] Tattered towels and linens may also lead to entanglement and constricting injury to the feet or limbs.

African pygmy hedgehogs normally walk with a slight waddle and are generally slow moving but are capable of bursts of speed. During normal ambulation the ventrum is lifted off the substrate.[29] They naturally seek small, dark crevices and hollows. Rooms must therefore be hedgehog-proofed; hedgehogs can easily get lost in the house and become lodged under furniture or appliances, behind baseboards, or in wall spaces.

Hedgehogs are good climbers and swimmers. Cages should be smooth walled in order to prevent escape. Hedgehogs have little fear of heights, and their spines are well suited to absorbing the shock of a blow or fall. A hedgehog's tendency to roll up when threatened may actually increase its risk of injury (e.g., traffic, automatic closing doors, getting stepped on). A shallow pan of warm water can be offered for swimming.[37,60]

Grooming Behaviors

Hedgehogs normally clean themselves every day. They lick and self-anoint, scratch regularly, and shake frequently, in order to rearrange their spines. Hedgehogs commonly self-anoint in response to exposure to leather items, tobacco, soaps, cosmetics, and plants containing volatile oils (Figure 7-22). Lack of grooming may be a sign of disease or stress. Subclinical mite infestations are commonplace in pet hedgehogs; however, easy epilation

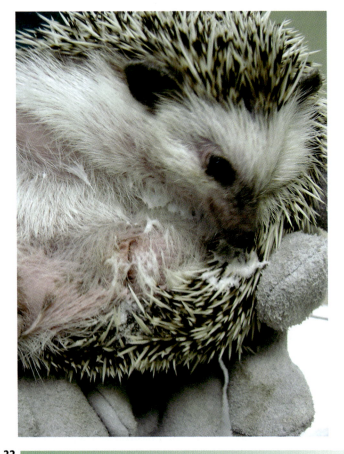

Figure 7-22
Hedgehogs may "self-anoint" in response to novel scents or flavors, applying thick, frothy saliva to their spines. This practice may play a role in defense or attracting a mate. (Courtesy Dan Johnson.)

of the spines and excessive seborrhea may be noted with quill mites (Figure 7-23). Infestations are not usually accompanied by a noticeable increase in scratching or grooming behavior, and this may be why cases are often advanced before the animal is presented and/or the condition is diagnosed.

Medical Implications of Abnormal Behaviors

Thorough physical examination of hedgehogs is difficult without sedation,[46] and anesthetizing with isoflurane or sevoflurane in an anesthetic chamber is recommended. Several methods have been documented for uncurling them[37] but these methods are not recommended in seriously ill patients or those with respiratory compromise. In cases of extreme obesity, hedgehogs may not be able to roll up in response to threatening stimuli (Figure 7-24). Likewise, a lack of response to stimuli may be a result of deafness, blindness, or weakness.

African pygmy hedgehogs do not hibernate, but they may enter dormancy if the environmental temperature falls below 18° C (65° F). Dormancy may also be triggered by systemic illness. Affected hedgehogs

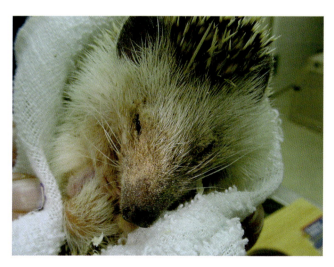

Figure 7-23
Mite infestations are very common in African pygmy hedgehogs and signs include dandruff and loose spines. Because they rarely exhibit pruritus, cases can become quite advanced before owners detect a problem, and patients may exhibit depression and anorexia. (Courtesy Dan Johnson.)

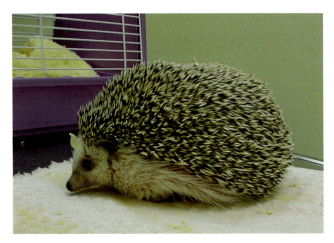

Figure 7-24
Obesity is common among captive hedgehogs, and affected individuals may not be able to completely roll into a defensive posture. Obesity can be prevented by limiting food intake, providing a hedgehog-safe running wheel, and encouraging natural hunting and foraging behaviors in captivity. (Courtesy Dan Johnson.)

are poorly responsive to stimuli, are hypothermic, and appear to be in shock. Even moribund patients may exhibit a dramatic response to fluid therapy, supplemental heat, and nutritional support. Aggressive nursing care may be needed for 24 hours or more before an accurate prognosis can be made.

Hedgehogs are susceptible to lodging of hard items against the palate.[29] Dental disease and oral tumors are common in African pygmy hedgehogs. Hypersalivation resulting from these conditions should be differentiated from normal self-anointing behavior. Nails can become overgrown and embedded in pads or tangled in cloth bedding. Necrosis of toes or feet is common if hair or string gets entangled around them (Figure 7-25).[46,60]

Behaviors Associated with Pain

Hedgehogs that experience pain or fear vocalize with a loud "ke-ke-ke" sound, or they may scream loudly. They quickly roll into a tight ball, protecting the feet, head, and underside. The spines become erect and point outward. Affected hedgehogs may exhibit lameness or a reluctance to move. Oral pain manifests as hypersalivation, difficulty prehending or chewing food, and anorexia.

How Behavior Relates to Captivity

- Hedgehogs are solitary by nature and should be housed individually.
- Provide supplemental heat for hedgehogs as needed in order to prevent dormancy.
- Provide a smooth-walled cage to prevent escape, and fill it with enough bedding to allow digging.
- Provide hedgehogs a hiding place for privacy and security.
- Allow hedgehogs to exercise outside of their cage, while observed, in a safe environment that has been hedgehog-proofed.
- In order to prevent foot and leg injuries, provide a solid-surface exercise wheel that is designed for hedgehogs.
- African pygmy hedgehogs are nocturnal by nature and should usually eat at night. To make hedgehogs more interactive, their activity cycle may be reversed, seemingly without causing them harm.
- Insects and other food items may be hidden in cage substrate for behavioral enrichment in order to encourage hunting and foraging behavior.

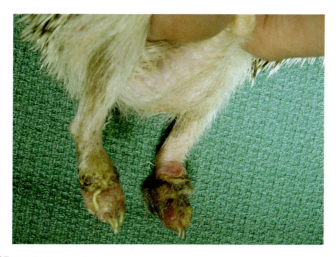

Figure 7-25
Frayed or tattered bedding can become entangled on a hedgehog's limbs and cause constricting injury and loss of extremities. (Courtesy Dan Johnson.)

Client Education Handout: African Pygmy Hedgehog *(Atelerix albiventris)*

Biologic Facts
- An insectivore related to moles and shrews.
- Are native to West and Central Africa and are the species most often encountered in the United States.
- Do *not* hibernate as European hedgehogs do.
- Have a very keen sense of smell, which they use to identify their surroundings.
- Will "self-anoint" if exposed to strong or unusual smell, foaming at the mouth then spreading the foam on their bodies.
- Nocturnal; more active at night than during the day.
- Need to be handled and well socialized when they are young in order to become well-adjusted pets. Some adult hedgehogs may not like to be handled regardless of socialization they receive when they are young.
- Average life span 3 to 5 years. Can live up to 10 years in captivity.

Housing
- Will range up to 300 m (325 yd) in the wild, so need adequate space to roam and explore (20 gal [75 L] or larger aquarium).
- Supervised time outside of the cage is advisable as long as the area has been hedgehog-proofed to prevent loss, injury, or escape.
- Enclosures with wire mesh bottoms not recommended, as these can cause foot and leg injuries.
- Enjoy privacy and require a box or other suitable hiding spot
- Shredded or pelleted recycled newspaper bedding is recommended (*not* pine or cedar shavings and *not* cat litter of any kind).
- Sipper bottle with fresh water should be available at all times and checked for patency daily.
- Average temperature should be maintained around 70° to 85° F (21° to 30° C). Provide supplemental heat (heat lamp, undertank heating pad) if necessary.
- Will use exercise wheels (provide a solid plastic wheel, not an open wire wheel).

Diet
- Commercial hedgehog diet (light or reduced-calorie, high-quality adult cat food may be used if hedgehog food is unavailable), approximately 3 teaspoons per day.
- 1 teaspoon daily of chopped mixed vegetables and/or fruits (beans, carrots, apples, pears, berries, squash, peas, potatoes, tomatoes).
- Offer live insects such as gut-loaded crickets, mealworms, earthworms, three or four times a week (avoid waxworms because of high fat content).
- Diet is extremely important, because obesity is one of the most common medical problems seen in pet hedgehogs.

Medical Care and Common Problems
- Twice yearly physical examinations* and fecal analysis for parasites recommended.
- Skin disease is common: mites, fungal disease, fleas.
- Dental disease and gum disease are common and can largely be prevented by feeding an appropriate diet. Routine brushing and scaling may be needed. Oral tumors are also common.
- All owners should be aware that hedgehogs can be carriers of *Salmonella*.
- Other problems include respiratory problems, nutritional problems, and tumors.
- A veterinarian should examine your hedgehog immediately if it is lethargic, has a decreased appetite, or has difficulty moving or if any unusual lumps or masses are seen.

*Locate a veterinarian who obtains continuing education about exotic pets and who has experience with African pygmy hedgehogs.

Prairie Dogs

Natural History and Behavior

The black-tailed prairie dog *Cynomys ludovicianus* is a stout, short-legged ground squirrel native to the Great Plains. It is diurnal, and its range extends from Montana and southern Saskatchewan to extreme northern Mexico.

Prairie dogs are named for the bark they use when threatened or excited, warning others in the colony of danger. The most prominent display is the "jump-yip," which combines a specialized leap with vocalization.

Prairie dogs exhibit a high degree of social organization. They are found in large colonies or towns, which are further divided into wards. Each ward is divided into several coteries, which contain eight to nine individuals on average. All individuals in a coterie are socially integrated and help to defend the territory against outsiders. The burrows of different coteries do not connect, and interactions between coteries are hostile. Prairie dogs do not store food in their burrows.

Coteries typically contain a single adult male, three to four adult females, and several yearling offspring. Young females remain with their coterie, whereas young males are eventually forced out. As a result, all the females of the unit are closely related. Bonds within the group are reinforced by friendly activities like kissing, nuzzling, grooming, playing together, and vocal communication.

Breeding usually does not begin until prairie dogs are 2 years old. A 7-year study on the Gunnison's prairie dog *(Cynomys gunnisoni)* in the wild indicated that the females who copulated with more than one male increased their probability of pregnancy and parturition; litter size was also increased.[26]

Some communal nursing of young will take place, but females tend to nest in isolation and while nesting are generally hostile toward the rest of the unit. They often seek to kill and devour the young of other mothers. Approximately 30% of all litters are eliminated by infanticide.[53] An adult male will not harm the young of his coterie and will seek to protect them.

Prairie dogs are considered an agricultural pest and are subject to intensive public and private poisoning programs. Capture or "harvesting" for the pet trade is accomplished through flooding and vacuuming of burrows and accounts for some of the medical conditions observed in newly acquired pups. Because most prairie dogs in the pet trade are wild-caught, the potential for zoonotic disease exists (e.g., tularema, plague, etc.).

Prairie dogs do not hibernate in the winter, but instead undergo torpor for 24 to 72 hours at a time under conditions of extreme cold and food deprivation.[28,39,37] As a native species, they are illegal to keep in some states. They are slated to be added to the United States Federal endangered species list, pending sufficient funding for enforcement.

Communicative Behaviors

Nine vocalizations have been described for prairie dogs.[53] Prairie dog communication has been studied in detail, and their vocalizations have been shown to correlate with specific activities.[61] The "jump-yip," which combines a leap and a vocalization, appears to be preliminary to territorial defense. Prairie dogs will vocalize in response to some human noises such as coughing and clearing the throat.

Anti-predator calls have been studied in the Gunnison's prairie dog, and it was found that females with related kin in the area were more likely to call if danger was present, especially if offspring were nearby.[25] The frequency of male antipredator calls was not related to the presence of nearby kin.[25]

Social and Antisocial Behaviors

Prairie dogs are active during the daytime and are social by nature. They require companionship and attention and do well in groups of two or three. If they do not get enough human interaction as solitary pets they can develop behavioral abnormalities such as excessive grooming, self-mutilation, or aggressiveness.[37]

If they are socialized at a young age they generally enjoy human contact and will interact with people. When approached, prairie dogs will often sit on their haunches, open their mouths, and bare their teeth as a greeting (Figure 7-26). This display may look like a threat but is usually an invitation to nuzzle. Most prairie dogs enjoy having their muzzle and eyes gently stroked.

Although the majority of pet prairie dogs are friendly, most also vigorously resist examination. Only exceptionally well-socialized prairie dogs will allow a complete physical examination without some form of restraint. Prairie dogs generally vocalize a warning before aggressive behavior, lunging forward and barking in a threatening manner. They generally bite as a last resort, but these injuries can be severe (Figure 7-27).

Prairie dogs lack loose skin over the scruff and cannot be restrained in this manner. Instead, place one hand under the rump and encircle the neck with the other. They may also be held bilaterally under the axilla. Most prairie dogs will tolerate this position if their haunches are supported and they will tuck their head into their chest. The use of a towel

Miscellaneous Small Mammal Behavior 307

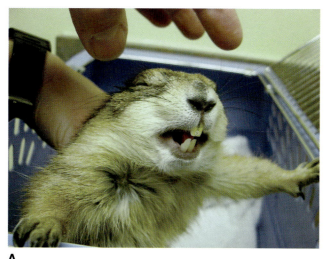

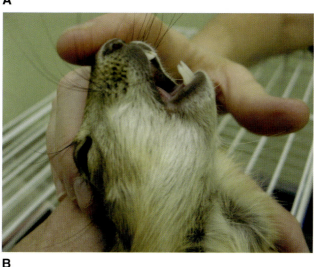

Figure 7-26
A, Prairie dogs usually greet handlers with their mouths open and their teeth bared. This may look intimidating, but is usually an invitation to nuzzle. **B,** Most prairie dogs enjoy having the muzzle stroked. (Courtesy Dan Johnson.)

or leather gloves is advisable with fractious individuals. None of these restraint techniques, however, is conducive to a thorough physical examination. Therefore most diagnostic and treatment procedures on prairie dogs will require anesthesia (see Medical Implications of Abnormal Behaviors).

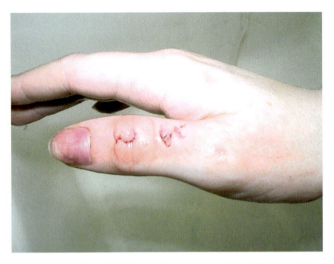

Figure 7-27
Prairie dog bites can be very severe. In the author's experience, prairie dogs vocalize before they bite and rarely bite without provocation. (Courtesy Dan Johnson.)

Reproductive Behaviors

Prairie dogs commonly become aggressive during the breeding season, also known as "rut." Prairie dogs are often presented for castration and ovariohysterectomy, as this helps to eliminate, minimize, or prevent aggressive behavior. Surgery between 6 and 9 months of age is preferable, as body fat is less and sexual aggression has not yet developed. However, the testicles at this age are small and readily retracted into the abdomen. Also, inguinal herniation, as with any species with open inguinal canals, can occur in prairie dogs. Postsurgical self-mutilation can also be a problem especially if preoperative, perioperative, and postoperative analgesics are not used. An abdominal approach is generally used for orchiectomy, especially when castration is done prior to sexual maturity. Prairie dogs reach sexual maturity at 2 to 3 years of age.

Breeding occurs in late winter and early spring (January to March). Females are monestrous, seasonal breeders for 2 to 3 weeks and have one litter per year. Breeding within a group is synchronous, with each adult female producing one litter annually. Gestation is 34 to 37 days, and litter size is one to eight; however, an average of only three pups survive to emerge above ground. Pups are approximately 15 g ($1/2$ oz) at birth, develop fur at approximately 3 weeks, and reportedly open their eyes at approximately 5 weeks.

Pups appear aboveground at approximately 5 to 6 weeks and are weaned at approximately 5 to 7 weeks. The majority of prairie dog pups in the pet trade are "harvested" each spring from the wild (see Natural History and Behavior). Prairie dogs have not consistently bred successfully in captivity.

Eating Behaviors

Prairie dogs normally sit upright and hold food between their front paws to eat (Figure 7-28). Prairie dogs are herbivorous and ferment cellulose in their cecum. Like other herbivorous small mammals, they are unable to regurgitate or eructate. They have hypsodont incisors and brachydont cheek teeth. In their natural habitat they eat primarily grasses and occasionally roots and insects. Pet prairie dogs should receive unlimited timothy grass hay and a limited amount of pellets each day. Prairie dog pellets are preferred, but rodent block or rabbit pellets are suitable. Alfalfa, fresh greens, and vegetables can be offered as treats.

Once prairie dogs reach adulthood, pelleted diets should no longer be fed on an ad libitum basis, as obesity is extremely common in older pets. Prairie dogs also should not get dog biscuits, nuts, breads, cereals, "junk food," or table foods, as these can lead to obesity and begging behaviors.[39] Provide fresh water daily in a bowl or sipper bottle.

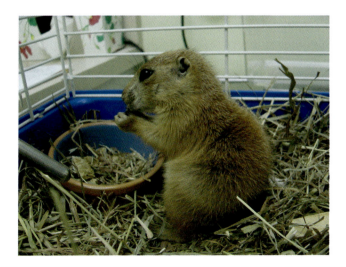

Figure 7-28
Like other members of the squirrel family, prairie dogs sit upright to eat and hold food in their hands. (Courtesy Dan Johnson.)

Elimination Behaviors

Prairie dogs are indiscriminate with regard to elimination. In response to fear they will often defecate during examination. Straining and/or vocalization during elimination may indicate constipation, colitis, urolithiasis, or blockage by a preputial plug. As with cats, owners and less-experienced veterinarians may interpret any of the above as "constipation." As hindgut fermenters, prairie dogs need a high-fiber diet and are sensitive to dietary changes[46] that can create an imbalance of intestinal bacterial flora and lead to diarrhea (Figure 7-29).[45]

Prairie dogs have a triad of perianal scent gland papillae[45] situated at the 2, 6 and 10 o'clock positions around the anus (Figure 7-30). Prairie dogs will rhythmically evert and contract these glands in a "winking" fashion whenever they are being handled for examination or struggling against restraint. When they do this, the glandular papillae strongly resemble fly larvae and have been mistaken by many owners (and veterinarians) as "internal parasites." The glands produce a musky scent but perianal sac removal is not necessary or routinely performed in prairie dogs.

Locomotor Behaviors and Activities

Prairie dogs are a diurnal species. They have no innate fear of heights and they like to climb but are not very agile.[39] Falls from beds, stairway landings, and even balconies occur frequently, resulting in injury to the teeth, lips, long bones, and vertebrae (Figure 7-31). Intervertebral disk disease has been reported. Diagnosis and treatment are the same as for other species. They also like to dig, so bedding such as recycled newspaper pellets or fiber products should be provided for them to do so.[39]

Lameness in prairie dogs will manifest as it does in other species. Lameness caused by pododermatitis occurs as a result of poor husbandry including a rough cage floor, wet bedding, and poor sanitation. This leads to secondary bacterial infections with *Staphylococcus* and other bacteria. Correct husbandry and treat infections based on results of bacterial culture and sensitivity.

Grooming Behaviors

Alopecia is a frequent occurrence in prairie dogs, stemming from many causes including rostral trauma, dermatophytosis, malnutrition, ectoparasites, poor ventilation or sanitation, and barbering, as well as hormonal and seasonal influences (Figure 7-32). Prairie dogs are susceptible to ectoparasites such as fleas, ticks, mites, and lice, and they may exhibit excessive

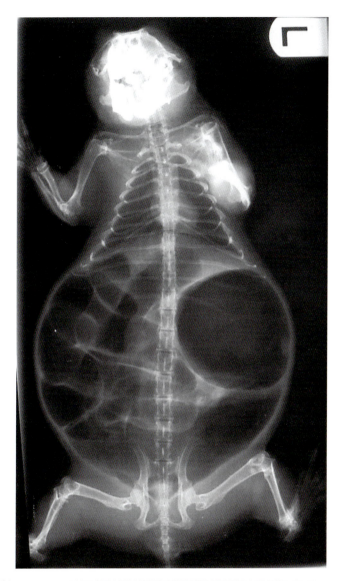

Figure 7-29
Prairie dogs have a functional cecum and are susceptible to gastrointestinal dysbiosis. Dietary change, stress, and inappropriate antibiotic use can lead to diarrhea, ileus, and bloat as illustrated in this radiograph. (Courtesy Dan Johnson.)

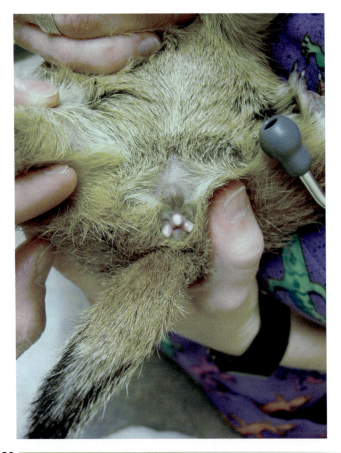

Figure 7-30
When excited, prairie dogs repeatedly "flash" the perianal scent gland papillae, and handlers occasionally mistake these for parasites or fly larvae. (Courtesy Dan Johnson.)

grooming as a result. Excessive grooming may also be a sign of stress or boredom. Some prairie dogs will use a dust bath, and this may help to prevent skin diseases.[4] Prairie dogs that do not have sufficient opportunities to dig will need their toenails trimmed frequently.

Medical Implications of Abnormal Behaviors

Many prairie dogs are handled frequently and are tame enough to be examined while awake, but others must be anesthetized, preferably by isoflurane induction in an anesthetic chamber. When a prairie dog is

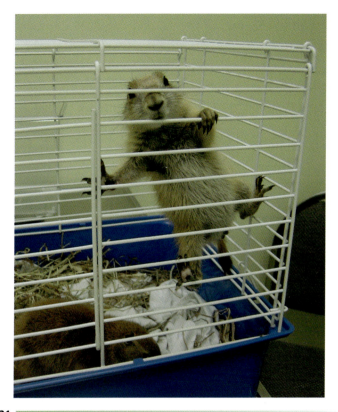

Figure 7-31
Prairie dogs have no fear of heights. They are good climbers; however, they frequently injure themselves by falling. (Courtesy Dan Johnson.)

anesthetized, it is important to elevate the head and thorax, as respiration can be compromised by the weight of the abdomen against the relatively smaller thorax, especially in obese patients.[39,44] Because prairie dogs have a very short, thick neck, e-collars are not useful.

One of the most common diseases of pet prairie dogs is obesity (Figure 7-33). Excessive fat promotes respiratory, heart, gallbladder, and liver disease. Avoid seeds, nuts, dog food, junk food, lack of exercise, and unlimited pelleted feed. Once prairie dogs reach adulthood, reduce the alfalfa content in the diet and increase the amount of grass hay. Offer free-choice timothy hay, limit pellets, give greens as treats, and offer plenty of opportunities for exercise.

Prairie dogs are obligate nasal breathers; therefore even mild impairment of nasal airflow can result in open-mouth breathing. Prairie dog

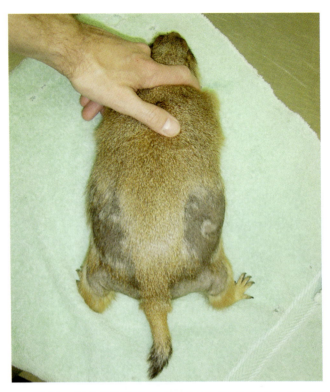

Figure 7-32
Alopecia is a common presenting sign in prairie dogs and may have many different causes, including parasitic or hormonal conditions, neoplasia, and infection. A skin biopsy can aid in the diagnosis of difficult cases. (Courtesy Dan Johnson.)

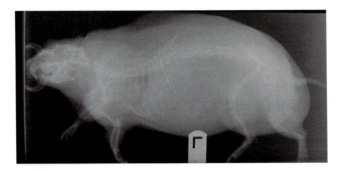

Figure 7-33
Obesity is very common in pet prairie dogs. If offered high-energy treats such as seeds, grains, and nuts, prairie dogs may consume these to the exclusion of grass hay and commercial prairie dog pellets. (Courtesy Dan Johnson.)

Miscellaneous Small Mammal Behavior

respiratory symptoms have many causes, many of which are related to husbandry and captivity. These include bacterial infection, foreign body, poor ventilation, excessive dust, improper humidity, allergy, obesity, dental disease, neoplasia, and heart disease. Open-mouth breathing will ultimately have a negative affect on appetite, activity, and sleep schedule. Dyspnea, lethargy, and anorexia may be associated with cardiomyopathy in prairie dogs older than 2 to 3 years of age.[45]

Odontoma and pseudoodontoma are forms of dental neoplasia and hyperplasia, respectively, and are commonly seen in prairie dogs.[39,44] These conditions are associated with chronic dental disease or tooth root trauma (Figures 7-34 and 7-35). Owners usually note that their prairie dog is having respiratory difficulty, as evidenced by open-mouth breathing and excessive abdominal movement with respiration. Lethargy and anorexia occur because individuals are unable to eat, drink, and breathe at the same time. Varying degrees of exophthalmia may be observed. These conditions are progressive. Trauma to the tooth roots caused by falling or chewing on metal or hard plastic cage bars is the most likely cause.[54]

Radiographs readily demonstrate these conditions. Surgical extraction of the incisors is difficult because of the thickness and hypercalcification of the tooth roots and the extensive vascularity of the hard palate. Placement of a stent over the frontal sinus may provide increased airflow,

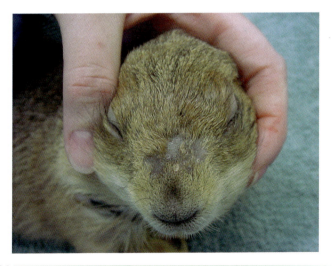

Figure 7-34
This photo shows nasal alopecia which may be associated with cage bar rubbing. Damage to the teeth has been associated with tooth root thickening. (Courtesy Teresa Bradley Bays.)

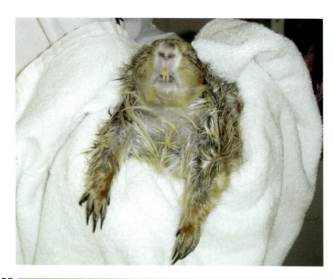

Figure 7-35
This patient displayed hypersalivation as a result of heat stress. Prairie dogs may also hypersalivate as a result of dental disease, gastrointestinal disease, and any condition that causes nausea. (Courtesy Dan Johnson.)

but the relief is usually temporary. These conditions are not recognized in wild prairie dogs.

True hibernation does not occur in prairie dogs; however, they do experience brief periods of torpor, especially in inclement weather.[37,39] Dormancy may be induced inadvertently in captive prairie dogs by the combination of obesity, a drop in environmental temperature below 16° C (60° F), and low light levels. A dormant prairie dog may be lethargic, cool to the touch, and poorly responsive. An affected prairie dog will appear to be seriously ill; however, it will show a dramatic response to warmth and rehydration. Illness can also trigger dormancy in prairie dogs; therefore supportive care may need to be given for 24 hours or more before an accurate assessment of a prairie dog's condition can be made. Provide warm subcutaneous fluids and a warm cage environment to rouse prairie dogs from dormancy.

Ataxia, torticollis, and stumbling can be attributed to *Baylisascaris* species infection. This zoonotic nematode can be acquired from skunk or raccoon feces, either from exposure in the wild or exposure through outside cages or from fecal residue on an old cage. Differential diagnoses include neoplasia, trauma, infectious agents, and toxin or heavy metal ingestion.

Prairie dogs that do not get adequate companionship and social interaction may become aggressive, self-mutilate, or groom excessively. Prairie dogs that roam freely are susceptible to electrocution as a result of chewing on electrical cables and wires. Lead intoxication can result from chewing on stained glass, lead paint, and other household sources. Zinc intoxication can result from chewing on galvanized cage wire.

Sick prairie dogs often do not eat or drink on their own. Apparent lack of appetite is a sign of many different illnesses in prairie dogs and is accompanied by diminished fecal production. Anorexia may be due to dental, metabolic, parasitic, gastrointestinal, or neoplastic disease. Supplemental fluids, nutritional support such as syringe-feeding Critical Care (Oxbow Pet Products, Murdock, NE), and prokinetics are indicated. Continue supportive care measures until appetite, defecation, and urination return to normal.

Wild caught prairie dogs can be reservoirs of many zoonotic diseases, and the veterinary clinician should discourage clients from keeping them as pets.[39,44] These diseases include *Yersinia pseudotuberculosis*, *Yersinia pestis*, *Baylisascaris procyonis*, and hantavirus.[46]

Behaviors Associated with Pain

Prairie dogs are generally hardy and more tolerant of discomfort than rabbits, guinea pigs, and chinchillas. A prairie dog that is experiencing pain and discomfort will be withdrawn and reluctant to move and will sit with its head tucked in toward its belly. Attempts to rouse such a patient will be met with an apathetic open-mouth display, and minimal vocalization, and the patient will tend to keep its eyes closed. Postoperatively, prairie dogs are prone to chewing sutures and causing incisions to dehisce. Subcuticular sutures and tissue adhesive are recommended, as well as judicious use of preoperative, perioperative, and postoperative analgesics. Complications are rare if adequate analgesia is used.

Behavioral Enrichment

Prairie dogs should be housed in large, solid-floored cages suitable for rabbits or guinea pigs. These are usually constructed of heavy-gauge wire, which provides good ventilation and gnawing resistance. Provide a deep layer of bedding substrate, such as pelleted fiber, shredded paper, or similar litter, to allow for digging behavior. Avoid clay litter and cedar or pine shavings. Recommended cage furnishings include PVC pipe sections buried in the bedding and a hide box for sleeping and security. Prairie dogs also enjoy chew toys and dust baths. Prairie dogs need a safe perch or shelf for standing "lookout." They will attempt to climb but are not graceful and will easily fall.

Prairie dogs normally investigate and chew on their cages, furnishings, and everything else in their environment. Rostral abrasions are the result of cage design. Affected prairie dogs spend much of their time pushing their noses through openings in the cage and chewing the wire. This behavior increases the risk of odontoma formation and the development of obstructive respiratory disease.[54] Prevent these problems by using cages constructed with smaller openings (e.g., "hardware cloth") or using cages that have a smooth-walled design (e.g., Plexiglas), without exposed wire or hardware that can be gnawed on. Cages need to be sturdy enough to resist chewing; therefore some wood or plastic cage designs would be inappropriate for housing prairie dogs.

Prairie dogs kept in captivity do best in a cool, dry, well-ventilated location. The ideal temperature is 18° to 27° C (65° to 80° F), and the ideal relative humidity is 40% to 60%.

How Behavior Relates to Captivity

- Prairie dogs are social animals that prefer to live in pairs or small groups.
- Prairie dogs have no fear of heights and must be prevented from situations in which they can fall and injure themselves.
- Lack of exercise in captivity will lead to obesity.
- Most pet prairie dogs are wild-caught, and potential for zoonoses exists.
- Although most prairie dogs become very tame, even a "friendly" prairie dog may not want to be held.
- To treat prairie dogs, practitioners will need to become familiar with the natural history, behaviors, nutritional requirements, and common conditions of this species.

Client Education Handout: The Black-tailed Prairie Dog *(Cynomys ludovicianus)*

Biologic Facts
- Life span: up to 7 years
- Adult body weight: 0.5 to 2.2 kg (1 to 5 lb)
- Sexual maturity: 2 to 3 years

Behaviors
- Most prairie dogs are wild-caught in the spring while they are still 2 to 3 months old.
- Prairie dogs are diurnal (active during the day).
- They do not hibernate but may become less active for several days in cold weather.
- They "bark" when excited or alarmed or as a greeting.
- Open-mouth greeting is not a threat; they greet each other and humans in this way.
- They are very social animals and need lots of attention.
- They like to climb but are very clumsy and fall easily.
- They need lots of deep bedding for digging.
- They can become aggressive during the mating season if not altered.

Diet
- Should be fed unlimited timothy grass hay and limited commercial pelleted diet (e.g., Oxbow Prairie Delight, rodent chow). *Do not* feed monkey chow or dog food.
- Alfalfa cubes may be added to the diet of young prairie dogs but should be eliminated from the diet as they age to prevent obesity
- Fresh fruit and vegetables, seeds, and nuts can be offered occasionally as treats.
- *Provide a large sipper bottle of clean fresh water; change it daily.*

Housing
- Large rodent or rabbit enclosure; provide some solid flooring if wire mesh floor
- Deep bedding for digging (recycled paper fiber bedding or pellets)
- Tunnels, boxes for hiding, toys, PVC pipe
- Chinchilla dust to "bathe" in
- Temperature 65 to 80° F (18° to 27° C), 40% to 60% humidity

Common Medical Conditions Requiring Veterinary Attention
- Dental problems (malocclusion, odontoma)
- Obesity
- Respiratory problems
- Trauma and fractures
- Heart disease
- Skin problems
- Liver disease

Preventive Care
- Twice yearly physical and dental examinations*, including a dental examination at a veterinary hospital where the doctor and staff have knowledge and experience with prairie dogs
- Annual fecal analysis
- Blood tests as needed
- Nail trimming as needed
- Spay or neuter (best before 12 months old, in May through October)
- No vaccinations required

*Locate a veterinarian who obtains continuing education about exotic pets and who has experience with prairie dogs.
Check state and local regulation regarding the maintenance of prairie dogs in captivity.

Short-Tailed Opossums

Natural History and Behavior

The short-tailed opossum *Monodelphis domestica* is native to eastern and central Brazil, Bolivia, and Paraguay. They are found in forests, open areas, and high moisture areas close to water sources. Nests are usually built in hollow logs, in fallen trees, along streams, and among rocks. Short-tailed opossums are also commonly found in dwellings, where they are a welcome means of pest control, as they eat rodents, insects, spiders, and scorpions.[52]

In the tropical extent of its range, short-tailed opossums are able to breed continuously, having up to four litters per year. Short-tailed opossums reach sexual maturity at 4 to 5 months of age. Gestation is 14 to 15 days, and litter size ranges from 5 to 12. Neonates are dependent on the mother for approximately 50 days; offspring cling to the nipple initially and hang onto the mother's back and flanks later on. Short-tailed opossums may live up to 4 to 6 years.[35,37]

Sensory Behaviors

Short-tailed opossums are very sensitive to light and noise. Excessive ultraviolet light exposure may lead to retinal melanoma. Short-tailed opossums have well-developed olfactory systems and rely heavily on their sense of smell.

Short-tailed opossums are sensitive to high frequencies, yet relatively insensitive to sound. At 60 dB sound pressure level (SPL), the hearing of *Monodelphis* extends from 3.6 kHz to 77 kHz, with a range of best sensitivity from 8 to 64 kHz. They are not particularly sensitive to tones, with the lowest threshold near 20 dB SPL.[18] Ears of short-tailed opossums are thin, hairless, and subject to desiccation; the pinnae will shrivel under prolonged exposure to low humidity.[55]

These opossums demonstrate less fear of new objects and investigate them more intensely than rats.[65] This may be because short-tailed opossums are nomadic and therefore routinely come in contact with objects that are new to them.

Communicative Behaviors

Both sexes communicate through a complex system of urine and scent gland marking behaviors. Studies suggest the use of glandular secretions is more common and more effective than urine for intraspecific communication among short-tailed opossums. Researchers believe that in the semiarid locations inhabited by the opossums, glandular secretions are less volatile and are effective for longer periods than urine. Also, because these opossums are nomadic and meet one another infrequently in the wild, these less-volatile glandular secretions would be of greater value.[66]

When short-tailed opossums investigate a new person or object, they typically "nuzzle" it by rubbing their snout over the object and depositing saliva.[55] It is believed that nuzzling dissolves odors and scent marks, allowing more chemical information about them to be obtained and improving the intake of chemical stimuli into the vomeronasal organ.[56] Nuzzling appears to be especially important in the recognition of conspecifics.

Males scent-mark using glands on the chin, neck, chest, and cloaca. Which scent gland a male uses is at least partially dependent on the substrate being marked. The marking odor is unpleasant to other male *M. domestica*. When a male encounters another male's scent mark, he will usually nuzzle it, then he in turn will exhibit scent-marking behavior.[57]

Short-tailed opossums also communicate using a variety of vocalizations, hissing, and chatter. When they feel threatened, the opossums exhibit an open-mouth threat, baring their sharp teeth.

Social and Antisocial Behaviors

The short-tailed opossum has been used extensively as a laboratory animal. Its primary use is in the study of photodermatology. It breeds well in captivity and is reasonably tame. *M. domestica* is largely nocturnal but in captivity will become active during the day.

South American short-tailed opossums are highly solitary. They are nomadic and rarely encounter others in the wild. They are highly intolerant of others and therefore should be caged individually. If two adults are introduced, violent aggression may ensue. Same-sex encounters are the worst, but conflicts rarely result in serious injury.

If handled from a very early age, young short-tailed opossums will lose their natural fear of people and can become very tame for the rest of their lives (Figure 7-36). In order to give them time to acclimate, however, newly acquired opossums should not be handled for the first week after purchase. Short-tailed opossums are curious by nature and will eventually come to investigate an extended hand, sniffing and nuzzling it. Once opossums are more secure and at ease they can easily be petted and picked up.

Offspring should be housed individually at approximately 2 to 3 months of age. If they are not separated, more dominant individuals will begin to nip at and exclude subordinates from the nest box. Tail-biting injuries may occur at this time. True fighting will be observed at approximately 4 months of age with the onset of sexual maturity. Mothers and sisters may

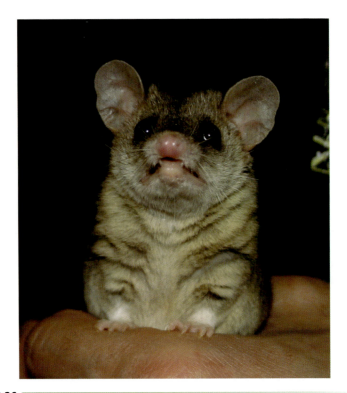

Figure 7-36
If they are handled from an early age, short-tailed opossums lose their natural fear of humans and become tame. *Monodelphis* are highly intolerant of other short-tailed opossums, however, and should be housed individually. (Courtesy CLAWS, Inc., Kindra D. Mammone.)

be kept together for longer periods in some situations; however, minor aggression and stress are likely to occur.

Reproductive Behaviors

Male Reproductive Behaviors

Male short-tailed opossums exhibit scent-marking by rubbing the chest and flanks against objects. Castration results in decreased marking behavior. Treatment with testosterone stimulates chest marking in these castrates, and those treated with either estradiol or testosterone display increased flank or hip marking.[13] Also, female aggression toward males was increased when the males had received testosterone.[13]

The scrotum of *M. domestica* hangs from a ventral abdominal stalk, away from body heat. At temperatures above 27° C (80° F), males will start "fanning" their testicles. To improve airflow and cool the testes, a male will lift its rump and lean on objects for support. This behavior should prompt owners to lower the cage temperature.

Males investigate the body odors (flank and urine odors) of diestrous females significantly more than the odors of juvenile females or those that are already in heat. Because *M. domestica* females have an induced estrus, it is advantageous for males to investigate and follow the odors of urine of diestrous females, which become receptive in proximity to males.[66]

The male and his nest box should be introduced into the female's cage, or both are introduced into a larger, neutral territory cage. Aggression between the breeding pair is normal within the first few days after introduction, and injury is possible. Therefore, it is advisable to monitor the pair and separate them if injuries occur. Chirping sounds and chasing are normal. The nest boxes of both animals need to be available as a place of refuge in the breeding cage. The pair will eventually start to exchange nest boxes as courtship progresses and they become accustomed to each other's odors. Males will actively investigate the female's odor deposits in the cage and emit rapid, faint (mostly ultrasonic) clicking sounds. The male will engage in elaborate face-rubbing ("nuzzling") and scent-marking behavior around the breeding cage.

Breeding pairs should be chosen carefully. Females prefer males who are close to their own age and will reject males who are either too young or too old. A successful breeding male is forceful and not easily deterred by the female's hissing and open-mouth threats.

Female Reproductive Behaviors

Female opossums are induced into estrus by direct exposure to a nonvolatile pheromone in male scent marks. Female opossums actively investigate the scent-markings of males, but not their urine markings.[66] Immature females that are continuously exposed to male scent-markings before sexual maturity reach estrus earlier, grow larger, and have greater uterine and ovarian development (greater size and number of follicles) than females that are not exposed to scent marks.[21] Intact females show a preference for intact males over castrated males, whereas ovariectomized females do not.[11]

The female will become receptive to the male and actively engage in courtship behavior approximately 5 days after pairing.[10] Aggression will temporarily cease, and the pair will be friendly and tolerant of each other. Estrus occurs after 6 to 8 days of continuous exposure to the male or his odor and lasts 3 to 12 days.[10,55] Breeding occurs during this time. Females will normally exhibit anogenital dragging just before mating, and a sex lock occurs during copulation.[12,15] The pair should be separated approximately 12 days after pairing, when after a period of peaceful cohabitation aggression resumes.

The pouch is not developed in short-tailed opossums. Instead, 11 to 17 mammae are arranged in a circle on the abdomen. Both males and females build nests using the mouth, forelegs, hind legs, and tail, and it has been found that at 24° C (75° F), both males and females used more nesting material and built larger nests of better quality than at 27° C (80° F).[14] Optimal temperature conditions are especially important for nursing females and their young. Marsupial babies are poor at regulating their own temperature, so the nest is woven tightly with only a very small opening, to conserve heat and humidity. Hypothermia can be fatal, as mothers may not be able to sustain lactation and thermoregulation.[55]

Mothers should not be disturbed during the first 2 to 3 weeks postpartum. During that period, mothers will rarely venture out of the nest box except to eat, drink, and eliminate. Average litter size is eight to nine. Very old or young mothers with a small litter of two to three may cannibalize the litter. Stressed mothers may also cannibalize their young.

Weaning occurs after 7 to 8 weeks. Lactating females and their young can be supplied with a shallow dish (to avoid drowning) of whole milk, half and half, or kitten milk replacer in order to make weaning easier.[55]

Eating Behaviors

Monodelphis usually seek food on the ground, foraging in the evening. The diet in the wild consists of small rodents, insects, scorpions, worms, carrion, seeds, and fruits. Short-tailed opossums are usually fed commercial fox diet or insectivore diet as a staple. Live foods (e.g., gut-loaded crickets, mealworms, earthworms, and pinkie mice) can be let loose in the cage, and fresh fruit can be placed throughout the cage to supplement the diet and encourage foraging behavior and exercise. Short-tailed opossums sit upright to eat. They are highly dexterous and use their fingers for complex food manipulation. In the wild *M. domestica* has been observed to catch flying insects in midair with its paws.

Short-tailed opossums dehydrate easily and therefore need a ready water supply. They can drink from a bowl or bottle; however, the jaw musculature of short-tailed opossums is relatively weak. To prevent dehydration, bottle spouts need to be free-flowing (without metal ball), and bottles should not be completely filled so that a vacuum does not form. Hang water bottles low enough that babies can also reach them.

Elimination Behaviors

Short-tailed opossums, especially lactating females, tend to use one corner of the cage as a latrine while keeping the nest area very clean. The bedding in this area should be removed and replaced with fresh bedding daily.

Short-tailed opossums like the presence of their own odors. When transferring animals to a clean cage it may be advisable to mix some of the soiled bedding with the fresh bedding to provide a background of familiar odor. Weekly cage cleaning is considered by some to be stressful for the opossum; therefore a biweekly cleaning schedule is recommended.[55] When cleaning the cage, especially the cage of a mother and her litter, it is important not to disturb the opossum and to leave its nest intact.

Locomotor Behaviors and Activities

Short-tailed opossums are most active during the first few hours after full darkness. They are among the least well-adapted opossums for arboreal life and usually dwell on the ground (Figure 7-37). Nonetheless, they can climb fairly well; therefore rocks and branches should be offered for climbing, jumping, and perching activity. *Monodelphis* will use running wheels for exercise and have incredible dexterity with their forefeet. The tail is weakly prehensile and can carry small items.

Grooming Behaviors

Healthy short-tailed opossums have smooth, silky, gray to brown fur. In general, short-tailed opossums are relatively clean and odorless.

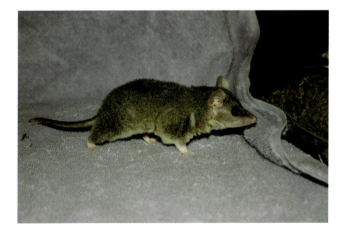

Figure 7-37
Short-tailed opossums are nocturnal. They are poorly adapted to arboreal life, preferring instead to forage close to the ground for insects, worms, fruit, seeds, and a variety of other food items. (Courtesy CLAWS, Inc., Kindra D. Mammone.)

Medical Implications of Abnormal Behaviors

Short-tailed opossums that are exposed to prolonged stress may groom less and develop a shaggy, unkempt appearance. Repetitive behaviors such as running in circles around the cage may also develop. Stress resulting from overbreeding can result in uterine prolapse.[55]

Common medical conditions that are seen in veterinary practice include the following:
- Rectal prolapse secondary to gastrointestinal infection
- Gastroenteritis, bloat, diarrhea
- Neoplasia: liver, pancreas, pituitary, uterine, skin, adrenal
- Kidney infection
- Renal failure
- Endocrine alopecia
- Ectoparasites
- Heart disease: cardiomyopathy, atherosclerosis
- Injuries and trauma
- Desiccation and necrosis of ear pinnae and tail tip if humidity is below 50%

Behaviors Associated with Pain

Short-tailed opossums react to pain in a manner similar to other small mammals. If injury to a limb occurs, lameness may result. While in pain, short-tailed opossums may become withdrawn, anorexic, and/or reluctant to move. Opossums that are normally easy to handle are more likely to display an open-mouth threat and to bite when experiencing pain.

How Behavior Relates to Captivity

Short-tailed opossums are solitary and should be housed individually except during breeding. They require a large enclosure (15-gallon terrarium or larger), with at least 1 in (2.5 cm) of bedding (e.g., recycled paper products), a nest box, food dish, and paper towel strips for nesting material.

Short-tailed opossums will be least stressed if the nest box has a small opening so that it can be easily defended. One author[55] recommends a lightweight upside-down plastic dog bowl, because it is safe, dark, and easy to defend. If a dog bowl is used, it should be plastic, not ceramic or glass, to allow the opossum to get in and out easily.

Loud noise, excess light, extreme temperature, low humidity or water intake, and excessive breeding all cause stress. Opossums have a lower body temperature than similar-sized rodents and other euthermic mammals. Short-tailed opossums are prone to chilling, and supplemental heat may be indicated.

Client Education Handout: South American Short-Tailed Opossum (Monodelphis domestica)

Biologic Facts
- Weight: male 90 to 150 g (3.1 to 5.2 oz); female 80 to 100 g (2.8 to 3.5 oz)
- Length: head and body 110 to 200 mm (4.3 to 7.9 in); tail 45 to 80 mm (1.8 to 3.2 in)
- Sexual maturity: 4 to 5 months
- Gestation: 14 to 15 days
- Litter size: 5 to 12
- Weaning: 60 to 90 days
- Longevity: 4 to 6 years
- Marsupial without a pouch; offspring attach to nipples and are easily observed during development
- Males have a prominent scrotal sac hanging from the ventral abdomen on a seminal stalk; the penis lies in the floor of the cloaca
- Primarily nocturnal

Diet
- Pelleted fox diet, pelleted insectivore diet
- Insects, insect larvae, worms, pinkie mice
- Fruit

Behaviors
- Nocturnal
- Solitary
- Nomadic
- Offer food in the evening

Housing
- Require high humidity (>50%) and ready access to water
- May require supplemental heat; ideal temp 24° C (75° F)
- Prefer a large cage with branches, perches, and rocks for exploring and hiding
- Provide plastic hide box with small opening

Conditions Requiring Veterinary Attention
- Prolapsed tissue protruding from anus
- Diarrhea, abdominal distension, bloating
- Cancer is common; look for bumps or masses on the skin or felt in the abdomen
- Little or no urine, urinating more, drinking to excess
- Hair loss, lesions on skin, dandruff, fleas, or mites
- Difficulty breathing, coughing, or exercise intolerance (easy exertion)
- Discharge from the eyes or nose
- Weakness or lameness
- Not eating and/or decreased or no stool production

Preventive Care
- Twice yearly complete physical examinations*
- Diet and husbandry review
- Fecal examination for parasites
- Dental and oral examination (may require anesthesia)
- Complete blood count and chemistry

*Locate a veterinarian who obtains continuing education about exotic pets and who has experience with short-tailed opossums.

Sugar Gliders

Natural History and Behavior

Sugar gliders *(Petaurus breviceps)* are native to northern and eastern Australia, New Guinea, and the surrounding islands. They inhabit woodlands and forests and are arboreal and largely nocturnal.[52] In the wild the density of sugar gliders in continuous forested areas is approximately one animal per 4 hectares (ha) (9.9 acres), and one animal per 2 ha (4.9 acres) in fragmented areas.[30] They shelter by day in leaf-lined nests inside of tree hollows. The natural range in New Guinea extends from sea level to 3000 meters (9900 feet) in altitude.[16]

Sugar gliders have a large gliding membrane extending from ankle to forefoot. They are capable of gliding flight for up to 70 m (230 ft) and have been observed to leap at and catch insects in flight. While sugar gliders are in flight they use the flattened tail as a rudder. The tail is also weakly prehensile and can coil around nesting material for transport. Gliders are mainly insectivorous, feeding on insects, larvae, arachnids, and small vertebrates for most of the year and sap, blossoms, and nectar only during the wet season (which is winter).[37]

Sugar gliders are social and produce a variety of sounds. Wild groups nest in colonies of up to seven adult males, females, and their young. During the winter gliders huddle together to conserve energy. They may simultaneously enter a daily torpor during cold weather when food and water are scarce. Groups are exclusive and territorial: established members may attack newly introduced individuals. The exportation of sugar gliders has been banned in Australia since 1959. Sugar gliders breed readily in captivity, and they gained popularity in the United States in the late 1990s.

Sensory Behaviors

Like most nocturnal species, sugar gliders have excellent night vision and a keen sense of hearing. Bright light can be stressful for gliders, and direct sunlight can result in retinal damage. As owls are a major predator of gliders in the wild, they may become stressed if placed in proximity to birds and loud bird noises.

Communicative Behaviors

Sugar gliders have a complex system of chemical communication based on the scents produced by the frontal, sternal, and paracloacal glands of males, and by the pouch and paracloacal glands of females (Figure 7-38). Each group has its own unique smell that identifies it to other individuals,

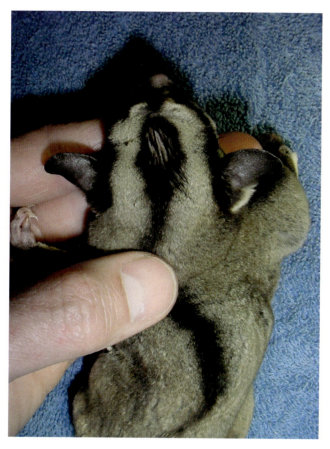

Figure 7-38
Male sugar gliders use the sternal scent gland, the frontal gland, and urine to mark their territory and other members of their group. The frontal gland is shown here. (Courtesy Dan Johnson.)

and is passively spread around the group's territory. The dominant male actively marks other members of the group with his scent. Gliders will also urine-mark their territory.

Sugar gliders are very vocal. Their repertoire includes a variety of yapping, buzzing, droning, hissing, and screaming sounds. Gliders may quietly chatter for attention, and they have an alarm call similar to the yapping of a small dog. The high-pitched cry of anger made when they are startled is known as "crabbing." When frightened, sugar gliders may also express their paracloacal glands, producing a white oily secretion with an odor resembling spoiled fruit.

Social and Antisocial Behaviors

Because of their highly social nature, captive sugar gliders should be kept in groups of two or more. They have been known to become clinically depressed when housed alone.[37] However, even in large captive enclosures, fighting between females and between males and abuse of mates and young are common. They are most active in the evenings and early mornings, and should get most of their social interaction during this period. Activity is usually highest shortly after the lights are turned out, and a light-dark cycle of 12 and 12 hours, or slightly shorter nights, has been suggested.[31]

Singly housed sugar gliders that are stressed by boredom, small cage size, and lack of a hiding space can develop aberrant behavior problems including eating and drinking excessively, pacing, screaming, and chewing on bars.[45] Solitary gliders require socialization periods of at least 2 hours a day.[51] Placing the glider cage in a high-traffic area such as the family room will provide additional human contact. Handling should be done at night when they are most active, as they tend to be irritable when awakened during the day.[51]

Sugar gliders bond readily with their owners, who frequently carry their pets around in fleece "glider-pouches," or close to the body, under clothing (see Locomotor Behaviors and Activities). Captive-bred joeys that are adopted at 7 to 12 weeks "out-of-pouch" (OOP) are the easiest to socialize. Baby gliders have no fear of humans and like to be held. They can be handled as soon as their eyes open (7 to 10 days OOP) to socialize them, and the parents do not seem to mind.

Sugar gliders are generally territorial and are aggressive toward new arrivals. Males establish territories and require adequate space between nest boxes to prevent fighting. New introductions should be made during the day when gliders are less active. Most established gliders will complain when a new member is introduced. If the enclosure is not of adequate size, fighting may be severe. Observe for signs of aggression, and if the new glider is rejected, it should be set up in a cage adjacent to the established group.

Nightly exchange of nest boxes between the cages will allow the scent of the established gliders and the new one to intermix. After several days the new glider should be able to be successfully introduced. Recently weaned sugar gliders may try to cling to the backs of older individuals in the group, and these adults may respond aggressively. Therefore, weanlings should be at least $^3/_4$ of their adult weight before they are introduced to a cage containing adults.

Research has indicated that dominant male sugar gliders are larger, faster, and more active and scent-mark more than socially subordinate males. They also have been found to have higher plasma testosterone and lower cortisol concentrations. When transferred into a foreign stable colony, dominant behavior decreases and a concomitant decrease in concentration of plasma testosterone and increase in cortisol levels is noted for at least the first 3 weeks of observation.[48]

Socialized sugar gliders are usually friendly and curious; they will readily jump from their owners and investigate strangers. However, sugar gliders that have been disturbed in the nest box or carry pouch will generally make a huge fuss and try to resist examination (but usually only bite as a last resort). Care should be taken not to injure a glider, while at the same time taking care not to be bitten.

Reproductive Behaviors

Male Reproductive Behaviors

Sugar gliders breed readily in captivity and are able to reproduce throughout the year. In the wild, males are polygynous, whereby one or two dominant, older males are usually responsible for most of the territorial maintenance and fathering of the young.[51] Co-dominant males are generally siblings or a father-son pair. Dominant males perform paternal care such as babysitting, huddling, and grooming the young while the female is out of the nest. However, in captive populations only one adult male is usually reproductively active.[31]

Sugar glider males reach sexual maturity at 12 to 14 months of age. The scent gland becomes increasingly developed with age. Three levels of glandular activity have been described.[31]

- Little or no activity, when no obvious scent gland production can be seen
- Medium level of activity, in which mildly waxy glandular products can be seen, with hair loss starting over the gland
- High level of glandular activity, in which total hair loss over the gland is visible and staining of the fur around the gland is obvious

Males have a prominent midabdominal scrotal sac that may increase in size during the breeding season. The distal extent of the penis is bifid. Manipulation and cleaning of the genitalia are normal behaviors, but excessive grooming and self-trauma may be signs of disease or a response to pain (see Grooming Behaviors).

Female Reproductive Behaviors and Neonatal Behaviors

The natural breeding season for wild sugar gliders in Australia is June to November.[51] Females are polyestrous, cycling every 29 days. A female produces a litter of one or two joeys and may produce a second litter during the breeding season if the first is lost; however, in tropical habitats and in captivity there seems to be no definite breeding season. Up to four litters per year are possible in captivity, but this intensive breeding can lead to numerous medical problems and is not recommended. In the wild, hierarchies develop among females in a nesting group. Subordinate females are harassed by the dominant one and often lose their young within the first few weeks after birth.[28]

Females reach sexual maturity at 8 to 12 months of age. The females of this species do not have a postpartum estrus or embryonic diapause, as other marsupials exhibit.[31] Longevity may be 12 to 14 years in captivity, and breeding for up to 10 years has been reported.

Mating usually occurs in the evening. Females exhibit readiness to breed by increasing their marking activity.[36] Gestation is 16 days, and the sugar glider joey weighs only 0.19 g (0.01 oz) and is 5 mm (0.2 in) long at birth. It crawls to the pouch (marsupium), where it stays attached to the nipple for 40 days. It first releases the nipple at 40 days but stays inside for 60 to 70 days, when it first emerges. From 70 days on, the joey leaves the pouch for longer periods of time. The eyes generally open at 75 to 80 days. Weaning occurs at 110 to 120 days of age, and joeys are independent by 17 weeks of age.

Prolapse of the pouch occasionally occurs as a result of overzealous pouch cleaning by the female. Differential diagnoses to consider include mastitis, bacterial infection, or yeast infection.

Eating Behaviors

Sugar gliders should be fed in the early evening when they are most active. Food and water should be placed high in the cage to promote their natural, arboreal feeding habits. This will limit the soiling of food dishes by urine and feces as well.

Sugar gliders are omnivorous and must consume a wide variety of food items in the wild in order to survive. Their natural diet consists of invertebrates, birds, eggs, small mammals, sap, nectar, and blossoms. Their incisors are specialized for gouging the bark of trees.[51] In captivity, food preferences can develop and lead to obesity and other nutritional problems.

A diet consisting of 50% protein (insects, egg with shell, pinkie mice, meat, high-quality cat food kibble, monkey chow) and 50% fructose and gum (nectar, maple syrup, honey, acacia gum, Arabica gum, lory diet, glider nectar) is recommended. In spite of published advice to the contrary, wild sugar gliders do not rely heavily on fruit, vegetables, nuts, grains, or seeds.[37] Pet gliders will readily accept these items to the exclusion of healthy foods; therefore these items should be provided only in limited quantities.

Sugar gliders are efficient hunters; therefore feeding live, gut-loaded insects and pinkie mice will add enrichment to their environment and provide variety in the diet. Gliders are dexterous, and they will manipulate food with their front feet. When sugar gliders chew an insect, they are able to gather the chitinous "pulp" into a pellet and spit this out rather than swallow it.

Elimination Behaviors

Sugar gliders urinate and defecate indiscriminately and cannot be litter trained. Gliders usually urinate while clinging to the side of the cage or running along branches. Fecal pellets normally resemble mouse droppings and quickly desiccate and fall to the cage bottom. Urine will build up as a whitish deposit on cage wire and will necessitate regular cleaning. Males have a bifid penis and urinate from the proximal portion of the penis rather than the forked tip[51] (see Medical Implications of Abnormal Behaviors).

Sugar gliders are naturally very clean, and they do not soil their nesting box under normal circumstances. Therefore, a soiled nest box may indicate medical or behavioral problems. Gliders frequently eliminate when they are frightened or handled during examination. Elimination is normally a passive process; therefore straining, vocalization, or evidence of a hunched posture while urinating or defecating may indicate disease.

Thermoregulatory Behaviors

During periods of cold or food scarcity in the wild, sugar gliders conserve energy by entering torpor for periods of up to 16 hours per day.[17] Sugar gliders can tolerate environmental temperatures of 18.3° to 32.2° C (65° to 90° F); however, the ideal range is 24° to 27° C (75° to 80° F). Gliders normally huddle together in the nest to conserve energy, so singly housed gliders are more susceptible to hypothermia than pairs or groups. Sugar gliders that are too cold will become torpid and difficult to rouse. Supplemental heat might be necessary in cool areas. Do not place gliders in drafty areas, in direct sunlight, or in areas where temperatures fluctuate widely.

Locomotor Behaviors and Activities

Sugar gliders are nocturnal and sleep in a nesting box or pouch during the day. They are most active in the early evening and throughout the night, so locomotor behaviors are best evaluated during that time. As gliders are arboreal, the nesting site should be placed high up in the cage, not on the cage bottom. They will jump from high places and glide to the owner's shoulder or to another perch.

While the gliding membrane of the sugar glider and flying squirrel are grossly similar in appearance, the sugar glider has substantial muscular control of its gliding membrane, which the flying squirrel lacks, and this may give sugar gliders some additional control over flight (Figure 7-39).[9] Sugar gliders have weakly prehensile tails that they can coil around items to carry them. The tail also acts as a rudder during flight. Limbs from nontoxic trees should be available for climbing.[36]

Sugar gliders feel safest when curled in carrying pouches, but placing them in tight-fitting clothes of the handler is not recommended because of the risk of injury.[51] Do not allow frayed fabric, string, rope, or towels to be placed in the cage, as gliders occasionally get tangled in these. Strangulation and constricting injury of limbs commonly occur (Figure 7-40). Sugar gliders can easily drown in toilets and tubs if they are allowed to roam freely.

Grooming Behaviors

Sugar gliders are fastidious groomers. Under normal conditions gliders keep themselves very clean and have almost no odor. Most of the odor associated with sugar gliders is from the urine in and around the cage. Sugar gliders may exhibit excessive grooming as a result of unsanitary conditions, ectoparasites, or skin infection and secondary to stress (see Medical Implications of Abnormal Behaviors) (Figure 7-41). Avoid pine

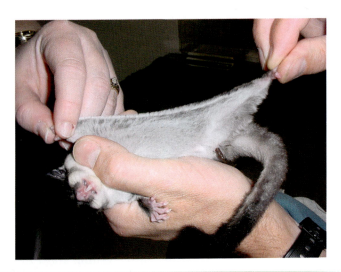

Figure 7-39
Sugar gliders possess a gliding membrane (patagium) that extends from the forefoot to the ankle. (Courtesy Dan Johnson.)

Miscellaneous Small Mammal Behavior 335

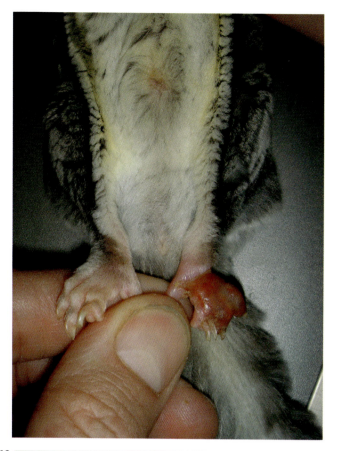

Figure 7-40
Tattered or frayed fabric can entangle extremities and cause strangulation. In severe cases amputation may be necessary. (Courtesy Dan Johnson.)

and cedar shavings, as these may be irritating. The cage, nest box, and bedding should be kept very clean in order to avoid fur pulling and self-mutilation. Bathing of sugar gliders is not generally recommended.

Medical Implications of Abnormal Behaviors

Sugar gliders can be difficult to examine, as they tend to cling to their pouches and "crab" while trying to get away. I frequently use a towel to assist in glider capture, and the examination can be accomplished in part with the glider in the towel, where it feels more secure. A cursory examination may be all that is possible while the sugar glider is awake, accom-

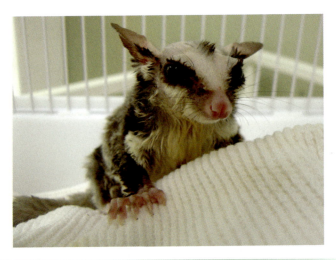

Figure 7-41
Alopecia, fur-pulling, and excessive grooming may occur as a result of stress. This female glider was presented for treatment of alopecia of the head and dorsal neck. The fur returned once the animal was placed in an appropriate environment. (Courtesy Dan Johnson.)

plished by exposing various parts of the sugar glider's body while the glider is held in a hand towel or by holding the glider gently around the neck.[41,45] Gliders produce a loud noise of protest that is between a scream and a chatter when restrained (see Communicative Behaviors). Although owners may be accustomed to short bursts of this vocalization at home, they may become alarmed when their pet loudly protests as it is being restrained.

The most accurate assessment of behavior will be possible in late afternoon or early evening. By keeping the examination room dimly lit (e.g., use the light from an x-ray view box), the practitioner may also be able to more accurately assess behavior. For a thorough physical examination, anesthesia may be necessary,[45] preferably using isoflurane (IsoFlo, Abbott Laboratories, North Chicago, IL) or sevoflurane (SevoFlo, Abbott Laboratories, North Chicago, IL).

A sick glider may sit apathetically in the corner of its cage and exhibit a reluctance to move. If severely ill or chilled, gliders may exhibit torporous behavior. Affected sugar gliders may appear to be in shock or moribund. If these patients are given aggressive supportive care (e.g., supplemental heat, fluid therapy, and nutritional support) they often dramatically improve. Therefore, sugar gliders that appear hypothermic and moribund should not be assumed to have a grave prognosis. Intensive care should be provided for 24 to 48 hours before the prognosis is determined.

Gliders can manifest stress in numerous ways including self-mutilation of the tail, limbs, or genitalia, aggressive behaviors, eating disorders (coprophagy, hyperphagia, polydipsia), cannibalism of young, fur pulling or alopecia, and stereotypic behavior or pacing (Figure 7-42). Such disorders may be associated with stressors such as isolation, overcrowding, unnatural social structure, sexual frustration, unsanitary conditions, or a perceived threat. Sugar glider males that are switched from one group in which they are dominant to another in which they are subordinate show a dramatic decrease in plasma testosterone and an increase in plasma cortisol.[48] Sugar gliders have been studied as a model for clinical depression in humans.[42]

Mature males that mutilate the penis or scrotum may require castration and scrotal ablation. If the forked distal aspect of the penis is severely damaged, it may be surgically removed, as well. The bifid portion of the penis lies distal to the urethral opening; therefore if it is damaged or surgically removed urethral stricture is unlikely to occur. Hypocalcemia has also been implicated in cases of penile prolapse.

Treatment and prevention of stress-related behavioral problems involve avoidance of causative factors. Keep cats, dogs, and pet birds out of the immediate cage vicinity. Provide proper nutrition and good hygiene, normal social grouping, adequate cage space, and appropriate nesting areas and cage accessories. Anecdotal success with antidepressants has been reported.

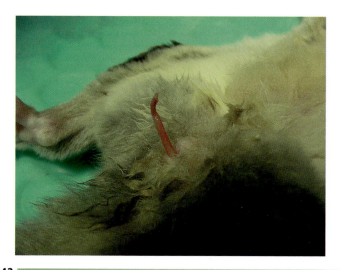

Figure 7-42
This male sugar glider mutilated his penis (note the bifurcated tip is abnormal). Self-mutilation in sugar gliders may be the result of stress, pain, or sexual frustration. (Courtesy Dan Johnson.)

A self-mutilation syndrome has been described that was associated with aberrant migration of a duodenal nematode.[40] CNS signs may result. Therefore, a fecal examination for parasites and anthelmintic therapy should be considered in cases of self-mutilation. Self-mutilation can also be seen in solitary gliders[37] as well as postsurgically, another reason why analgesia before and after surgery is an absolute necessity (see Behaviors Associated with Pain).

Weakness, tremors, and seizures can result from hypocalcemia resulting from improper diet, lactation, and excessive breeding. Hind limb paresis syndrome can cause a reluctance to move (Figure 7-43). Additional calcium should be provided during breeding and lactation. Gliders suffering from parasites, constipation, megacolon, prolapse, or urolithiasis may vocalize or strain while eliminating and may exhibit irritability or anorexia. Stressed or sick gliders should be provided supplemental heat that is carefully regulated to 26° to 29° C (80° to 85° F).

Behaviors Associated with Pain

Sugar gliders that are in pain may be withdrawn and reluctant to move. When forced to move, they frequently become more aggressive than usual and make loud "crabbing" vocalizations. Trauma such as cuts, punctures, and fractures are common. Falling may occur because of generalized weakness (e.g., from hypocalcemia or hind limb paresis syndrome), so a medical workup may be indicated in cases of trauma. Injuries and trauma are diagnosed and treated as for other small mammals.

Recovery from gas anesthesia in sugar gliders is usually rapid and violent. Gliders often immediately begin to vocalize and chew at skin

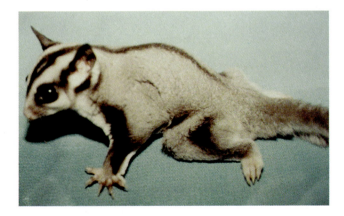

Figure 7-43
Hind limb weakness and reluctance to move ("hind limb paresis syndrome") may be the result of nutritional spinal osteodystrophy. (Courtesy Dan Johnson.)

incisions. Skin closure after surgery is best accomplished by placing subcutaneous sutures and using tissue adhesive (e.g., cyanoacrylate). It is imperative to provide preoperative, perioperative, and postoperative analgesics using multimodal therapy with a combination of analgesics; to monitor the patient carefully postoperatively; and to watch for self-trauma.

Behavioral Enrichment

Gliders will readily entertain themselves with bird toys such as swings, perches, ladders, and bells. They should be provided with nontoxic tree branches. They will chew on bone if it is provided, and they will climb in and out of pieces of pipe and other play items. Gliders will run on an exercise wheel, but this should be a solid-constructed wheel (without rungs) in order to prevent injuries.[51] They will also play and run in clear exercise balls; however, these should not be used where falls could occur. The provision of multiple opportunities for exercise is critical to preventing obesity and stereotypic behaviors in captive gliders. Nest boxes should be provided and cleaned at least once per week.[51]

How Behavior Relates to Captivity

- Sugar gliders are relatively difficult to keep and feed properly.
- Most problems are diet and husbandry related.
- Gliders are highly social animals that are best kept in pairs or groups of three or more; however, fighting between cage mates is common.
- Solitary gliders require a lot of attention and will bond readily with their owners.
- Gliders are susceptible to many household dangers: drowning (in toilets and tubs), burns (landing on light bulbs and other hot surfaces), electrocution (chewing on electric cords), toxic plants, other household chemicals and toxins, being stepped or sat on, and being shut in a window, door, or recliner chair.
- Because of the sugar glider's prominent eyes, corneal trauma can easily occur.
- Constricting injuries from frayed fabric are common; remove tattered or stringy fabric from the glider cage.
- Gliders should not be housed near birds or rodents due to the predator-prey situation, which can cause stress, injury, or death.
- Place food bowls and water or nectar sippers high in the cage, not on the cage floor.
- Feed sugar gliders in the evening.
- Sugar gliders that are cold will become torpid and difficult to rouse. Most collections will need some form of supplemental heat (e.g., infrared heat lamp, ceramic heat emitter) in order to prevent cold stress.

Client Education Handout: Sugar Glider *(Petaurus breviceps)*

Biologic Facts
- Arboreal, nocturnal marsupial from Australia and New Guinea
- Scent-marking allows recognition by group members
- Can glide up to 70 feet (21 m) using a thin membrane that stretches from wrists to ankles
- Adults weigh 80 to 160 g (4 to 6 oz) and are usually 30.5 cm (12 in) long
- Life span: up to 12 to 14 years in captivity
- Sexual maturity occurs at approximately 12 months for males, 8 to 12 months for females; can breed all year
- Exportation of sugar gliders has been banned in Australia since 1959

Diet
- Sugar gliders are highly insectivorous.
- Avoid preservatives, pesticides, and excessive fats.
- Diet should consist of 50% protein (insects, egg with shell, pinkie mice, meat, high-quality cat food kibble, monkey chow).
- Diet should also consist of 50% fructose and gum (nectar, maple syrup, honey, acacia gum, Arabica gum, lory diet, glider nectar).
- Leadbeater's mix provides a suitable mixture of the above and can be fed to gliders as a staple diet.
- Vegetables, fruits, seeds, and nuts should be limited.
- Food supplements—Repcal, Herptivite, Glideraide—and especially calcium may be needed for breeding females.

Housing
- Sugar gliders need as large an enclosure as possible to allow space to climb, run, jump, and glide. A large, tall, aviary-type wire cage is best. It is difficult if not impossible to provide a cage large enough for normal activity in captivity.
- Wire cages are best with the wire spacing no greater than 15 mm (1/2 in) for babies to 19 mm (3/4 in) for adults.
- Avoid putting the cage near a window or bright light; sunlight can seriously damage a glider's eyesight.
- Nest boxes should be provided and placed near the top of the enclosure (some people use pouches). Corn cob, recycled paper, and aspen bedding are suitable cage litter.
- Avoid pine and cedar litters, as they may cause problems.
- The environment should be draft free. Ideal temperatures range from 75° to 80° F (23° to 26° C). Supplemental heat might be necessary.
- The cage, nest box, and bedding should be kept *very clean* to avoid excessive grooming, fur-pulling, and self-mutilation.

Behaviors
- Sugar gliders are *highly social animals* and are best kept in pairs or groups of three or more.
- Solitary gliders require *a lot of attention* and will bond readily with their owners.
- Captive-bred joeys are the easiest to be socialized; it is best to adopt when they are 7 to 12 weeks out of the pouch.
- They are nocturnal and most active in the evenings and early mornings.
- They make loud screeching and "crabbing" noises when frightened or excited.
- They may "bark" or quietly "chatter" for attention.

Common Problems Requiring Veterinary Attention
- Malnutrition and its consequences: rear-limb paralysis, rickets, blindness, cataracts
- Pneumonia, coughing, sneezing, discharge from the eyes or nose
- Diarrhea, little or no stool production, decreased or no appetite
- Stress-related diseases including self-mutilation, cannibalism of young, eating disorders
- Hair loss
- Neutering of males will prevent reproduction and is less invasive than spaying of females

Preventive Care
- Twice yearly physical examinations*
- An examination should be performed by a veterinarian knowledgeable in small mammal exotics within 1 week of acquisition
- Annual examination of the stool
- Review of diet and husbandry
- Nails—may need periodic trimming
- Blood work (complete blood count, chemistry) and radiographs as recommended by veterinarian
- No vaccines currently required, although tetanus toxoid may be considered

*Locate a veterinarian who obtains continuing education about exotic pets and who has experience with sugar gliders.

References

1. Alderton D: *Foxes, wolves and wild dogs of the world,* New York, 1999, Sterling. 1999.
2. Bedford JM, Mock OB, Nagdas SK, Winfrey VP, Olson GE: Reproductive characteristics of the African pygmy hedgehog, Atelerix albiventris, *J Reprod Fertil* 120:143-150, 2000.
3. Bekoff M: Social behavior and ecology of the African Canidae: a review. In Fox MW, editor: *The wild canids,* Malabar, Fla., 1983, Krieger.
4. Bennett RA: Husbandry and medicine of prairie dogs. Proceedings of the Association of Avian Veterinarians Exotic Small Mammal Medicine and Management Program, Portland, Ore., August, 2000.
5. Bertschinger HJ, Asa CS, Calle PP, et al: Control of reproduction and sex related behaviour in exotic wild carnivores with the GnRH analogue deslorelin: preliminary observations, *J Reprod Fertil* 57(suppl):275-283, 2001.
6. Brodie ED Jr: Hedgehogs use toad venom in their own defense, *Nature* 68:627, 1977.
7. Catania KC, Collins CE, Kaas JH: Organization of sensory cortex in the East African Hedgehog *(Atelerix albiventris), J Comp Neurol* 421(2):256-274, 2000.
8. Donnelly TM: Disease problems of chinchillas. In Quesenberry KE, Carpenter JW, editors: *Ferrets, rabbits, and rodents: clinical medicine and surgery,* ed 2, St. Louis, 2003, Saunders.
9. Endo H, Yokokawa K, Kurohmaru M, et al: Functional anatomy of gliding membrane muscles in the sugar glider *(Petaurus breviceps), Ann Anat* 180(1):93-96, 1998.
10. Fadem BH: Evidence for the activation of female reproduction by males in a marsupial, the gray short-tailed opossum *(Monodelphis domestica), Biol Reprod* 33(1):112-116, 1985.
11. Fadem BH, Dziadosz DR, Jackson LM, Harder JD: Partner preference of intact and ovariectomized female gray short-tailed opossums *(Monodelphis domestica), Horm Behav* 38(3):187-192, 2000.
12. Fadem BH, Erianne DC: Male gray short-tailed opossums *(Monodelphis domestica)* receive penile intromissions when treated with estrogen and progesterone in adulthood, *Horm Behav* 31(3):289-295, 1997.
13. Fadem BH, Erianne GS, Karen LM: The hormonal control of scent marking and precopulatory behavior in male gray short-tailed opossums *(Monodelphis domestica), Horm Behav* 23(3):381-392, 1989.
14. Fadem BH, Kraus DB, Sheffet RH: Nest-building in gray short-tailed opossums: temperature effects and sex differences, *Physiol Behav* 36(4):667-670, 1986.
15. Fadem BH, Taylor-Ali L, Erianne DC: The hormonal induction of mating behavior in female gray short-tailed opossums *(Monodelphis domestica), Horm Behav* 30(1):44-49, 1996.
16. Flannery T: *Mammals of New Guinea,* New York, 1995, Cornell University Press.
17. Flemming MR: Thermoregulation and torpor in the sugar glider, *Petaurus breviceps, Aust J Zool* 28:521, 1980.
18. Frost SB, Masterton RB: Hearing in primitive mammals: *Monodelphis domestica* and *Marmosa elegans, Hear Res* 76(1-2):67-72, 1994.
19. Graffam WS, Fitzpatrick MP, Dierenfield ES: Fiber digestion in the African white-bellied hedgehog *(Atelerix albiventris):* a preliminary evaluation, Bronx, NY, 1999, Nutrition Department, Wildlife Conservation Society.

20. Hall L: *Fennec fox: a guide to care and breeding,* Camarillo, CA, 1997, Lynn Hall.
21. Harder JD, Jackson LM: Male pheromone stimulates ovarian follicular development and body growth in juvenile female opossums *(Monodelphis domestica), Reprod Biol Endocrinol* 1(1):21, 2003.
22. Heffner RS, Heffner HE: Behavioral hearing range of the chinchilla, *Hear Res* 52(1):13-16, 1991.
23. Hillyer EV, Quesenberry KE, Donnelly TM: Biology, husbandry and clinical techniques. In Hillyer EV, Quesenberry KE, editors: *Ferrets, rabbits, and rodents: clinical medicine and surgery,* Philadelphia, 1997, Saunders.
24. Hoefer HL, Crossley DA: Chinchillas. In Merideth A, Redrobe S (editors): *BSAVA Manual of Exotic Pets,* ed 4, Gloucester, 2002, British Small Animal Veterinary Association.
25. Hoogland JL: Why do Gunnison's prairie dogs give anti-predator calls? *Anim Behav* 51:871-880, 1996.
26. Hoogland JL: Why do female Gunnison's prairie dogs copulate with more than one male? *Anim Behav* 55:351-359, 1998.
27. Hutchins M, editor: *Grzimek's animal life encyclopedia,* vol 13, Mammals II, ed 2, Farmington Hills, MI, 2002, Gale Group.
28. Hutchins M, editor: *Grzimek's animal life encyclopedia,* vol 16, Mammals V, ed 2, Farmington Hills, MI, 2004 gale Group.
29. Ivey E, Carpenter JW: African hedgehogs. In Quesenberry KE, Carpenter JW, editors: *Ferrets, rabbits, and rodents: clinical medicine and surgery,* ed 2, St. Louis, 2003, Saunders.
30. Jackson SM: Population dynamics and life history of the mahogany glider, *Petaurus gracilis,* and the sugar glider, *Petaurus breviceps,* in north Queensland, *Wildl Res* 27(1):21-37, 2000.
31. Jackson SM: *Australian mammals: biology and captive management,* Collingwood, Victoria, Australia, 2003, CSIRO.
32. Johnson D: Introduction to fennec foxes, *Exotic DVM Magazine* 5(4):42, 2003.
33. Johnson SD: Orchiectomy of the mature sugar glider *(Petaurus breviceps), Exotic Pet Practice,* 2:71, 1997.
34. Johnson-Delaney CA: Hedgehogs. In *Exotic companion medicine handbook for veterinarians,* Lake Worth, Fla., 1998, Zoological Education Network.
35. Johnson-Delaney CA: Marsupials: short-tailed opossum *(Monodelphis domestica).* In *Exotic companion medicine handbook for veterinarians,* Lake Worth, FL, 1998, Zoological Education Network.
36. Johnson-Delaney CA: Marsupials: sugar gliders. In *Exotic companion medicine handbook for veterinarians,* Lake Worth, FL, 1998, Zoological Education Network.
37. Johnson-Delaney CA: Other small mammals. In Merideth A, Redrobe S: *BSAVA manual of exotic pets,* ed 4, Gloucester, 2002, British Small Animal Veterinary Association.
38. Johnson-Delaney CA: Special rodents: chinchillas. In *Exotic companion medicine handbook,* Lake Worth, FL, 1998, Zoological Education Network.
39. Johnson-Delaney CA: Special rodents: prairie dogs. In *Exotic companion medicine handbook,* Lake Worth, FL, 1996, Zoological Education Network.
40. Johnson-Delaney CA: The marsupial pet: sugar gliders, exotic possums, and wallabies. *Proceedings of the Association of Avian Veterinarians,* St. Paul, Minn., August, 1998.
41. Johnson-Delaney CA: Therapeutics of common exotic marsupials, *Vet Clin North Am Exot Anim Pract* 3(1):173-181, 2000.

42. Jones IH, Stoddart DM, Mallick J: Towards a sociobiological model of depression. A marsupial model *(Petaurus breviceps)*, *Br J Psychiatry* 166(4):475-479, 1995.
43. Larsen RS, Carpenter JW: Husbandry and medical management of African Hedgehogs, *Vet Med* 94:877-890, 1999.
44. Lightfoot TL: Clinical techniques of selected exotic species: chinchilla, prairie dog, hedgehog, and chelonians, *Semin Avian Exot Pet Med* 6(3):97-99, 1997.
45. Lightfoot TL: Clinical examination of chinchillas, hedgehogs, prairie dogs, and sugar gliders, *Vet Clin North Am Exot Anim Pract* 2(2):447-464, 1999.
46. Lightfoot TL: Therapeutics of African pygmy hedgehogs and prairie dogs. *Vet Clin North Am Exot Anim Pract* 3(1):155-172, 2000.
47. Macdonald D, editor: *The encyclopedia of animals,* Oxfordshire, 2001, Barnes and Noble Books/Andromeda Oxford.
48. Mallick J, Stoddart DM, Jones I, et al: Behavioral and endocrinological correlates of social status in the male sugar glider *(Petaurus breviceps,* Marsupialia: Petauridae), *Physiol Behav* 55(6):1131-1134, 1994.
49. Maloiy GMO, Kamau JMZ, Shkolnik A, et al: Thermoregulation and metabolism in a small desert carnivore: the fennec fox *(Fennecus zerda)* (Mammalia). *J Zool (Lond)* 198: 279-291, 1982.
50. Mammone K: Personal communication, March 15, 2005.
51. Ness R, Booth R: Sugar gliders. In Quesenberry K, Carpenter J, editors: *Ferrets, rabbits, and rodents: clinical medicine and surgery,* ed 2, St. Louis, 2004, Saunders.
52. Nowak RM, editor: Walker's mammals of the world, Vol I, ed 6, Baltimore, 1999, Johns Hopkins University Press.
53. Nowak RM, editor: Walker's mammals of the world, Vol II, ed 6, Baltimore, 1999, Johns Hopkins University Press.
54. Phalen DN, Antinoff N, Fricke ME: Obstructive respiratory disease in prairie dogs with odontomas, *Vet Clin North Am Exot Anim Pract* 3(2):513-517, 2000.
55. Poran N: Just playin' opossum: The South American short-tailed opossum *(Monodelphis domestica).* Naomie Poran, Ph.D., 1999.
56. Poran NS: Vomeronasal organ and its associated structures in the opossum *Monodelphis domestica, Microsc Res Tech,* 43(6):500-510, 1998.
57. Poran NS, Tripoli R, Halpern M: Nuzzling in the gray short-tailed opossum. II: Familiarity and individual recognition, *Physiol Behav* 53(5):969-973, 1993.
58. Quesenberry KE, Donnelly TM, Hillyer EV: Biology, husbandry, and clinical techniques of guinea pigs and chinchillas. In Quesenberry K, Carpenter J, editors: *Ferrets, rabbits, and rodents: clinical medicine and surgery,* ed 2, St. Louis, 2003, Saunders.
59. Sheldon JW: *Wild dogs: The natural history of the nondomestic Canidae,* New York, 1992, Academic Press.
60. Simone-Freilicher EA, Hoefer HL: Hedgehog care and husbandry, *Vet Clin North Am Exot Anim Pract* 7(2):257-267, 2004.
61. Smith WJ, Smith SL, Oppenheimer EC, et al: Vocalizations of the black-tailed prairie dog, *Cynomys ludovicianus, Anim Behav* 25(1):152-164, 1977.
62. Tisljar M, Janic D, Grabarevic Z, et al: Stress-induced Cushing's syndrome in fur-chewing chinchillas, *Acta Vet Hung* 50(2):133-142, 2002.
63. Vreinds MM, Heming-Vriends TM: *Hedgehogs: a complete owner's manual.* Happauge, NY, 2000, Barons Educational Series.
64. Wheler CL, Grahn BH, Pocknell AM: Unilateral proptosis and orbital cellulitis in eight African hedgehogs *(Atelerix albiventris), J Zoo Wildl Med* 32(2): 236-241, 2001.

65. Wesierska M, Walasek G, Kilijanek J, et al: Behavior of the gray short-tailed opossum *(Monodelphis domestica)* in the open field and in response to a new object, in comparison with the rat, *Behav Brain Res* 143(1):31-40, 2003.
66. Zuri I, Su W, Halpern M: Conspecific odor investigation by gray short-tailed opossums *(Monodelphis domestica)*, *Physiol Behav* 80(2-3):225-232, 2003.

Index

A

Abnormal behaviors, medical implications.
  See also under individual topics.
  of ferrets, 199-203, 201f
  of guinea pigs, 228-231, 228f, 230f,
  of psittacines, 74-88
  of rabbits, 34-38, 35f
  of reptiles, 151-155, 151f-152f
  of small mammals,
    chinchillas, 274-278, 275f-276f
    fennec foxes, 289
    hedgehogs, 301-302, 301f-302f
    prairie dogs, 312-317, 312f
    short-tailed opossums, 326
    sugar gliders, 335-338, 335f-338f
  of small rodents, 247f, 256-257
Abyssinian guinea pig behaviors. *See* Guinea pig behaviors.
Activities and locomotive behaviors, *See also under individual topics.*
  of ferrets, 172-173
  of guinea pigs, 213-216, 214f, 216f
  of rabbits, 24-29, 24f-25f, 26b-27b
  of reptiles, 139-141
  of small mammals
    chinchillas, 272
    fennec foxes, 287-288
    hedgehogs, 299
    prairie dogs, 310
    sugar gliders, 333-334, 334f
  of small rodents, 251-253, 253f
Acupuncture, psittacines, 88
Adrenal disease, ferrets, 200-202, 201f
African Grey behaviors, 94-95, 95f. *See also* Psittacine behaviors.
African pygmy hedgehog behaviors, 293-304. *See also* Hedgehog behaviors.
African spurred tortoise behaviors, 106-108, 121. *See also* Reptile behaviors.
Agapornis roseicollis behaviors, 55-56. *See also* Psittacine behaviors.
Aggressive behaviors. *See also* Antisocial *vs.* social behaviors.

Aggressive behaviors *(Continued)*
  of ferrets, 189-197
  of reptiles, 117-121, 114f, 118f
Agonistic behaviors, reptiles, 117-121, 114f, 118f
Aldabra tortoise behaviors, 122. *See also* Reptile behaviors.
Allergies, psittacines, 82
Alligator snapping turtle behaviors, 132-133. *See also* Reptile behaviors.
Alopecia, small rodents, 256, 257f
Amazona species behaviors, 51-102. *See also* Psittacine behaviors.
American guinea pig behaviors. *See* Guinea pig behaviors.
Amitriptyline (Elavil), 85
Anolis carolinensis behaviors, 103-104, 103-162, 111. *See also* Reptile behaviors.
Anorexia
  in psittacines, 71
  in rabbits, 35-36
Antisocial *vs.* social behaviors. *See also under individual topics.*
  of ferrets, 177-179
  of guinea pigs, 208-210, 209b
  of psittacines, 74-88
  of rabbits, 7-12, 8f-9f, 9, 10b-11b
  of reptiles, 108-112, 108b-111b, 109f
  of small mammals
    chinchillas, 265-267, 265f-266f
    fennec foxes, 283-285, 284f-285f
    hedgehogs, 295-296
    prairie dogs, 306-308, 307f-308f
    short-tailed opossums, 321-322, 322f
    sugar gliders, 330-331
  of small rodents, 243-246, 244f-245f
Ara species behaviors, 51-102. *See also* Psittacine behaviors.
Aspic viper behaviors, 138. *See also* Reptile behaviors.
Ateletix albiventris behaviors, 293-304. *See also* Hedgehog behaviors.

Page numbers followed by b indicate boxes; f, figures.

B

Ball python behaviors, 121, 135-136. *See also* Reptile behaviors.
Barking, ferrets, 171
Basilicus vittatus behaviors, 118. *See also* Reptile behaviors.
Bearded dragon behaviors, 103-162. *See also* Reptile behaviors.
Behavioral enrichment considerations
   for guinea pig behaviors, 226-227
   for prairie dogs, 317-318
   for rabbits, 31-34, 33f-34f
   for reptile behaviors, 148-151
   for sugar gliders, 339
Behaviors of exotic pets. *See also* under individual topics.
   ferret behaviors, 163-206
   guinea pig behaviors, 207-238
   psittacine behaviors, 51-102
   rabbit behaviors, 1-50
   reptile behaviors, 103-162
   small mammal behaviors, 263-344
   small rodent (mouse, rat, gerbil, and hamster) behaviors, 239-263
Birds (exotic) behaviors, 51-102. *See also* Psittacine behaviors.
Biting behaviors. *See* Antisocial *vs.* social behaviors.
Black-footed ferret behaviors, 165. *See also* Ferret behaviors.
Blindness, psittacines, 68-69, 69f
Blood spurting, reptiles, 121
Bonaire whiptail lizard behaviors, 127. *See also* Reptile behaviors.
Bonding processes, guinea pigs, 210-212, 211f
Bordetella bronchiseptica, 12
Box turtle behaviors, 129-130, 138-139. *See also* Reptile behaviors.
Broad-headed snake behaviors, 124. *See also* Reptile behaviors.
Budgerigar behaviors, 53-54. *See also* Psittacine behaviors.
Burmese python behaviors, 134. *See also* Reptile behaviors.
Burrowing behaviors, reptiles, 147

C

C position, rabbits, 38-40, 39f
Cacatua alba behaviors, 63-64. *See also* Psittacine behaviors.
Caique behaviors, 51-102. *See also* Psittacine behaviors.
Calyptorhynchus lathami behaviors, 63-64. *See also* Psittacine behaviors.
Cannibalism, small rodents, 243
Caparinia tripilis, 296
Captivity-related considerations
   of chinchillas, 278-279
   of fennec foxes, 289-291, 289f, 291f
   of hedgehogs, 303
   of prairie dogs, 318
   of psittacines, 57-62, 71-74
   of reptiles, 108b-111b
   of short-tailed opossums, 326
Categoric class formation, psittacines, 97
Cataracts, psittacines, 68-69, 69f
Catatus moluccensis behaviors, 79-80. *See also* Psittacine behaviors.
Caudal autotomy (tail shed), reptiles, 118-119
CAV-1 (canine adenovirus), 289
Cavia porcellus behaviors, 207-238. *See also* Guinea pig behaviors.
Chamaeleo [Furcifer] pardalis behaviors, 107. *See also* Reptile behaviors.
Chameleons, 103-162. *See also* Reptile behaviors.
Chelonian behaviors, 103-162. *See also* Reptile behaviors.
Chelydra serpentina behaviors, 105-108. *See also* Reptile behaviors.
Chinchilla behaviors. *See also* Small mammal behaviors.
   abnormal behaviors, medical implications of, 274-278, 275f-276f
   captivity-related considerations, 278-279
   client education for, 280b
   communicative behaviors, 265
   eating behaviors, 271
   elimination behaviors, 271-272
   euthanasia considerations and, 278
   grooming behaviors, 272-274, 273f-274f
   locomotor behaviors and activities, 272
   natural history and, 263
   pain-associated behaviors, 278
   reproductive behaviors
      female reproductive behaviors, 268-271, 269f-270f
      male reproductive behaviors, 267-271, 269f-270f
   sensory behaviors, 263-265, 264f

Chinchilla behaviors *(Continued)*
  social *vs.* antisocial behaviors, 265-267, 265f-266f
Chinese water dragon behaviors, 154-155. *See also* Reptile behaviors.
Chlamydosarus kingii behaviors, 113. *See also* Reptile behaviors.
Chortling, small rodents, 242
Chuckwalla behaviors, 118. *See also* Reptile behaviors.
Clemmys insculpta behaviors, 146. *See also* Reptile behaviors.
Client education
  for chinchilla behaviors, 280b
  for fennec fox behaviors, 292b
  for hedgehog behaviors, 304b
  for prairie dog behaviors, 319b
  for short-tailed opossum behaviors, 327b
  for sugar glider behaviors, 340f
Clomipramine (Clomicalm), 85, 88
Clucking, small rodents, 241
Cnemidophorus murinus behaviors, 127. *See also* Reptile behaviors.
Cockatiel and cockatoo behaviors, 51-102. *See also* Psittacine behaviors.
Coiling up, reptiles, 121
Coloration considerations, reptile behaviors and, 142-143, 143f
Communicative behaviors. *See also under individual topics.*
  of ferrets, 168-172, 168f-170f, 172f
  of guinea pigs, 213b
  of psittacines, 96-98
  of rabbits, 4-7, 5b-6b
  of reptiles, 141f
  of small mammals
    chinchillas, 265
    fennec foxes, 282-283, 283f
    hedgehogs, 295
    prairie dogs, 306
    short-tailed opossums, 320-321
    sugar gliders, 328-329, 329f
  of small rodents, 241-243
Conure behaviors. *See* Psittacine behaviors.
Corucia zebrata behaviors, 131. *See also* Reptile behaviors.
Croalus durissus behaviors, 134. *See also* Reptile behaviors.
Crocodilian behaviors, 103-162. *See also* Reptile behaviors.
Crypsis, reptiles, 117

Cuterebra organisms, 28
Cynomys ludovicianus behaviors, 305-319. *See also* Prairie dog behaviors.

D

Dacryocystitis, rabbits, 36
Deafness, rabbits, 4
Defensive behaviors. *See* Antisocial *vs.* social behaviors.
Depo-Lupron, 88, 116
Depo-Provera, 87, 116
DermCaps, 88
Desert lizard and tortoise behaviors, 144. *See also* Reptile behaviors.
Diazepam, 85
Diet- and nutrition-related behaviors. *See* Eating behaviors.
Diffenbachia seguine, 32
Domestication-related considerations,. *See also under individual topics.*
  of ferret behaviors, 163-166
  of guinea pig behaviors, 207-208, 208f
  of rabbits, 1-2
Dooking, ferrets, 171
Dusky Pionus parrots, 57-58. *See also* Psittacine behaviors.

E

Eastern hog-nosed snake behaviors, 119. *See also* Reptile behaviors.
Eating behaviors. *See also under individual topics.*
  of guinea pigs, 219-223, 220f-221f
  of rabbits, 17-20, 20f
  of reptiles, 132-138, 133f, 136f-137f
  of small mammals
    chinchillas, 271
    fennec foxes, 286-287
    hedgehogs, 298
    prairie dogs, 309, 309f, 311f
    short-tailed opossums, 324
    sugar gliders, 332-333
  of small rodents, 250-251
Eclectus behaviors, 82-83, 93-94. *See also* Psittacine behaviors.
Education, client. *See* Client education.
Egg yolk stroke, psittacines, 70
Egyptian hedgehog behaviors, 293-304. *See also* Hedgehog behaviors.
Elavil, 87
Elimination behaviors. *See also under individual topics.*

Elimination behaviors *(Continued)*
  of ferrets, 173-174, 175b
  of guinea pigs, 223-224
  of rabbits, 20-23, 22b, 23
  of reptiles, 138-139
  of small mammals
    chinchillas, 271-272
    fennec foxes, 287
    hedgehogs, 299
    prairie dogs, 310
    short-tailed opossums, 324-325
    sugar gliders, 333
  of small rodents, 251
Encephalitozoon cuniculi, 28
Endoparasites, psittacines, 81
English guinea pig behaviors. *See* Guinea pig behaviors.
Environmental enrichment considerations. *See also under individual topics.*
  for ferret behaviors, 188-189, 189f-190f, 191b
  for guinea pig behaviors, 226-227
  for psittacine behaviors, 58-61, 59f, 61f
  for rabbit behaviors, 31-34, 33f-34f
  for reptile behaviors, 148-151
  for small mammal behaviors
    prairie dogs, 317-318
    sugar gliders, 339
Epilepsy, small rodents, 256
Erinaceus europaeus behaviors, 293-304. *See also* Hedgehog behaviors.
Essential fatty acids, psittacines, 88
Estivation, reptiles, 146-147
Ethograms, 51-52
European hedgehog behaviors, 293-304. *See also* Hedgehog behaviors.
European polecat behaviors, 163-206. *See also* Ferret behaviors.
European rabbit behaviors, 1-50. *See also* Rabbit behaviors.
Euthanasia-related considerations. *See also under individual topics.*
  for chinchillas, 278
  for guinea pigs, 236
  for rabbits, 42-44
  for reptiles, 155-156
Exotic pet behaviors. *See also under individual topics.*
  ferret behaviors, 163-206
  guinea pig behaviors, 207-238
  psittacine behaviors, 51-102

Exotic pet behaviors *(Continued)*
  rabbit behaviors, 1-50
  reptile behaviors, 103-162
  small mammal behaviors, 263-344
  small rodent (mouse, rat, gerbil, and hamster) behaviors, 239-263
Exploratory behaviors, ferrets, 182-183

F

Feeding behaviors. *See also under individual topics.*
  of ferrets, 180-191
Female reproductive behaviors. *See also under individual topics.*
  of ferrets, 176-177
  of guinea pigs, 225-226
  of rabbits, 13-15, 16f
  of reptiles, 130-131
  of small mammals
    chinchillas, 268-271, 269f-270f
    fennec foxes, 285-286
    hedgehogs, 296-298, 297f-298f
    prairie dogs, 308-309
    short-tailed opossums, 323-324
  of small rodents, 246-249
Fennec fox behaviors. *See also* Small mammal behaviors.
  abnormal behaviors, medical implications of, 289
  captivity-associated behaviors, 289-291, 290f, 291f
  CAV-1 (canine adenovirus), 289
  client education for, 292b
  communicative behaviors, 282-283, 283f
  eating behaviors, 286-287
  elimination behaviors, 287
  female reproductive behaviors, 286
  grooming behaviors, 288
  locomotor behaviors and activities, 287-288
  Mazuri Exotic Canine Diet for, 287
  natural history and, 281
  pain-associated behaviors, 289
  reproductive behaviors
    female reproductive behaviors, 285-286
    male reproductive behaviors, 286
  sensory behaviors, 281-282, 282f
  social *vs.* antisocial behaviors, 283-285, 284f-285f
Fennecus zerda behaviors. *See* Fennec fox behaviors.

Ferret behaviors
  abnormal behaviors, medical implications of
    adrenal disease, 200-202, 201f
    descriptions of, 199-200
    insulinoma, 202-203
  aggressive behaviors
    biting behaviors and, 193-197, 194b-196b
    causes of, 195b
    fear-related aggression, 195b
    maternal aggression, 195b
    medical condition-related aggression, 195b
    nonspecific aggression, 189-193
    play aggression, 195b
    predatory aggression, 195b
    prevention and management of, 196b
    questionnaire for, 194b
    redirected aggression, 195b
    sexual aggression, 195b
  communicative behaviors
    barking, 171
    body language and visual displays, 171-172, 172f
    dooking, 171
    hissing, 171
    olfactory communications, 168-170, 168f-169f
    screaming, 171
    vocalizations, 170-171
  domestication considerations and, 163-166
  elimination behaviors
    descriptions of, 173-174
    litter box training, 175b
  environmental enrichment considerations and
    descriptions of, 188-189, 191b
    suggestions for, 191b
  exploratory behaviors, 182-183
  feeding behaviors, 180-191
  grooming behaviors, 179-180, 180f
  locomotive behaviors and activities, 172-173
  natural history and
    descriptions of, 163-166
    introgression and, 165
  pain-associated behaviors, 203
  play behaviors, 184-188, 184f-187f
  prey-catching behaviors, 181-182

Ferret behaviors *(Continued)*
  reproductive behaviors
    descriptions of, 174-175
    female reproductive behaviors, 176-177
    male reproductive behaviors, 175-176
  sensory behaviors
    hearing, 166-167, 167f
    olfactory behaviors, 167-168
    vision, 166
  sleep behaviors, 197-199, 198f
  social *vs.* antisocial behaviors, 177-179
Filoerections, psittacines, 54
Florida box turtle behaviors, 138-139. *See also* Reptile behaviors.
Fluoxetine (Prozac), 85
Folliculitis, psittacine behaviors, 82
Food-related behaviors. *See* Eating behaviors.
Fox (fennec) behaviors, 281-292. *See also* Fennec fox behaviors.
Frill-necked lizard behaviors, 113. *See also* Reptile behaviors.
Fundamental topics. *See* Overviews and summaries.

G

Gallotia caesaris behaviors, 127. *See also* Reptile behaviors.
Garter snake behaviors, 106-108, 123-124. *See also* Reptile behaviors.
Gastrointestinal stasis, rabbits, 36
Gecko behaviors, 103-162. *See also* Reptile behaviors.
Geochelone denticulata and *geochelone carbonaria* behaviors, 134-135. *See also* Reptile behaviors.
Geochelone species behaviors, 103-108, 122. *See also* Reptile behaviors.
Gerbil behaviors. *See also* Small rodent (mouse, rat, gerbil, and hamster) behaviors.
  abnormal behaviors, medical implications of, 247f, 256-257
  communicative behaviors, 241-243
  eating behaviors, 250-251
  elimination behaviors, 251
  grooming behaviors, 253-255, 254f-
  locomotor behaviors and activities, 251-253, 253f
  natural history and, 239-240

350 Index

Gerbil behaviors *(Continued)*
  pain-associated behaviors, 258-260, 259f-260f
  reproductive behaviors, 246-249, 252f
  sensory behaviors, 240-241, 241f-242f
  social *vs.* antisocial behaviors, 243-246, 244f-245f
  temperature sensitivity and, 256
GnRH agonists, 88
Gold macaw behaviors, 93. *See also* Psittacine behaviors.
Grass snake behaviors, 119, 120. *See also* Reptile behaviors.
Great ape similarities, psittacines, 96-97
Green anole lizard behaviors, 103-104, 111. *See also* Reptile behaviors.
Green iguana behaviors, 103-162. *See also* Reptile behaviors.
Gritching, small rodents, 242
Grooming behaviors. *See also* under individual topics.
  of ferrets, 179-180, 180f
  of guinea pigs, 216-219, 217f-219f
  of rabbits, 29-31, 29f
  of reptiles, 141-142
  of small mammals
    chinchillas, 272-274, 273f-274f
    fennec foxes, 288
    hedgehogs, 300-301, 300f
    prairie dogs, 310-312
    sugar gliders, 333-334, 336f
  of small rodents, 253-255, 254f-255f
Guinea pig behaviors, 207-238
  abnormal behaviors, medical implications of, 228-231, 229b
  behavioral enrichment considerations and, 226-227
  ls and, 207-208, 208f
  ication-related considerations and, 08, 208f
  iors, 219-223, 220f-221f
  haviors, 223-224
  d considerations and,
  16-219, 217f-219f
  siderations and
  ctivities,
  8, 208f
  7f

Guinea pig behaviors *(Continued)*
  pain-associated behaviors 235f
    clinical signs of, 234b
    descriptions of, 234-235, 235f
  reproductive behaviors
    female reproductive behaviors and parental care, 225-226
    male reproductive behaviors, 224
  sensory behaviors, 212-213
    auditory behaviors, 213
    visual behaviors, 212
    vocalization behaviors, 212-213, 213b
  social *vs.* antisocial behaviors, 208-210, 209b
    descriptions of, 208-210
    taming and bonding processes and, 210-212, 211f
Gustation, reptiles, 127

H

Hairless guinea pigs, 207, 208f. *See also* Guinea pig behaviors.
Haloperidol (Haldol), 85
Hamster behaviors. *See also* Small rodent (mouse, rat, gerbil, and hamster) behaviors.
  abnormal behaviors, medical implications of, 247f, 256-257
  communicative behaviors, 241-243
  eating behaviors, 250-251
  elimination behaviors, 251
  grooming behaviors, 253-255, 254f-255f
  locomotor behaviors and activities, 251-253, 253f
  natural history and, 239-240
  pain-associated behaviors, 258-260, 259f-260f
  reproductive behaviors, 246-249, 252f
  sensory behaviors, 240-241, 241f-242f
  social *vs.* antisocial behaviors, 243-246, 244f-245f
  temperature sensitivity and, 256
Hand-raised psittacine behaviors, 51-102. *See also* Psittacine behaviors.
Hatchling and juvenile behaviors, reptiles, 131-132
Hearing. *See* Sensory behaviors.
Heavy metal toxicity, psittacines, 69-70
Hedgehog behaviors. *See also* Small mammal behaviors.
  abnormal behaviors, medical implications of, 301-302, 301f-302f

Hedgehog behaviors *(Continued)*
  captivity-associated behaviors and considerations, 303
  client education for, 304b
  communicative behaviors, 295
  eating behaviors, 298
  elimination behaviors, 299
  grooming behaviors, 300-301, 300f
  locomotor behaviors and activities, 299
  natural history and, 293-294
  pain-associated behaviors, 302
  reproductive behaviors
    female reproductive behaviors, 296-298, 297f-298f
    male reproductive behaviors, 296
  sensory behaviors, 294-295
  social vs. antisocial behaviors, 295-296
Height dominance, psittacines, 75-76
Hemiechinus auritus behaviors, 293-304. *See also* Hedgehog behaviors.
Hepatic encephalopathy, psittacines, 69
Heterodon platirhinos behaviors, 119. *See also* Reptile behaviors.
Hibernation, reptiles, 146-147, 147b
Hissing, ferrets, 171
History, natural. *See* Natural history.
Hog-nosed snake behaviors, 119. *See also* Reptile behaviors.
Hoplocephalus bungaroides behaviors, 124. *See also* Reptile behaviors.
Horned lizard behaviors, 121. *See also* Reptile behaviors.
Hospital environment considerations
  for guinea pigs, 231-234
  for psittacines, 89-96
  for rabbit, 38-40, 39f
House ferret behaviors, 163-206. *See also* Ferret behaviors.
Husbandry considerations, psittacines, 65-68
Hypnosis, 42

I

Iguana behaviors, 103-162. *See also* Reptile behaviors.
Insulinoma, ferrets, 202-203
Intraspecies contacts, 54-56

J

Japanese natricine snake behaviors, 107-108. *See also* Reptile behaviors.
Juvenile behaviors, reptiles, 131-132

K

Kingsnake behaviors, 114. *See also* Reptile behaviors.
Komodo dragon behaviors. *See* Reptile behaviors.

L

Leopard gecko behaviors, 106-108, 111, 115. *See also* Reptile behaviors.
Leporids. *See* Rabbit behaviors.
Leuprolide acetate (Depo-Lupron), 88
Litter box training
  of ferret behaviors, 175b
  of rabbits, 22b
Lizard behaviors, 103-162. *See also* Reptile behaviors.
Locomotor behaviors and activities. *See also under individual topics.*
  of ferrets, 172-173
  of guinea pigs, 213-216, 214f, 216f
  of rabbits, 24-29, 24f-25f, 26b-27b
  of reptiles, 139-141
  of small mammals
    chinchillas, 272
    fennec foxes, 287
    hedgehogs, 299
    prairie dogs, 310
    sugar gliders, 333-334, 334f
  of small rodents, 251-253, 253f
Long-eared Egyptian hedgehog behaviors, 293-304. *See also* Hedgehog behaviors.
Lovebird behaviors, 55-56. *See also* Psittacine behaviors.

M

Macaw behaviors, 51-102. *See also* Psittacine behaviors.
Male reproductive behaviors. *See also under individual topics.*
  of ferrets, 175-176
  of guinea pigs, 224
  of rabbits, 12-13
  of reptiles, 129-130
  of small mammals
    chinchillas, 267-268
    fennec foxes, 286
    hedgehogs, 296
    prairie dogs, 308-309
    short-tailed opossums, 322-3´
    sugar gliders, 331
  of small rodents, 246-247

352 Index

Mammal (small) behaviors, 263-344. *See also* Small mammal behaviors.
Mazuri Exotic Canine Diet, 287
Medical implications of abnormal behaviors. *See also under individual topics.*
  of ferrets, 199-203, 201f
  of guinea pigs, 228-231, 229b
  of psittacine behaviors, 74-88
  of rabbits, 34-38, 35f
  of reptiles, 151-155, 151f-152f
  of small mammals
    chinchillas, 274-278, 275f-276f
    fennec foxes, 289
    hedgehogs, 301-302, 301f-302f
    prairie dogs, 312-317, 312f
    short-tailed opossums, 326
    sugar gliders, 335-338, 335f-338f
  of small rodents, 247f, 256-257
Medroxyprogesterone acetate (Depo-Provera), 87
Melopsittacus undulates behaviors, 53-54. *See also* Psittacine behaviors.
Meloxicam, 71
Mice behaviors. *See* Small rodent (mouse, rat, gerbil, and hamster) behaviors.
Miscellaneous small mammal behaviors, 263-344. *See also* Small mammal behaviors.
Moluccan cockatoo behaviors, 79-80. *See also* Psittacine behaviors.
Monitor lizard behaviors, 145-146. *See also* Reptile behaviors.
Monodelphis domestica behaviors, 320-328. *See also* Short-tailed opossum behaviors.
 behaviors. *See also* Small rodent use, rat, gerbil, and hamster) iors.
    ehaviors, medical implications 256-257
    behaviors, 241-243
    50-251
     s, 251
     3-255, 254f-255f
     activities,
     40
     258-260,
     -249, 252f
     241f-242f

Mouse behaviors *(Continued)*
  social *vs.* antisocial behaviors, 243-246, 244f-245f
  temperature sensitivity and, 256
Musk gland secretion, reptiles, 121
Mustela species behaviors, 163-206. *See also* Ferret behaviors.

N

Natrix natrix behaviors, 119, 120. *See also* Reptile behaviors.
Natural history. *See also under individual topics.*
  ferret behaviors and, 163-166
  rabbit behaviors and, 1-2
  small mammal behaviors and
    chinchillas, 263
    fennec foxes, 281
    hedgehogs, 293-294
    prairie dogs, 305-306
    short-tailed opossums, 320
    sugar gliders, 328
  small rodent behaviors and, 239-240
Neonatal behaviors
  of guinea pigs, 226, 227f
  of rabbits, 15-17
  of sugar gliders, 331-332
Nerium oleander, 32
Nile crocodile behaviors, 122. *See also* Reptile behaviors.
Niveoscincus ocellatus behaviors, 146. *See also* Reptile behaviors.
Nomadic psittacine behaviors, 52. *See also* Psittacine behaviors.
Nutrition- and diet-related behaviors. *See* Eating behaviors.
Nymphicus hollandicus behaviors, 51-102. *See also* Psittacine behaviors.

O

OCD (obsessive-compulsive disorder) and OCD-like alterations, 86-87
Oedura lesueurii behaviors, 124. *See also* Reptile behaviors.
Olfactory communications, ferrets, 168-170, 168f-169f
Omnivorous lizard behaviors, 127. *See also* Reptile behaviors.
Opossum (short-tailed) behaviors, 320-328. *See also* Short-tailed opossum behaviors.
Oryctolagus cuniculus behaviors, 1-50. *See also* Rabbit behaviors.

P

Pain-associated behaviors. *See also under individual topics.*
  of ferrets, 203
  of guinea pigs, 234-235, 234b, 235f
  of rabbits, 41-42, 43b
  of reptiles, 148, 149b-150b, 150f
  of small mammals
    chinchillas, 278
    fennec foxes, 289
    hedgehogs, 302
    prairie dogs, 317
    short-tailed opossums, 326
    sugar gliders, 338-339, 338f
  of small rodents, 258-260, 259f-260f
Pair-bonded Glossy Black cockatoo behaviors, 63-64. *See also* Psittacine behaviors.
Panther chameleon behaviors, 107, 134-135. *See also* Reptile behaviors.
Parental care behaviors
  of guinea pigs, 225-226
  of rabbits, 13-15, 16f
  of reptiles, 130-131
Parrot behaviors, 51-102. *See also* Psittacine behaviors.
Pasturella, 12
Peach-faced lovebird behaviors, 55-56. *See also* Psittacine behaviors.
Perireferential communication, psittacines, 97
Peruvian guinea pig behaviors. *See* Guinea pig behaviors.
Pet (exotic) behaviors. *See also under individual topics.*
  ferret behaviors, 163-206
  guinea pig behaviors, 207-238
  psittacine behaviors, 51-102
  rabbit behaviors, 1-50
  reptile behaviors, 103-162
  small mammal behaviors, 263-344
  small rodent (mouse, rat, gerbil, and hamster) behaviors, 239-263
Petarus breviceps behaviors, 328-340. *See also* Sugar glider behaviors.
Photoperiods, psittacines, 66
Photo-pollution, reptiles, 108
Phyrnosoma species behaviors, 121. *See also* Reptile behaviors.
Physignathus concincinus behaviors, 154-155. *See also* Reptile behaviors.

Piled-on behaviors, small rodents, 244-245, 244f
Pionus fucus behaviors, 57-58. *See also* Psittacine behaviors.
Pituitary adenoma, psittacines, 68-69
Play behaviors, ferrets, 184-188, 184f-187f
Pogona vitticeps behaviors, 105, 108. *See also* Reptile behaviors.
Polecat behaviors, 163-206. *See also* Ferret behaviors.
Polygynandrous/polygamous behaviors, rabbits, 13
Prairie dog behaviors. *See also* Small mammal behaviors.
  abnormal behaviors, medical implications of, 312-317, 312f
  behavioral enrichment for, 317-318
  captivity-associated behaviors and considerations, 318
  client education for, 319b
  communicative behaviors, 306
  eating behaviors, 309, 309f, 311f
  elimination behaviors, 310
  grooming behaviors, 310-312
  locomotor behaviors and activities, 310
  natural history and, 305-306
  pain-associated behaviors, 317
  reproductive behaviors
    female reproductive behaviors, 308-309
    male reproductive behaviors, 308-309
  social *vs.* antisocial behaviors, 306-308, 307f-308f
Prehensile-tailed skink behaviors, 131. *See also* Reptile behaviors.
Prey-catching behaviors, ferrets, 181-182
Prozac, 87
Pseudopregnancies, rabbits, 14
Psittacine behaviors
  abnormal behaviors, medical implications of, 74-88
  captivity-related considerations and, 57-62, 71-74
    acceptable behaviors, substitution of, 72-73
    behavior analyses and, 71-72
    behavior modification and, 60-6, 72-74
    descriptions of, 57-58, 71
    desired behaviors, reinforcem
    inactivity, consequences of,
    initiation and, 62

Psittacine behaviors *(Continued)*
  new behaviors, teaching of, 72-73
  normal behaviors, exaggeration of, 60-61
  positive reinforcement and, 61-62
  punishment impacts on, 62
  socialization, 58
  stimulation, 58-59, 59f, 61f
  toys and, 60, 61f
  undesirable behaviors, extinction of, 73-74
 disease considerations and
  anorexia, 71
  blindness, sudden, 68-69, 69f
  cataracts, 68-69, 69f
  egg yolk stroke, 70
  heavy metal toxicity, 69-70
  hepatic encephalopathy, 69
  meloxicam and, 71
  NSAIDs (nonsteroidal antiinflammatory drugs) and, 71
  neurologic diseases, 68-69
  neuropathies, miscellaneous, 70
  pain-associated behaviors, 71
  pituitary adenoma, 70
  retinal detachments, 68-69
 environment enrichment considerations and, 58-61, 59f, 61f
 hospital environment considerations and
  aggressive behaviors, 89-96, 92f, 95f
  caiques, 95
  conures, 90-91
  descriptions of, 89
  Eclectus species, 93-94
  macaws (Ara species), 92-93
  miscellaneous species, 95-96
  gray parrots, 95
  lories, 95-96
  normal behaviors, 89
  cockatoos, 90-92, 92f
  environment considerations,

Psittacine behaviors *(Continued)*
  perches, 65
  photoperiods, 66
  wing trimming, 67-68
 intelligence, cognition, and communication considerations
  categoric class formation, 97
  descriptions of, 96
  great ape similarities, 96-97
  perireferential communication, 97
  sentinel behaviors, 97-98
  significance of, 99
 medication considerations for
  acupuncture and, 88
  amitriptyline (Elavil), 85
  clomipramine (Clomicalm), 85
  DermCaps, 88
  descriptions of, 84-85
  diazepam, 85
  essential fatty acids and, 88
  fluoxetine (Prozac), 85
  GnRH agonists, 88
  haloperidol (Haldol), 85
  hCG (human chorionic gonadotropin), 87-88
  hormonal medications, 87-88
  leuprolide acetate (Depo-Lupron), 88
  medroxyprogesterone acetate (Depo-Provera), 87
  psychotropic medications, 85-87
  SSRIs (selective serotonin reuptake inhibitors), 87
  TCAs (tricyclic antidepressants), 87-88
 problem behaviors and syndromes
  aggressive dominant behaviors, 77
  allergies, 82
  associated medical conditions of, 81-82
  biting, 77-78
  cockatoo prolapse syndrome, 79-80, 79f
  coelomic cavity granulomas and masses, 82
  dermatitis, 82
  dominance-related considerations, 74-77
  endocrine abnormalities, 82
  endoparasites, 81
  environmental factors and, 82-88
  feather destruction, 81-82
  folliculitis, 82
  heavy metal toxicity, 82
  height dominance, 75-76

Psittacine behaviors *(Continued)*
  hepatic disease, 81
  innate (true) dominant behaviors, 76-77
  learned dominant behaviors, 77
  medical modifications of, 84-88
  neuroses, 78-79
  nutritional factors and, 82-88
  OCD (obsessive-compulsive disorder) and OCD-like alterations, 86-87
  phobias, 78-79
  zinc toxicity, 82
 social *vs.* antisocial behaviors, 74-88
 taming and training considerations and, 71-74
 wild bird behaviors
  body language, 54, 55f-56f
  breeding behavior displays, 54
  communicative behaviors, 53
  descriptions of, 51-52
  ethograms and, 51-52
  filoerections, 54
  foraging behaviors, 54
  grooming, 53b
  intraspecies contacts and, 54-56
  of nomadic psittacines, 52
  parenting behaviors, 56
  posturing, 54
  species differences and variations and, 52, 54-56
  tail feather fanning, 54
  territoriality, 54
  time allocation and, 52-53, 53b
  vocalization, 53-54, 53b
  voluntary pupillary constrictions and dilations, 54
Psittacus erithacus behaviors, 51-102. *See also* Psittacine behaviors.
Psychotropic medications, psittacines, 85-87
Pup cannibalism, small rodents, 243
Pygmy hedgehog behaviors, 293-304. *See also* Hedgehog behaviors.
Python behaviors, 121. *See also* Reptile behaviors.

R

Rabbit behaviors
 abnormal behaviors, medical implications of
  anorexia, 35-36
  dacryocystitis, 36

Rabbit behaviors *(Continued)*
  descriptions of, 34-38
  gastrointestinal stasis, 36
  morbidity and mortality, 36-37
  renal failure, 37
  routine well-care visits and, 34
  stress, 35
 adoption considerations and, 42-44, 44f
 behavioral enrichment and, 31-34, 33f-34f
 communicative behaviors, 4-7, 5b-6b
 domestication-related considerations and, 1-2
 eating behaviors, 17-20, 20f
 elimination behaviors
  descriptions of, 20-23
  litter box training, 22b
 euthanasia considerations and, 42-44
 grooming behaviors, 29-31, 29f
 hospital environment considerations and
  C position and, 38-40, 39f
  descriptions of, 38-40
 hypnosis and, 42
 locomotive behaviors and activities
  descriptions of, 24-29
  negative behavior modification and prevention, 26b-27b
 natural history of, 1-2
 neonatal behaviors, 15-17
 outdoor enclosure considerations and, 31
 pain management considerations and
  associated behaviors, 41-42
  clinical signs of, 43b
  descriptions of, 41
 reproductive behaviors, 12-15, 16f
  descriptions of, 12
  female reproductive and maternal behaviors
  male, 12-13
  nest building, 14-15
  ovariohysterectomies and, 14, 16f
  polygamous behaviors, 13
  polygynandrous/polygamous behaviors, 13
  pseudopregnancies and, 14
  spaying and, 15
 sensory behaviors
  hearing, 3
  olfactory behaviors, 3-4
  touch, 3
  vision, 2-3

Rabbit behaviors *(Continued)*
  social *vs.* antisocial behaviors
    abnormal repetitive behaviors, 8-9
    aggressive behaviors, 9-12
    bonding, 8f, 10b-11b
    descriptions of, 7-12
    destructive behaviors, 11-12
  urinary behaviors, 23
Rat behaviors. *See also* Small rodent (mouse, rat, gerbil, and hamster) behaviors.
  abnormal behaviors, medical implications of, 247f, 256-257
  communicative behaviors, 241-243
  eating behaviors, 250-251
  elimination behaviors, 251
  grooming behaviors, 253-255, 254f-255f
  locomotor behaviors and activities, 251-253, 253f
  natural history and, 239-240
  pain-associated behaviors, 258-260, 259f-260f
  reference resources for, 261
  sensory behaviors, 240-241, 241f-242f
  social *vs.* antisocial behaviors, 243-246, 244f-245f
  temperature sensitivity and, 256
Rattlesnake behaviors, 134. *See also* Reptile behaviors.
Red-footed tortoise behaviors, 134-135. *See also* Reptile behaviors.
-directed aggression, ferrets, 195b
 sided garter snake behaviors,
   -108, 128-129. *See also* Reptile
    viors.
     n, reptiles, 120
      abbits, 37
       aviors. *See also under*

Reproductive behaviors *(Continued)*
  of small mammals
    chinchillas (female), 268-271, 269f-270f
    chinchillas (male), 268-271, 269f-270f
    fennec foxes (female), 285-286
    fennec foxes (male), 286
    hedgehogs (female), 296-298, 297f-298f
    hedgehogs (male), 296
    prairie dogs (female), 308-309
    prairie dogs (male), 308-309
    short-tailed opossums (female), 323-324
    short-tailed opossums (male), 322-323
    sugar gliders (female), 331-332
    sugar gliders (male), 331
  of small rodents, 246-249, 252f
    female, 246-249
    male, 246-247
Reptile behaviors
  abnormal behaviors, medical implications of, 151-155, 151f-152f
  agonistic (defensive and aggressive) behaviors
    antipredator behaviors, defensive, 117-121, 114f, 118f
    blood spurting, 121
    caudal autotomy (tail shed), 118-119
    coiling up, 121
    death display, 119
    defensive behaviors, active, 119-121
    defensive behaviors, miscellaneous, 121
    Depo-Lupron and, 116
    Depo-Provera and, 116
    descriptions of, 112-121, 116f, 118f
    detection avoidance (crypsis), 117
    escape behavior (direct evasion), 117-118, 118f
    mating combat, 115-117
    musk gland secretion and elimination, 121
    passive defensive behaviors (avoidance), 117-119
    regurgitation, 120
    retraction into shell, 121
    self-inflation and vocalization, 119
    symbolic bite and biting, 119-120
    tail flicking and whipping, 120-121
    territorial defense, 114-115
    threat displays, 114f
  behavioral enrichment considerations and, 148-151

Reptile behaviors *(Continued)*
  coloration considerations and, 142-143, 143f
  communicative behaviors, 141f
  developmental aspects of, 104-105
  eating behaviors, 132-138, 133f, 136f-137f
  elimination behaviors, 138-139
  environmental considerations of
    descriptions of, 105-108
    environmental pollution, 107-108
    photo-pollution, 108
    UV (ultraviolet light), 106-108
  euthanasia-related considerations and, 155-156
  grooming behaviors, 141-142
  gustation and, 127
  hatchling and juvenile behaviors, 131-132
  locomotor behaviors and activities, 139-141
  pain-associated behaviors
    clinical signs of, 149b-150b
    descriptions of, 148
  reproductive behaviors
    descriptions of, 127-129
    female reproductive behaviors, 130-131
    male reproductive behaviors, 129-130
  sensory behaviors
    auditory behaviors, 125-127
    descriptions of, 123
    olfactory behaviors, 123-124
    somatic hearing, 126
    vibration responses, 125-127
    vision, 125
    vocalizations, 125-127
    VOs (vomeronasal organs) and, 123
  sneezing behaviors, 142
  social *vs.* antisocial behaviors
    captivity-related considerations and, 108b-111b
    descriptions of, 108-112
    multiple species housing and, 109f
    taming and training considerations and, 122-123
  thermoregulatory behaviors
    burrowing behaviors, 147
    descriptions of, 143-146
    estivation, 146-147
    hibernation, 146-147, 147b
Retinal detachments, psittacines, 68-69
Retraction into shell, reptiles, 121

Rodent (small) behaviors, 239-262. *See also* Small rodent (mouse, rat, gerbil, and hamster) behaviors.

S

Salmonella species, 135-136
Sauromalus obesus behaviors, 118. *See also* Reptile behaviors.
Scanning, rabbits, 5b
Screaming
  of ferrets, 171
Self-inflation, reptiles, 119
Senegals, 95-96. *See also* Psittacine behaviors.
Sensory behaviors. *See also under individual topics.*
  of ferrets, 166-168
  of guinea pigs, 212-213
  of rabbits, 2-4
  of reptiles, 123-127
  of small mammals
    chinchillas, 263-265, 264f
    fennec foxes, 281-282, 282f
    hedgehogs, 294-295
    short-tailed opossums, 320
    sugar gliders, 328
  of small rodents, 240-241, 241f-242f
Sentinel behaviors, psittacines, 97-98
Short-tailed opossum behaviors. *See also* Small mammal behaviors.
  abnormal behaviors, medical implications of, 326
  captivity-associated behaviors and considerations, 326
  client education for, 327b
  communicative behaviors, 320-321
  eating behaviors, 324
  elimination behaviors, 324-325
  natural history and, 320
  pain-associated behaviors, 326
  reproductive behaviors
    female reproductive behaviors,
    male reproductive behaviors, ?
  sensory behaviors, 320
  social *vs.* antisocial behaviors,
    322f
Side-blotched lizard behaviors,
Skink behaviors, 131. *See also*
  behaviors.
"Skinny" pig behaviors, 208
  Guinea pig behaviors.

Sleep behaviors, ferrets, 197-199, 198f
Small mammal behaviors
　of chinchillas
　　abnormal behaviors, medical implications of, 274-278, 275f-276f
　　captivity-related considerations, 278-279
　　client education for, 280b
　　communicative behaviors, 265
　　eating behaviors, 271
　　elimination behaviors, 271-272
　　euthanasia considerations and, 278
　　female reproductive behaviors, 268-271, 269f-270f
　　grooming behaviors, 272-274, 273f-274f
　　locomotor behaviors and activities, 272
　　male reproductive behaviors, 267-268
　　natural history, 263
　　pain-associated behaviors, 278
　　reproductive behaviors, 267-271, 269f-270f
　　sensory behaviors, 263-265, 264f
　　social *vs.* antisocial behaviors, 265-267, 265f-266f
　of fennec foxes
　　abnormal behaviors, medical implications of, 289
　　captivity-associated behaviors, 289-291, 291f
　　CAV-1 (canine adenovirus), 290
　　client education for, 292b
　　communicative behaviors, 282-283, 283f
　　eating behaviors, 286-287
　　elimination behaviors, 287
　　female reproductive behaviors, 285-286
　　grooming behaviors, 288
　　locomotor behaviors and activities, 287-288
　　male reproductive behaviors, 286
　　Mazuri Exotic Canine Diet for, 287
　　natural history, 281
　　pain-associated behaviors, 289
　　reproductive behaviors, 285-286
　　sensory behaviors, 281-282, 282f
　　social *vs.* antisocial behaviors, 283-285, 284f-285f
　of hedgehogs
　　abnormal behaviors, medical implications of, 301-302, 301f-302f
　　captivity-associated behaviors, 303

Small mammal behaviors *(Continued)*
　　client education for, 304b
　　communicative behaviors, 295
　　eating behaviors, 298
　　elimination behaviors, 299
　　female reproductive behaviors and parental care considerations, 296-298, 297f-298f
　　grooming behaviors, 300-301, 300f
　　locomotor behaviors and activities, 299
　　male reproductive behaviors, 296
　　natural history, 293-294
　　pain-associated behaviors, 302
　　reproductive behaviors, 296-298, 297f-298f
　　sensory behaviors, 294-295
　　social *vs.* antisocial behaviors, 295-296
　of prairie dogs
　　abnormal behaviors, medical implications of, 312-317, 312f
　　behavioral enrichment for, 317-318
　　captivity-associated behaviors and considerations, 318
　　client education for, 319b
　　communicative behaviors, 306
　　eating behaviors, 309, 309f, 311f
　　elimination behaviors, 310
　　female reproductive behaviors, 308-309
　　grooming behaviors, 310-312
　　locomotor behaviors and activities, 310
　　male reproductive behaviors, 308-309
　　natural history, 305-306
　　pain-associated behaviors, 317
　　reproductive behaviors, 308-309
　　social *vs.* antisocial behaviors, 306-308, 307f-308f
　of short-tailed opossums
　　abnormal behaviors, medical implications of, 326
　　captivity-associated behaviors and considerations, 326
　　client education for, 327b
　　communicative behaviors, 320-321
　　eating behaviors, 324
　　elimination behaviors, 324-325
　　female reproductive behaviors, 323-324
　　grooming behaviors, 325
　　locomotor behaviors and activities, 325, 325f
　　male reproductive behaviors, 322-323
　　natural history, 320

Small mammal behaviors *(Continued)*
   pain-associated behaviors, 326
   reproductive behaviors, 322-324
   sensory behaviors, 320
   social *vs.* antisocial behaviors, 321-322, 322f
   of sugar gliders
      abnormal behaviors, medical implications of, 335-338, 335f-338f
      behavioral enrichment considerations for, 339
      captivity-associated behaviors and considerations, 339
      client education for, 340b
      communicative behaviors, 328-329, 329f
      eating behaviors, 332-333
      elimination behaviors, 333
      female reproductive behaviors, 331-332
      grooming behaviors, 333-334, 336f
      locomotor behaviors and activities, 333-334, 334f
      male reproductive behaviors, 331
      natural history, 328
      neonatal behaviors, 331-332
      pain-associated behaviors, 338-339, 338f
      reproductive behaviors, 331-332
      sensory behaviors, 328
      social *vs.* antisocial behaviors, 330-331
      thermoregulatory behaviors, 333

Small rodent (mouse, rat, gerbil, and hamster) behaviors
   abnormal behaviors, medical implications of, 247f, 256-257
   alopecia, 256, 257f
   cheek pouches and, 257
   descriptions of, 256-257
   epilepsy, 256
   tumors, 257
   communicative behaviors
      chortling, 242
      clucking, 241
      descriptions of, 241-243
      gritching, 242
      squeaking and squealing, 241-242
      vocalizations, 241-243
   eating behaviors, 250-251
   elimination behaviors, 251
   grooming behaviors, 253-255, 254f-255f

Small rodent (mouse, rat, gerbil, and hamster) behaviors *(Continued)*
   locomotor behaviors and activities, 251-253, 253f
   natural history and, 239-240
   pain-associated behaviors, 258-260, 259f-260f
   reproductive behaviors
      copulation/mating plugs and, 248
      female reproductive behaviors, 247-249
      male reproductive behaviors, 246-247
      nesting, 252f
      nesting behaviors, 252f
   sensory behaviors
      scent marking, 240-241, 241f-242f
      smell, 240-241
   social *vs.* antisocial behaviors
      aggressive behaviors, 243-246
      descriptions of, 243-246
      piled-on behaviors, 244-245, 244f
      pup cannibalism, 243
      temperature sensitivity and, 256
Snake behaviors, 103-162. *See also* Reptile behaviors.
Snapping turtle behaviors, 105-108. *See also* Reptile behaviors.
Social *vs.* antisocial behaviors. *See also under individual topics.*
   of ferrets, 177-179
   of guinea pigs, 208-210, 209b
   of psittacines, 74-88
   of rabbits, 7-12, 8f-9f, 9, 10b-11b
   of reptiles, 108-112, 108b-111b, 109f
   of small mammals
      chinchillas, 265-267, 265f-266f
      fennec foxes, 283-285, 284f-285f
      hedgehogs, 295-296
      prairie dogs, 306-308, 307f-308f
      short-tailed opossums, 321-322, 322f
      sugar gliders, 330-331
   of small rodents, 243-246, 244f-245f
Somatic hearing, reptiles, 126
South American rattlesnake behaviors, 134. *See also* Reptile behaviors.
SSRIs (selective serotonin reuptake inhibitors), 87
Steppe polecat behaviors, 165. *See also* Ferret behaviors.
Sugar glider behaviors. *See also* Small mammal behaviors.

Sugar glider behaviors *(Continued)*
  abnormal behaviors, medical implications of, 335-338, 335f-338f
  behavioral enrichment considerations for, 339
  client education for, 340f
  communicative behaviors, 328-329, 329f
  eating behaviors, 332-333
  elimination behaviors, 333
  grooming behaviors, 333-334, 336f
  locomotor behaviors and activities, 333-334, 334f
  natural history and, 328
  neonatal behaviors, 331-332
  pain-associated behaviors, 338-339, 338f
  reproductive behaviors
    female reproductive behaviors, 331-332
    male reproductive behaviors, 331
  sensory behaviors, 328
  social *vs.* antisocial behaviors, 330-331
  thermoregulatory behaviors, 333
Symbolic biting, reptiles, 119-120

T

Tail flicking and whipping, reptiles, 120-121
Tail shed, reptiles, 118-119
Taming and training considerations
  for guinea pigs, 210-212, 211f
  for psittacine behaviors, 71-74
  for reptiles, 122-123
TCAs (tricyclic antidepressants), 87-88
Temperature sensitivity, small rodents, 256
Terrapene carolina bauri behaviors, 138-139. *See also* Reptile behaviors.
Thamnophis sirtalis parietalis behaviors, 106-108. *See also* Reptile behaviors.
Thermoregulatory behaviors
  of reptiles, 143-147
  of sugar gliders, 333
Tortoise behaviors, 103-162. *See also* Reptile behaviors.
Turtle behaviors, 103-162. *See also* Reptile behaviors.

U

Umbrella cockatoo behaviors, 63-64, 76-77, 79-80. *See also* Psittacine behaviors.
Urinary behaviors, rabbits, 23
Uta stansburiana behaviors, 140-141. *See also* Reptile behaviors.

V

Varanus varius behaviors, 145. *See also* Reptile behaviors.
Velvet gecko behaviors, 124. *See also* Reptile behaviors.
Vibration responses, reptiles, 126
Viper behaviors, 138. *See also* Reptile behaviors.
Vipiparous lizard behaviors, 146. *See also* Reptile behaviors.
Vision. *See* Sensory behaviors.
Vocalizations. *See* Communicative behaviors.
Volpes zerda behaviors. *See* Fennec fox behaviors.
VOs (vomeronasal organs), reptiles, 123

W

White-fronted amazon behaviors, 64-65. *See also* Psittacine behaviors.
Wild bird behaviors. *See also* Psittacine behaviors.
  body language, 54, 55f-56f
  breeding behavior displays, 54
  communicative behaviors, 53
  descriptions of, 51-52
  ethograms and, 51-52
  filoerections, 54
  foraging behaviors 54
  intraspecies contacts and, 54-56
  of nomadic psittacines, 52
  parenting behaviors, 56
  posturing, 54
  species differences and variations and, 52, 54-56
  tail feather fanning, 54
  territoriality, 54
  time allocation and, 52-53, 53b
  vocalization, 53-54
  voluntary pupillary constrictions and dilations, 54
Wing trimming, psittacines, 67-68
Wood turtle behaviors, 146. *See also* Reptile behaviors.

Y

Yellow-footed tortoise behaviors, 134-135. *See also* Reptile behaviors.
Yellow-naped amazon behaviors, 73. *See also* Psittacine behaviors.